2000
YEAR BOOK OF
ANESTHESIOLOGY AND
PAIN MANAGEMENT™

Statement of Purpose

The YEAR BOOK Series

The YEAR BOOK series was devised in 1901 by health professionals who observed that the literature of medicine and related disciplines had become so voluminous that no one individual could read and place in perspective every potential advance in a major specialty. That has never been more true than it is today.

More than merely a series of books, YEAR BOOK volumes are the tangible results of a unique service designed to accomplish the following:

- to *survey* a wide range of journals
- to *select* from those journals papers representing significant advances and statements of important clinical principles
- to provide *abstracts* of those articles that are readable, convenient summaries of their key points
- to provide *informed commentary* about their relevance

These publications grow out of a unique process that draws on the talents of outstanding authorities in clinical and fundamental disciplines, trained literature specialists, and professional writers—all supported by the resources of Mosby, the world's preeminent publisher for the health professions.

The Literature Base

Mosby and its editors survey approximately 500 journals published worldwide, covering the full range of the health professions. On an annual basis, the publisher examines usage patterns and polls its expert authorities to add new journals to the literature base and to delete journals that are no longer useful as potential YEAR BOOK sources.

The Literature Survey

More than 250,000 peer-reviewed articles per year are scanned systematically—including title, text, illustrations, tables, and references—by the publisher's team of literature specialists. Each scan is compared, article by article, to the search strategies that the publisher has developed in consultation with the nearly 200 outside experts who form the pool of YEAR BOOK editors. A given article with broad scientific or clinical implications may be reviewed by any number of YEAR BOOK editors, from one to a dozen or more, regardless of the discipline for which the paper was originally published. In turn, each editor who receives the article reviews it to determine whether it should be included in his or her volume. This decision is based on the article's inherent quality, its relevance to readers of that YEAR BOOK, and the editor's goal to represent a comprehensive picture of a given field in each volume of the YEAR BOOK. In addition, the editor indicates when to include figures and tables from the article to help the YEAR BOOK reader better understand the information.

Of the quarter million articles scanned each year, only 5% are selected for publication within the YEAR BOOK series, thereby assuring readers of the high value of every selection.

The Abstract

The publisher's abstracting staff is headed by a seasoned medical editing professional and includes individuals with extensive experience in writing for the health professions. When an article is selected for inclusion in a YEAR BOOK, it is assigned to a member of the abstracting staff. The abstractor, guided in many cases by notations supplied by the physician editor, writes a structured, condensed summary designed to rapidly communicate to the reader the essential information contained in the article.

The Commentary

The YEAR BOOK editorial boards, sometimes assisted by guest contributors, write comments that place each article in perspective. This provides the reader with insights from authorities in each discipline that point out the value of the article and that often reflect the authority's thought processes in assessing the article.

Additional Editorial Features

The editorial boards of each YEAR BOOK organize the abstracts and comments to provide a logical and satisfying sequence of information. To enhance the organization, editors also provide introductions to sections or individual chapters, comments linking a number of abstracts, citations to additional literature, and other features.

The published YEAR BOOK contains enhanced bibliographic citations for each selected article, including extended listings of multiple authors and identification of author affiliations. Each YEAR BOOK contains a Table of Contents specific to that year's volume. From year to year, the Table of Contents for a given YEAR BOOK may vary, depending on developments within the field.

Every YEAR BOOK contains a list of the journals from which articles have been selected. This list represents a subset of approximately 500 journals surveyed by the publisher and occasionally reflects a particularly pertinent article from a journal that is not surveyed routinely.

Finally, each volume contains a comprehensive subject index and an index to authors of each selected article.

The 2000 Year Book Series

Year Book of Allergy, Asthma, and Clinical Immunology™: Drs Rosenwasser, Boguniewicz, Milgrom, Routes, and Spahn

Year Book of Anesthesiology and Pain Management™: Drs Tinker, Abram, Chestnut, Roizen, Rothenberg, and Wood

Year Book of Cardiology®: Drs Schlant, Collins, Gersh, Graham, Kaplan, and Waldo

Year Book of Chiropractic®: Dr Lawrence

Year Book of Critical Care Medicine®: Drs Parrillo, Balk, Calvin, Franklin, and Shapiro

Year Book of Dentistry®: Drs Zakariasen, Boghosian, Dederich, Hatcher, Horswell, and McIntyre

Year Book of Dermatology and Dermatologic Surgery™: Drs Thiers and Lang

Year Book of Diagnostic Radiology®: Drs Osborn, Birdwell, Dalinka, Groskin, Maynard, Oestreich, Pentecost, Ros, Smirniotopoulos, and Young

Year Book of Emergency Medicine®: Drs Burdick, Cydulka, Cone, Hamilton, Loiselle, and Niemann

Year Book of Endocrinology®: Drs Mazzaferri, Fitzpatrick, Horton, Kannan, Meikle, Molitch, Morley, Osei, Poehlman, and Rogol

Year Book of Family Practice®: Drs Berg, Bowman, Davidson, Dexter, Morrison, and Scherger

Year Book of Gastroenterology™: Dr Lichtenstein

Year Book of Hand Surgery®: Drs Amadio and Hentz

Year Book of Medicine®: Drs Barkin, Frishman, Jett, Klahr, Loehrer, Malawista, Mandell, and Mazzaferri

Year Book of Neonatal and Perinatal Medicine®: Drs Fanaroff, Maisels, and Stevenson

Year Book of Nephrology, Hypertension, and Mineral Metabolism: Drs Schwab, Bennett, Emmett, Moe, and Textor

Year Book of Neurology and Neurosurgery®: Drs Bradley and Gibbs

Year Book of Nuclear Medicine®: Drs Gottschalk, Blaufox, Coleman, Strauss, and Zubal

Year Book of Obstetrics, Gynecology, and Women's Health®: Drs Mishell, Herbst, and Kirschbaum

Year Book of Oncology®: Drs Loehrer, Eisenberg, Glatstein, Gordon, Johnson, Pratt, and Thigpen

Year Book of Ophthalmology®: Drs Wilson, Cohen, Eagle, Grossman, Laibson, Maguire, Nelson, Penne, Rapuano, Sergott, Shields, Spaeth, Tipperman, Ms Gosfield, and Ms Salmon

Year Book of Orthopedics®: Drs Morrey, Beauchamp, Currier, Swiontkowski, Tolo, and Trigg

Year Book of Otolaryngology–Head and Neck Surgery®: Drs Paparella, Holt, and Otto

Year Book of Pathology and Laboratory Medicine®: Drs Raab, Dabbs, Olson, Silverman, and Stanley

Year Book of Pediatrics®: Dr Stockman

Year Book of Plastic, Reconstructive, and Aesthetic Surgery®: Drs Miller, Bartlett, Garner, McKinney, Ruberg, Salisbury, and Smith

Year Book of Psychiatry and Applied Mental Health®: Drs Talbott, Ballenger, Frances, Jensen, Meltzer, Simpson, and Tasman

Year Book of Pulmonary Disease®: Drs Jett, Castro, Maurer, Peters, Phillips, and Ryu

Year Book of Rheumatology, Arthritis, and Musculoskeletal Disease™: Drs Panush, Hadler, Hellmann, LeRoy, Pisetsky, and Simon

Year Book of Sports Medicine®: Drs Shephard, Alexander, Kohrt, Nieman, Torg, and Mr George

Year Book of Surgery®: Drs Copeland, Bland, Deitch, Eberlein, Howard, Luce, Seeger, Souba, and Sugarbaker

Year Book of Urology®: Drs Andriole and Coplen

Year Book of Vascular Surgery®: Dr Porter

2000

The Year Book of ANESTHESIOLOGY AND PAIN MANAGEMENT™

Editor-in-Chief
John H. Tinker, MD

Associate Editors
Stephen E. Abram, MD
David H. Chestnut, MD
Michael F. Roizen, MD
David M. Rothenberg, MD, FCCM
Margaret Wood, MD

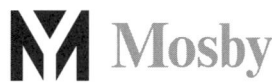 Mosby

St. Louis Baltimore Boston Carlsbad Naples New York Philadelphia Portland London
Madrid Mexico City Singapore Sydney Tokyo Toronto Wiesbaden

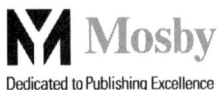

Mosby
Dedicated to Publishing Excellence

Publisher: Susan Patterson
Associate Publisher: Gretchen C. Murphy
Developmental Editor: Jennifer Richardet
Manager, Periodical Editing: Kirk Swearingen
Production Editor: Stephanie M. Geels
Project Supervisor, Production: Joy Moore
Production Assistant: Karie House
Manager, Literature Services: Idelle L. Winer
Illustrations and Permissions Specialist: Steve Ramay

2000 EDITION
Copyright © 2000 by Mosby, Inc

Printed in the United States of America
Composition by Thomas Technology Solutions, Inc
Printing/binding by Maple-Vail

Editorial Office:
Mosby, Inc
11830 Westline Industrial Dr
St Louis, MO 63146
Customer Service: periodical.service@mosby.com
           www.mosby.com/periodicals/

International Standard Serial Number: 1073-5437
International Standard Book Number: 0-323-00646-9

Editorial Board

Table of Contents

Journals Represented

Mosby and its editors survey approximately 500 journals for its abstract and commentary publications. From these journals, the editors select the articles to be abstracted. Journals represented in this YEAR BOOK are listed below.

Acta Anaesthesiologica Scandinavica
American Industrial Hygiene Association Journal
American Journal of Cardiology
American Journal of Emergency Medicine
American Journal of Obstetrics and Gynecology
American Journal of Surgery
American Surgeon
Anaesthesia
Anaesthesia and Intensive Care
Anesthesia and Analgesia
Anesthesiology
Annals of Internal Medicine
Annals of Surgery
Annals of Thoracic Surgery
Archives of Surgery
British Journal of Anaesthesia
British Journal of Surgery
Canadian Journal of Anaesthesia
Canadian Journal of Anesthesia
Chest
Circulation
Clinical Journal of Pain
Critical Care Medicine
Diseases of the Colon and Rectum
European Respiratory Journal
Gastroenterology
Infection Control and Hospital Epidemiology
International Journal of Obstetric Anesthesia
Journal of Clinical Anesthesia
Journal of General Internal Medicine
Journal of Pain and Symptom Management
Journal of Pediatric Surgery
Journal of Pharmacology and Experimental Therapeutics
Journal of Thoracic and Cardiovascular Surgery
Journal of Trauma: Injury, Infection, and Critical Care
Journal of Urology
Journal of the American Medical Association
Lancet
New England Journal of Medicine
Obstetrics and Gynecology
Pain
Pharmacotherapy
Regional Anesthesia and Pain Medicine
Scandinavian Journal of Rehabilitation Medicine
Science
Southern Medical Journal
Stroke

STANDARD ABBREVIATIONS

The following terms are abbreviated in this edition: acquired immunodeficiency syndrome (AIDS), cardiopulmonary resuscitation (CPR), central nervous system (CNS), cerebrospinal fluid (CSF), computed tomography (CT), deoxyribonucleic acid (DNA), electrocardiography (ECG), health maintenance organization (HMO), human immunodeficiency virus (HIV), intensive care unit (ICU), intramuscular (IM), intravenous (IV), magnetic resonance (MR) imaging (MRI), ribonucleic acid (RNA), ultrasound (US), and ultraviolet (UV).

NOTE

The YEAR BOOK OF ANESTHESIOLOGY AND PAIN MANAGEMENT™ is a literature survey service providing abstracts of articles published in the professional literature. Every effort is made to ensure the accuracy of the information presented in these pages. Neither the editors nor the publisher of the YEAR BOOK OF ANESTHESIOLOGY AND PAIN MANAGEMENT™ can be responsible for errors in the original materials. The editors' comments are their own opinions. Mention of specific products within this publication does not constitute endorsement.

To facilitate the use of the YEAR BOOK OF ANESTHESIOLOGY AND PAIN MANAGEMENT™ as a reference tool, all illustrations and tables included in this publication are now identified as they appear in the original article. This change is meant to help the reader recognize that any illustration or table appearing in the YEAR BOOK OF ANESTHESIOLOGY AND PAIN MANAGEMENT™ may be only one of many in the original article. For this reason, figure and table numbers will often appear to be out of sequence within the YEAR BOOK OF ANESTHESIOLOGY AND PAIN MANAGEMENT™.

1 Studies of Outcomes, Risks, Costs, and Benefits

Epidural Catheter Tip Position and Distribution of Injectate Evaluated by Computed Tomography
Hogan Q (Med College of Wisconsin, Milwaukee)
Anesthesiology 90:964-970, 1999   1–1

Objective.—Asymmetric epidural blockade is common, occurring in as many as 21% of patients. Patterns of asymmetric distribution have not been studied. Catheter positions and patterns of circumferential distribution of solution injected during routine epidural anesthesia were assessed by means of CT.

Methods.—A Tuohy needle was inserted into the epidural space in 20 women, average age 55 years, who were undergoing brachytherapy for cervical cancer. An 18-gauge radiopaque catheter with lateral sideports at 14, 10, and 6 mm from the tip was inserted 3 cm into the epidural space of 17 patients, and a 19-gauge, soft-tip, spring-wound epidural catheter with a 4-mm-long open area beginning 2.5 mm from the tip was used in 3 patients. A continuous epidural infusion of bupivacaine (0.125%) and fentanyl (3 μg/mL) was provided postoperatively and adjusted to provide relief throughout the course of brachytherapy. The level of analgesia was determined by pin scratch, and ability to flex ankles, knees, and hips was documented twice daily. Four hours after surgery, CT was performed to guide placement of radiation sources. The tip of the catheter was identified, contrast material was injected, and a series of images was obtained. Images were examined by evaluators who were blinded to the extent of analgesia.

Results.—Air was found in all spinal cords. The catheter was placed where desired in 8 patients, higher than intended in 11, and through posterior epidural fat in 1. Eight catheter tips were in or near the posterior epidural space, 9 were found in the intervertebral foramina, and 2 were located in the paravertebral tissues lateral to the intervertebral foramina. Patterns of spread were not consistent, although most showed spread anterior to the dura, and most showed posterior and lateral spread. In most patients, contrast material left asymmetrically through an intervertebral foramina, mainly into the psoas muscle. Air bubbles and fat arrested distribution of analgesia in 2 patients. Layering of the solution without foraminal spread was observed in 9 of 15 patients after a 4-mL injection and in 5 of 19 patients after a 10-mL injection. Subdural accumulation was noted in 1 patient, and leakage through the ligamentum flavum was observed in 2. Whereas most patients had left and right block levels that differed by 2 or fewer segments, 2 patients had a maximum difference of 4 segments and 1 had a difference of 5 segments.

Conclusion.—Catheter position and analgesia distribution vary greatly from patient to patient, but adequate analgesia is provided in most cases.

▶ This is a neat study, but, it was performed in only 20 female patients. As might be expected, the pattern of spread was highly variable. These are not easy or inexpensive studies to do and so probably will never be done in a large patient population. I would have been interested in the use of CT to evaluate possible hematoma in patients receiving drugs that may affect hemostasis; perhaps then we would know just when is the best time to pull (ie, remove) the epidural catheter.

M. Wood, MD

Preoperative Fasting Practices in Pediatrics
Ferrari LR, Rooney FM, Rockoff MA (Harvard Med School, Boston; Children's Hosp, Boston)
Anesthesiology 90:978-980, 1999   1–2

Objective.—Preoperative fasting practices were determined in major pediatric medical centers in the United States and Canada.

Methods.—One pediatric anesthesiologist at each of 51 hospitals listed in the second edition of the *Directory of Pediatric Anesthesiology Fellowship Programs* was asked to provide preoperative fasting guidelines used at his or her institution.

Results.—There were 44 responders (86%). Ad libitum ingestion of clear liquids up to 2 hours before anesthesia was permitted in children younger than 6 months of age by 64% of the hospitals and in children age 6 months or older by 48% of the hospitals. One hospital limited the volume of clear liquids to 8 ounces. Ingestion of breast milk was permitted up to 4 hours before anesthesia in all children. In children younger than 6 months of age, 39% of the institutions permitted ingestion up to 4 hours before anesthesia and 39% permitted ingestion up to 6 hours before anesthesia. Half of the institutions permitted ingestion of formula up to 6 hours before anesthesia in children age 6 months or older. Half of the institutions required a 6-hour fast for solid foods, and half required fasting after midnight. Breast milk was considered a clear fluid by 36% of the hospitals, a solid by 34%, and "something else" by the remaining hospitals. Only 23% of the hospitals allowed ingestion of breast milk less than 4 hours before anesthesia. Formula was categorized as a solid food by 43%, not specified by 36%, and considered neither a solid nor a clear fluid by 20%. Solid food was restricted to at least 4 hours before anesthesia by 34% and was restricted after midnight by 32% in children younger than 6 months of age.

Conclusion.—There are no standard guidelines for fasting before anesthesia in pediatric hospitals.

▶ There is controversy regarding preoperative fasting guidelines for both pediatric and adult anesthetic practice. This study showed that there are no uniform evidence-based fasting guidelines in place in pediatric hospitals in the United States. This may be because there are insufficient data to establish such guidelines. Although pediatric anesthesiologists are clearly more concerned about formula and breast milk than about clear fluids, the authors recommend further discussion. However, it is apparent that, at least in pediatrics, the old practice of making patients eat nothing after midnight has disappeared.

M. Wood, MD

Morbidity and Mortality in Cirrhotic Patients Undergoing Anesthesia and Surgery

Ziser A, Plevak DJ, Wiesner RH, et al (Mayo Clinic and Found, Rochester, Minn; Univ of Pittsburgh, Pa; Univ of Iowa Hosps and Clinics, Iowa City)
Anesthesiology 90:42-53, 1999   1–3

Objective.—Patients with cirrhosis who undergo anesthesia and surgery have an increased mortality rate. Factors that might predict perioperative complications and death in such patients were retrospectively investigated.

Methods.—Records of all 733 adult patients with cirrhosis (338 women), aged 18 to 87 years, undergoing surgery between January 1980 and January 1991 were reviewed for demographic information and concurrent medical conditions. Patients were followed up for 2.7 to 13.7 years. A questionnaire was mailed to living patients at the time of the last follow-up, asking about their health and whether or not there had been a liver transplantation. Patients who had undergone a liver transplantation were excluded from the study.

Results.—Postoperative complications, most commonly pneumonia, occurred in 222 patients (30.1%). Multivariate analysis identified 10 variables associated with occurrence of perioperative complications. There were 72 in-hospital deaths (9.8%) and 13 out-of-hospital deaths (1.8%) within 30 days of surgery, with most deaths occurring in the immediate postoperative period. Multivariate analysis identified 8 variables associated with death, including male sex, a high Child-Pugh score, ascites, cryptogenic cirrhosis, elevated creatinine level, preoperative infection, a high ASA status, and respiratory surgery.

Conclusion.—This investigation confirms that cirrhotic patients undergoing surgery and anesthesia have high morbidity and mortality rates.

▶ Patients with cirrhosis often require surgery and anesthesia, and of course many undergo transplantation surgery. It would be helpful for anesthesiologists to be able to give patients and families some idea of the risk involved. The perioperative mortality rate within 30 days of surgery was 11.6%, and the complication rate was 30%; note that these are figures from a large, well-respected academic health center. To put this number in perspective, overall mortality for all patients 48 hours after anesthesia and surgery is usually under a round 0.8% to 1.0%. This is an important retrospective study, and the next step will be to tease out the causes of the high morbidity and to find ways to prevent their occurrence.

M. Wood, MD

β-Adrenergic Blockers and Vasovagal Episodes During Shoulder Surgery in the Sitting Position Under Interscalene Block
Kahn RL, Hargett MJ (Hosp for Special Surgery, New York)
Anesth Analg 88:378-381, 1999   1–4

Objective.—Approximately 17% of patients undergoing shoulder surgery who are anesthetized with interscalene block in the sitting position experience vasovagal episodes. Because perioperative use of β-adrenergic

TABLE 1.—Patient Demographics and Results

	Group 1 (Event) (n = 20)	Group 2 (No Event) (n = 130)
Age (yr)	47 ± 17	46 ± 16
Sex (M/F)	15/5	89/41
Height (cm)	173 ± 9	171 ± 12
Weight (kg)	80 ± 22	90 ± 32
ASA physical status (%)		
I	50	54
II	45	39
III	5	7
Preoperative		
Systolic BP (mm Hg)	132 ± 19	134 ± 21
Diastolic BP (mm Hg)	73 ± 8	77 ± 11
Heart rate (bpm)	71 ± 11	72 ± 13
Intraoperative		
IV fluids (mL), median (range)	860 (500-1750)	938 (200-3000)
Patients taking β-adrenergic blockers, n (%)	4 (20)	24 (18)*

*$P = .95$.
Abbreviations: ASA, American Society of Anesthesiologists; BP, blood pressure.
(Courtesy of Kahn RL, Hargett MJ: β-adrenergic blockers and vasovagal episodes during shoulder surgery in the sitting position under interscalene block. *Anesth Analg* 88[2]:378-381, 1999.)

agents is associated with a much lower incidence of vasovagal episodes, a retrospective review was conducted to determine whether there was an association between β-adrenergic blockade and the incidence of vasovagal episodes.

Methods.—Of the 151 patients undergoing shoulder surgery between February 1995 and April 1995, 20 (13.3%) who had a vasovagal episode were assigned to group 1. Their charts were reviewed to determine whether they had received β-blockers; age, height, weight, sex, American Society of Anesthesiologists status, preoperative heart rate and blood pressure, type of surgery, total IV fluids, and intraoperative medications were also determined.

Results.—One patient who received atropine was excluded from the analysis. β-Blockers were administered to 20% of the patients in group I and 18% of those in group 2 (Table 1). There was no significant difference between groups.

Conclusion.—There was no association between use of β-blockers and the incidence of vasovagal episodes in this retrospective study. A randomized study is needed to determine incontrovertibly whether β-blockers are truly effective.

▶ This study highlights the high incidence of sudden decrease in heart rate or blood pressure during shoulder surgery performed on patients under interscalene block. It is important to determine the mechanism of these events, which require treatment with perhaps ephedrine or an anticholinergic because prophylaxis might be effective in their prevention. At the present time, it is not possible to determine whether β-blockers are effective in prophylaxis, and apparently a randomized trial is under way.

M. Wood, MD

Magnitude and Time Course of Impaired Primary Haemostasis After Stopping Chronic Low and Medium Dose Aspirin in Healthy Volunteers
Sonksen JR, Kong KL, Holder R (City Hosp, Birmingham, England; Univ of Birmingham, England)
Br J Anaesth 82:360-365, 1999   1–5

Objective.—Most clinicians recommend discontinuing aspirin 7 to 10 days before an invasive procedure, but many patients require aspirin to reduce mortality and morbidity from serious diseases. A few small studies have suggested that primary hemostasis normalizes 48 hours after aspirin ingestion. The changes in bleeding time in the 48 hours after stopping chronic low- or medium-dose aspirin were measured in a randomized, double-blind, placebo-controlled study.

Methods.—Bleeding time was determined in 52 healthy volunteers (42 women), aged 22 to 55 years, at baseline and at 2, 9, 24, and 48 hours after 7 days of 75 mg aspirin daily, 300 mg aspirin daily, or placebo.

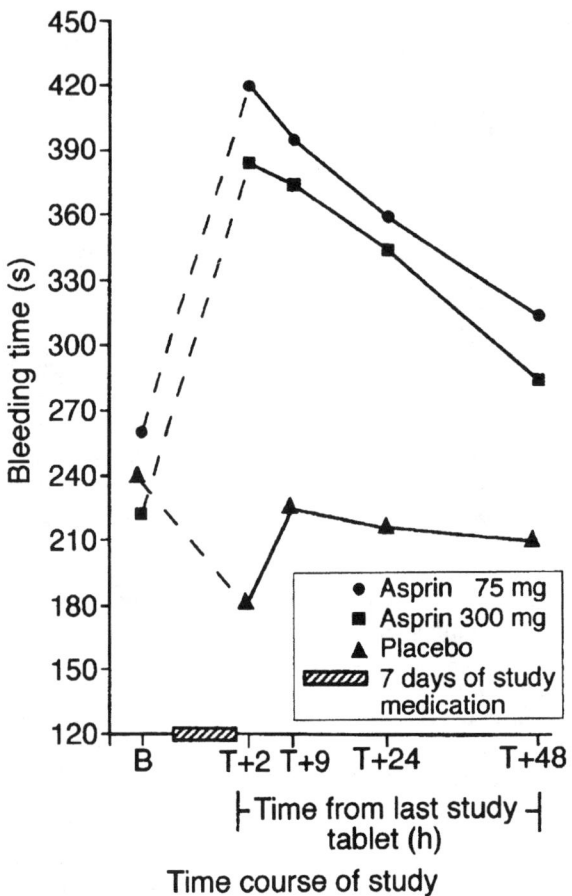

FIGURE 1.—Median bleeding times at each time in the aspirin 75-mg, 300-mg, and placebo groups. B, Baseline. (Courtesy of Sonksen JR, Kong KL, Holder R: Magnitude and time course of impaired primary haemostasis after stopping chronic low and medium dose aspirin in healthy volunteers. *Br J Anaesth* 82:360–365, 1999, by permission of Oxford University Press.)

Results.—Four patients were excluded from the analysis for protocol violations. Median bleeding times peaked before 9 hours in the aspirin groups and were significantly different from baseline values (Fig 1). Six (2 in the 75-mg group and 4 in the 300-mg group) of the 33 volunteers who took aspirin were considered hyperresponders because their bleeding times were extended by more than 5.9 minutes (Fig 2). Although there was a significant difference between baseline and 48-hour bleeding times for both the 75-mg aspirin group (49 seconds) and the 300-mg group (64 seconds), there was no significant difference between groups. There were no bleeding times of more than 10 minutes, which would be considered abnormal.

Conclusion.—Aspirin-induced primary hemostasis had resolved in all healthy volunteers by 48 hours.

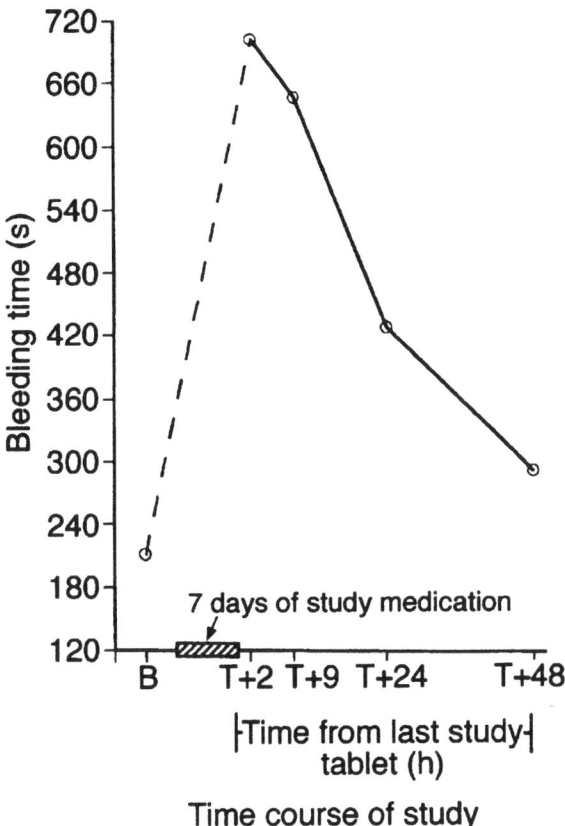

Time course of study

FIGURE 2.—Median bleeding time of hyperresponders at each time. (Courtesy of Sonksen JR, Kong KL, Holder R: Magnitude and time course of impaired primary haemostasis after stopping chronic low and medium dose aspirin in healthy volunteers. *Br J Anaesth* 82:360–365, 1999, by permission of Oxford University Press.)

▶ This study demonstrated that aspirin prolongs bleeding time (as expected) but that bleeding time had returned to nearly normal 48 hours after stopping aspirin. About 25% of patients are hyperresponders, making interindividual variability important, and, as usual, it is the "outliers" who give rise to complications and adverse effects. However, even in this group, primary hemostasis was nearly normal 48 hours after cessation of aspirin therapy. What are the clinical implications of a prolonged bleeding time? In contrast to other coagulation studies, bleeding time is not an easy test to do, and hence there is not a large database from which to estimate risk if bleeding time is prolonged beyond a certain limit. We do have an indication that aspirin increases the incidence and risk of bleeding, but we do not have a good handle on the relationship between bleeding time and risk of bleeding. However, the data regarding time course and primary hemostasis after stopping chronic medium- and low-dose aspirin therapy are very useful and a step in the right direction.

M. Wood, MD

The Value of Routine Preoperative Medical Testing Before Cataract Surgery

Schein OD, for the Study of Medical Testing for Cataract Surgery (Johns Hopkins Univ, Baltimore, Md; et al)

N Engl J Med 342:168-175, 2000   1–6

Introduction.—The rates of perioperative morbidity and mortality associated with cataract surgery are low, despite the fact that patients with cataracts tend to be elderly and have serious coexisting illnesses. These patients commonly undergo routine medical testing before cataract surgery. A prospective, randomized clinical trial was performed to determine whether routine medical testing before cataract surgery reduces the rate of complications in the perioperative period.

Methods.—A total of 19,557 elective cataract surgeries (18,189 patients) from 9 centers were randomly assigned to be preceded or not preceded by a standard battery of medical tests (electrocardiography, complete blood count, and measurement of serum levels of electrolytes, urea nitrogen, creatinine, and glucose), in addition to a history and phys-

TABLE 3.—Rates of Intraoperative and Postoperative Adverse Events

Event	No Testing (N = 9626)		Routine Testing (N = 9624)		Relative Risk (95% CI)†
	No. of Events	No./1000 Operations	No. of Events	No./1000 Operations	
Overall					
Death	2	0.2	1	0.1	2.00 (0.2-22.0)
Hospitalization	33	3.4	28	2.9	1.17 (0.7-2.0)
Other events	266	27.6	272	28.3	0.97 (0.8-1.2)
Total	301	31.3	301	31.3	1.00 (0.9-1.2)
Intraoperative					
Death	0		0		
Hospitalization‡	5	0.5	3	0.3	1.67 (0.4-7.0)
Other events	180	18.7	187	19.4	0.96 (0.8-1.2)
Total	185	19.2	190	19.7	0.97 (0.8-1.2)
Postoperative					
Death	2	0.2	1	0.1	2.00 (0.2-22.0)
Hospitalization	30	3.1	25	2.6	1.20 (0.7-2.0)
Other events	89	9.2	90	9.4	0.99 (0.7-1.3)
Total	121	12.6	116	12.1	1.04 (0.8-1.3)

*Two events occurred (1 intraoperative and 1 postoperative) in 5 operations in each group. Events that occurred before discharge were considered intraoperative.

†The relative risk for operations that were not preceded by routine testing, as compared with operations that were preceded by testing. CI denotes confidence interval.

‡For the intraoperative period, hospitalization was defined as an unplanned hospital admission.

Abbreviation: CI, confidence interval.

TABLE 4.—Diagnoses Associated with Adverse Events

Event	Intraoperative Events				Postoperative Events			
	No Testing (N = 9626)		Routine Testing (N = 9624)		No Testing (N = 9626)		Routine Testing (N = 9624)	
	No. of Events	No./1000 Operations	No. of Events	No./1000 Operations	No. of Events	No./1000 Operations	No. of Events	No./1000 Operations
Cardiovascular								
Myocardial infarction	0		0		3	0.3	5	0.5
Myocardial ischemia	7	0.7	4	0.4	3	0.3	3	0.3
Congestive heart failure	0		0		5	0.5	5	0.5
Arrhythmia*	60	6.2	65	6.8	13	1.4	10	1.0
Bradycardia	44	4.6	45	4.7	8	0.8	2	0.2
Atrial fibrillation	6	0.6	8	0.8	3	0.3	6	0.6
Ventricular tachycardia	1	0.1	0		0		1	0.1
Other arrhythmia	11	1.1	13	1.4	2	0.2	1	0.1
Hypertension	102	10.6	118	12.3	13	1.4	16	1.7
Hypotension	12	1.2	10	1.0	8	0.8	4	0.4
Cerebrovascular								
Stroke	0		0		2	0.2	4	0.4
Transient ischemic attack	0		0		0		1	0.1
Pulmonary								
Respiratory failure	0		0		1	0.1	1	0.1
Bronchospasm	7	0.7	1	0.1	2	0.2	0	
Oxygen desaturation	3	0.3	4	0.4	4	0.4	1	0.1
Upper respiratory tract infection	1	0.1	0		14	1.5	19	2.0
Pneumonia	0		0		5	0.5	6	0.6

(Continued)

TABLE 4 (cont.)

Event	Intraoperative Events				Postoperative Events			
	No Testing (N = 9626)		Routine Testing (N = 9624)		No Testing (N = 9626)		Routine Testing (N = 9624)	
	No. of Events	No./1000 Operations	No. of Events	No./1000 Operations	No. of Events	No./1000 Operations	No. of Events	No./1000 Operations
Metabolic†								
Hypoglycemia	2	0.2	0		0		0	
Treatment for hyperglycemia in patients with diabetes	0		0		3	0.3	3	0.3
Anemia	0		0		1	0.1	1	0.1
Hypokalemia	0		0		0		2	0.2
Other								
Musculoskeletal problem	0		0		24	2.5	15	1.6
Urinary tract infection	0		0		11	1.1	9	0.9
Dermatitis	0		0		7	0.7	7	0.7
Gastrointestinal disturbance	0		0		11	1.1	12	1.2
Atypical chest pain	1	0.1	1	0.1	2	0.2	2	0.2
Other‡	0		0		4	0.4	8	0.8

Note: The rate of bronchospasm differed significantly between the 2 groups. There were no other significant differences between the groups.

*Some patients had more than 1 type of arrhythmia.

†There were no cases of diabetic ketoacidosis or nonketotic hyperosmolarity.

‡In the no-testing group, chills, depression, syncope, and a vasovagal episode were each associated with 1 operation. In the routine-testing group, anxiety was associated with 2 operations, and dizziness, hyponatremia, amnesia, syncope, hyperventilation, and dyspnea were each associated with 1.

(Reprinted by permission of *The New England Journal of Medicine*, from Schein OD, for the Study of Medical Testing for Cataract Surgery: The value of routine preoperative medical testing before cataract surgery. *N Engl J Med* 342:168-175. Copyright 2000, Massachusetts Medical Society. All rights reserved.)

ical examination. Patients were followed up for adverse medical events and interventions on the day of surgery and during the 7 days after surgery.

Results.—In the no-test group, there were 9408 patients who underwent 9624 surgeries. In the group that had testing, there were 9411 patients who underwent 9624 surgeries. Treatment for hypertension and arrhythmia, especially bradycardia, accounted for the most common medical treatments in both groups. The overall perioperative rate of complications was the same for both groups (31.3 events/1000 surgeries). The no-testing and testing groups had similar rates of intraoperative events (19.2 and 19.7, respectively, per 1000) and postoperative events (12.6 and 12.1, respectively, per 1000) (Table 3). Analyses stratified by age, sex, race, physical status, and medical history showed that routine testing offered no benefit in reducing the rate of perioperative events (Table 4).

Conclusion.—Routine medical testing before cataract surgery does not improve the safety of the surgical procedure. It is estimated that the cost of routing medical testing before cataract surgery exceeds $150 million annually. It is likely that the cost of medical testing could be saved without any negative effect on patients' health or clinical outcomes. It is also reasonable to apply these findings to similar populations of patients undergoing surgeries associated with similar surgical risk and use of local anesthesia and IV sedation.

► This is a very important study. It shows that routine preoperative assessment and testing do not affect adverse outcome for cataract surgery. I think we have to ask the question: Why do preoperative testing? To prevent adverse outcome for that particular surgical event or to use it as an opportunity to evaluate the patient's health status and intervene if necessary? I think the health care industry has made this decision—they do not pay. But perhaps physicians have not yet decided. I also think that if we did the same study for postoperative events we would find the same results: no effect on outcome.

M. Wood, MD

Supplemental Perioperative Oxygen to Reduce the Incidence of Surgical-Wound Infection

Greif R, for the Outcomes Research Group (Donauspital, Vienna; et al)
N Engl J Med 342:161-167, 2000   1–7

Introduction.—One of the factors that influence the incidence of surgical-wound infection is the oxygen tension in the tissue. The bacterial activity of neutrophils is mediated by oxidative killing, a crucial defense against operative pathogens. Oxidative killing depends on the generation of bactericidal superoxide radicals from molecular oxygen. The rate of this reaction is subject to the partial pressure of oxygen in the tissue. A simple way to improve oxygen tension is to increase the concentration of inspired oxygen. The use of supplemental oxygen during the perioperative period

TABLE 2.—Outcomes in the 2 Study Groups

Characteristic	Patients Who Received 30% Oxygen (n = 250)	Patients Who Received 80% Oxygen (n = 250)	P Value
Infection — no. (%)	28 (11.2)	13 (5.2)	0.01
ASEPSIS score*	5±9	3±7	0.01
Collagen deposition — ng/mm†	267±109	258±118	0.38
Protein deposition — µg/mm†	163±74	153±91	0.31
First solid food — days after surgery	4.4±1.6	4.5±1.8	0.27
Staples removed — days after surgery	10.4±1.5	10.3±1.4	0.21
Duration of hospitalization after surgery — days	11.9±4.0	12.2±6.1	0.26

Note: Plus-minus values are means ± SD. All P values are 2-tailed.
*Higher scores indicate poorer healing and a greater likelihood of infection.
†Collagen deposition and protein deposition were measured in 32 patients who received 30% oxygen and 22 patients who received 80% oxygen.
(Reprinted by permission of *The New England Journal of Medicine*, from Greif R, for the Outcome Research Group: Supplemental perioperative oxygen to reduce the incidence of surgical-wound infection. *N Engl J Med* 342:161-167. Copyright 2000, Massachusetts Medical Society. All rights reserved.)

was examined for its ability to reduce the incidence of postoperative wound infections in patients undergoing elective colorectal resection.

Methods.—The age range of 500 patients undergoing elective open colorectal resection was 18 to 80 years. The reason for surgery was cancer or inflammatory bowel disease in most patients. Patients were randomly assigned to receive either 30% or 80% inspired oxygen during surgery and for 2 hours afterward. Anesthesia was standardized and all patients were given prophylactic antibiotics. A double-blind protocol was used to evaluate wounds daily until discharge and at a 2-week follow-up clinic visit. Timing of suture removal and date of discharge were determined by the surgeon, who was blinded to the patient's treatment-group assignment.

TABLE 3.—Outcome According to the Presence or Absence of Wound Infection

Characteristic	Infection (n = 41)	No Infection (n = 459)	P Value
ASEPSIS score*	25±13	2±4	<0.001
White-cell count ($\times 10^{-3}$/mm^3)			
Before surgery	8.1±3.0	7.5±2.8	0.19
First day after surgery	11.5±4.0	10.1±3.4	0.02
Third day after surgery	10.7±3.1	8.7±3.2	0.001
Sixth day after surgery	12.5±3.5	8.4±3.2	<0.001
Ninth day after surgery	11.7±4.9	9.0±3.5	0.003
Staples removed (days after surgery)	11.1±2.4	10.3±1.4	<0.001
Duration of hospitalization (days)	18.7±8.3	11.4±4.1	<0.001

Note: Plus-minus values are means ± SD. All P values are 2-tailed.
*Higher scores indicate poorer healing and a greater likelihood of infection.
(Reprinted by permission of *The New England Journal of Medicine*, from Greif R, for the Outcome Research Group: Supplemental perioperative oxygen to reduce the incidence of surgical-wound infection. *N Engl J Med* 342:161-167. Copyright 2000, Massachusetts Medical Society. All rights reserved.)

Results.—Both groups had normal oxygen saturation. The arterial and subcutaneous partial pressure of oxygen was significantly lower in patients who received 30% oxygen versus those who received 80% oxygen. Thirteen (5.2%) and 28 (11.2%) patients who received 80% and 30% oxygen, respectively, had surgical-wound infections (P = .01) (Table 2). The absolute difference between the 30% and 80% oxygen groups was 6.0% Patients with infections had significantly higher ASEPSIS scores and postoperative white-cell counts, had their staples removed 1 day later after surgery, and had prolonged hospital stay by 1 week (Table 3). The 2 groups had a similar duration of hospitalization.

Conclusion.—The administration of supplemental oxygen during colorectal surgery and for 2 hours after surgery reduced to half the incidence of surgical-wound infection. The costs and risks of this practice are minimal and may reduce the incidence of this dangerous and expensive complication.

▶ I have to admit that I was surprised at the results of this study. There is a move to not administer supplemental oxygen in some hospitals if the oxygen saturation measured on a pulse oximeter is above a certain level, especially in outpatient surgical patients—mainly because of cost. The authors mention, in their conclusions, that the cost of supplemental perioperative oxygen is trivial; that is not the case. Oximeter probes, mask, and other equipment may cost around $100, and in these days of cost cutting, this would not be considered insignificant by hospital administrators.

M. Wood, MD

The Effect of Bisoprolol on Perioperative Mortality and Myocardial Infarction in High-Risk Patients Undergoing Vascular Surgery
Poldermans D, for the Dutch Echocardiographic Cardiac Risk Evaluation Applying Stress Echocardiography Study Group (Erasmus Med Ctr, Rotterdam, The Netherlands; et al)
N Engl J Med 341:1789-1794, 1999   1–8

Introduction.—Patients undergoing major vascular surgery are at increased risk for serious perioperative cardiac complications, including nonfatal myocardial infarction and death. Drugs that block β-adrenergic receptors can prevent cardiac complications, including acute myocardial infarction, silent ischemia, and heart failure. It has been proposed that perioperative blockage of β-adrenergic receptors can decrease the risk of perioperative cardiac complications. An assessment was made of the effect of perioperative blockage of β-adrenergic receptors on the incidence of death from cardiac causes and nonfatal myocardial infarction within 30 days after major vascular surgery in patients at high risk for these events in a randomized, multicenter trial.

Methods.—Between 1996 and 1999, all patients undergoing elective abdominal aortic or infrainguinal arterial reconstruction at 7 participating centers were prospectively screened. Eligible patients were randomly assigned to receive either standard perioperative care or standard care plus perioperative β-blockade with bisoprolol.

Results.—Of 1351 patients screened, 846 had 1 or more cardiac risk factors. One hundred seventy-three had positive results on dobutamine echocardiography. Fifty-three patients who were already taking a β-blocker were excluded, as were 8 patients with extensive wall-motion abnormality at rest or during stress testing. Two (3.4%) of 59 patients randomized to receive bisoprolol died of cardiac causes, compared to 9 (17%) of 53 patients in the standard care group ($P = .02$). Nine (17%) patients in the standard care group experienced nonfatal myocardial infarction, compared with none in the standard care plus bisoprolol group ($P < .001$).

Conclusion.—Compared with high-risk patients receiving standard care for major vascular surgery, patients who received standard care plus bisoprolol had a decreased perioperative incidence of death from cardiac causes and nonfatal myocardial infarction.

▶ This is a major study demonstrating that β-adrenergic blockade reduces perioperative mortality and the incidence of myocardial infarction in patients who are undergoing vascular surgery. This is a particularly high-risk surgical group and the results are important. We have seen similar results from other studies reported over the last few years. Indeed, β-adrenergic blockade has been shown to reduce the incidence of sudden death in nonsurgical patients.

Why then, is this therapeutic perioperative intervention not routine? When will it be routine? Bisoprolol was started 37 days before surgery, on average, but the range was 7 to 89 days. Is the time required before surgery to initiate therapy a bar to intervention? Who should perform the intervention? I believe that there is an opportunity here for anesthesiologists to administer β-adrenergic antagonists as part of the continuum of perioperative care to patients who are at intermediate or high risk of cardiac complications—and really make a difference.

M. Wood, MD

Dexmedetomidine Failed to Block the Acute Hyperdynamic Response to Electroconvulsive Therapy
Fu W, White PF (Univ Texas, Dallas)
Anesthesiology 90:422-424, 1999   1–9

Introduction.—Several studies have shown clonidine, a mixed α_2-adrenergic agonist and antagonist, to have a beneficial effect on the hyperdynamic response to electroconvulsive therapy (ECT). Six patients undergoing ECT were studied to evaluate the acute hemodynamic effects of dexmedetomidine, an investigational α_2-adrenergic agonist with a more favorable pharmacokinetic profile than clonidine.

Methods.—The patients were undergoing a series of 3 to 6 consecutive ECT treatments. In the double-blind crossover design, patients were randomly assigned to receive dexmedetomidine, 0.5 or 1.0 µg/kg, or normal saline solution (in a total volume of 0.4 mL/kg). The IV infusions were given 10 to 30 minutes before induction of anesthesia for ECT. An electrical stimulus was administered 2 minutes after induction of anesthesia. To evaluate the effects of the timing of the drug, 3 patients received both doses of dexmedetomidine either 10 or 30 minutes before induction of anesthesia on separate occasions. All patients were monitored for cardiovascular variables, duration of seizure activity, degree of sedation, and time to discharge from the phase I recovery unit.

Results.—The mean age of the patients was 73 years. A total of 24 ECT treatments were evaluated. Mean arterial pressure and heart rate values were unchanged after the 5-minute infusion of the study drug, but these values increased significantly 1 to 2 minutes after administration of the electrical stimulus. Hemodynamic variables were similar in the pretreatments with dexmedetomidine and saline solution, both before and after ECT. The 3 pretreatment regimens did not differ in the times for peak mean arterial pressure and heart rate values to return to baseline values. Times to orientation and to discharge from the phase I unit were prolonged with both dexmedetomidine doses.

Conclusion.—The doses of dexmedetomidine administered to these patients resulted in an increased level of preanesthetic sedation and prolonged recovery compared with placebo and failed to alter the acute hyperdynamic response immediately after ECT. Findings of this pilot study do not support the drug's use as an anesthetic adjuvant during this procedure.

▶ Dexmedetomidine a selective α_2-adrenergic agonist is an extremely interesting drug looking for an indication. Perhaps its use may lie in the production of sedation in the ICU.

M. Wood, MD

Ulnar Neuropathy in Surgical Patients
Warner MA, Warner DO, Matsumoto JY, et al (Mayo Med School, Rochester, Minn; Mayo Clinic, Rochester, Minn)
Anesthesiology 90:54-59, 1999   1–10

Introduction.—Ulnar neuropathy may lead to severe motor disability in surgical patients. The mechanism of this perioperative complication is uncertain, although some studies have suggested that improper positioning or padding of the upper extremity can lead to ulnar nerve compression in the area of the medial epicondyle or cubital tunnel. The frequency, natural history, and risk factors of perioperative ulnar neuropathy were evaluated.

Methods.—The prospective study included 1502 adults undergoing elective noncardiac surgery during a 3-month period. Fifty-seven percent

TABLE 2.—Clinical Characteristics of Patients Who Developed Ulnar Neuropathy

Patient Number	Gender (M/F)	Age (yr)	Procedure	Anesthetic Type	Initial Symptoms	Side
1	M	56	Direct laryngoscopy	Gen	Paresthesia	Bilateral
2	M	60	Herniorrhaphy	Gen	Paresthesia	Right
3	M	74	TURP	Reg	Paresthesia	Left
4	F	50	Vaginal hysterectomy	Gen	Paresthesia	Left
5	M	57	Radical prostatectomy	Reg	Paresthesia	Right
6	M	69	Radical prostatectomy	Gen	Paresthesia	Left
7	M	53	Colostomy	Gen	Paresthesia	Right

Symptom Onset (Days After Surgery)	Neurologic Examination	Course
2	Normal	Resolved within 2 wk
3	Normal	Resolved within 5 wk
4	Normal	Improvement within 6 mo, but residual numbness
4	Normal	Resolved within 6 wk
5	Weakness FDI, ADM; reduced two point sensation 5th finger	Surgery, slight improvement at 2 yr; residual symptoms of numbness, pain, and grip weakness
6	Normal	Improvement within 6 mo, but residual numbness
7	Normal	Resolved within 6 wk

Note: Paresthesia = numbness 4 or 5 fingers.
Abbreviations: TURP, Transurethral resection of the prostate; *Gen,* general; *Reg,* regional (spinal or epidural); *FDI,* first dorsal interosseous muscle; *ADM* abductor digit quinti muscles.
(Courtesy of Warner MA, Warner DO, Matsumoto JY, et al: Ulnar neuropathy in surgical patients. *Anesthesiology* 90:54-59, 1999. Copyright American Society of Anesthesiologists, Inc. Used with permission of Lippincott-Raven Publishers.)

of the patients were women; the mean age was 54 years. Before surgery and every day during the first postoperative week, the patients were assessed using a study questionnaire and neurologic examination. Patients discharged from the hospital during the first postoperative week were followed up by telephone. The diagnosis of ulnar neuropathy was made on the basis of physical examination and symptoms, as well as electrophysiologic studies when indicated. Patients with ulnar neuropathy were followed up for 2 years to determine their long-term outcomes and disabilities.

Results.—Seven patients with ulnar neuropathy were identified, for a frequency of 0.5%. All but 1 of the affected patients were men. The first symptoms of ulnar neuropathy appeared at 2 to 7 days postoperatively, although patients tended to underestimate the time to onset on later questioning—some recalled noticing symptoms immediately on awakening from anesthesia. Six patients had mild ulnar neuropathy, causing only sensory deficits. In 4 of the 7 patients, symptoms resolved within 6 weeks. The other 3 still had symptoms 2 years postoperatively, including 1 patient with a persistent motor deficit (Table 2). The only significant risk factor was male sex; body weight was not a significant factor.

Conclusions.—Ulnar neuropathy is a rare complication of surgery. It affects mainly older men, with symptoms appearing several days after surgery. The male predominance suggests a relationship to certain differences in the anatomy of the ulnar nerve and elbow. In some cases, symptoms of carpal tunnel syndrome may mimic perioperative ulnar neuropathy.

▶ Although ulnar neuropathy is not a frequent complication in surgical patients, it can cause a great deal of discomfort to patients and is not easy to diagnose. The cause is unknown, which makes prevention difficult. In this study, types of procedure are mentioned, but the authors excluded patients undergoing cardiac surgery, in which there may be a very real risk. Men aged 50 to 70 years appear to be at increased risk.

M. Wood, MD

Dilution of Spinal Lidocaine Does Not Alter the Incidence of Transient Neurologic Symptoms
Pollock JE, Liu SS, Neal JM, et al (Virginia Mason Med Ctr, Seattle)
Anesthesiology 90:445-450, 1999   1–11

Background.—Previous researchers have suggested that the dilution of 5% hyperbaric lidocaine before injection for spinal anesthesia may reduce the incidence of transient neurologic symptoms. However, no decrease in incidence between 5% and 2% lidocaine has been reported. Whether further dilution of spinal lidocaine from 2% to 0.5% would reduce the incidence of transient neurologic symptoms was investigated.

Methods.—One hundred nine patients with ASA physical status 1 or 2 who were scheduled for outpatient knee arthroscopy were enrolled in a randomized, double-blind trial. The patients received 50 mg hyperbaric spinal lidocaine in a concentration of 2%, 1%, or 0.5%. On the third postoperative day, patients were interviewed about the incidence of post-operative complications, including transient neurologic symptoms, defined as pain or dysthesia in 1 or both buttocks or legs within 24 hours of surgery.

Findings.—Transient neurologic symptoms occurred in 15.8% of the patients who received 2% lidocaine, 22.2% of those who received 1% lidocaine, and 17.1% of those who received 0.5% lidocaine (Tables 3 and 4). The differences were not statistically significant.

TABLE 3.—Patients Reporting Transient Neurologic Symptoms

	Yes (N = 20)	No (N = 89)
Age (mean) (yr) SD	48.0	50.01
	12.79	12.49
Weight (mean) (kg) SD	67.7	68.0
	4.55	3.99
Sex (F) (N)	13 (*P* = 0.14)	52
(M) (N)	7	57

(Courtesy of Pollock JE, Liu SS, Neal JM, et al: Dilution of spinal lidocaine does not alter the incidence of transient neurologic symptoms. Anesthesiology 90:445-450, 1999. Copyright American Society of Anesthesiologists, Inc. Used with permission of Lippincott-Raven Publishers.)

TABLE 4.—Incidence of Transient Neurologic Symptoms

Licocaine	2% (n = 38)	1% (n = 36)	0.5% (n = 35)
Incidence of TNS*	6 (15.8)	8 (22.2)	6 (17.1)
Incidence of backpain without TNS*	6 (15.8)	6 (16.7)	6 (17.1)

Note: Values are number (%).
*Categories are mutually exclusive.
(Courtesy of Pollock JE, Liu SS, Neal JM, et al: Dilution of spinal lidocaine does not alter the incidence of transient neurologic symptoms. *Anesthesiology* 90:445-450, 1999. Copyright American Society of Anesthesiologists, Inc. Used with permission of Lippincott-Raven Publishers.)

Conclusions.—Reducing spinal lidocaine concentrations from 2% to 1% or 0.5% does not decrease the incidence of transient neurologic symptoms in ambulatory patients who are undergoing arthroscopy. The incidences of transient neurologic symptoms associated with all 3 concentrations are comparable to those reported for 5% lidocaine.

Repeated Transient Neurological Symptoms After Spinal Anaesthesia With Hyperbaric 5% Lidocaine

Panadero A, Monedero P, Fernandez-Liesa JI, et al (Univ of Navarra, Spain)
Br J Anaesth 81:471-472, 1998   1–12

Background.—A single injection of lidocaine for spinal anesthesia has been associated with transient neurologic symptoms. A patient with repeated pain after spinal lidocaine anesthesia was reported.

> *Case Report.*—Man, 74, with a superficial bladder tumor underwent cystoscopy. Three months earlier, the patient had undergone transurethral resection of the bladder tumor with spinal anesthesia. For the current procedure, spinal anesthesia was induced by injection of undiluted 5% hyperbaric lidocaine, 75 mg. No pain or paresthesia occurred during needle insertion or drug injection. Analgesia to T10 was obtained with no hypotension and without vasopressors. Surgery was performed with the patient in the lithotomy position. The duration of the procedure was 30 minutes. The following morning, the patient had no complaints. However, before discharge, the patient asked whether he would experience the same discomfort that he had after previous surgery. He described pain in the hips, buttocks, and legs, radiating to the toes, the day after his previous operation. His past medical record was reviewed, indicating that he had been given a spinal anesthetic consisting of 5% hyperbaric lidocaine, 75 mg, with a 24-gauge Sprotte needle. Thus, the current clinician decided to delay discharge; 30 hours after the spinal puncture, the patient reported a dull pain involving the hips, buttocks, and legs and radiating to the toes. He did not

have headache, fever, or sensory, motor, or muscle tendon reflex abnormalities. Also, he had no bladder or bowel dysfunction. Acetaminophen, 500 mg every 6 hours, partially alleviated his symptoms, which disappeared completely after 18 hours. The patient was then discharged. Six months later, he underwent two 30-minute cytoscopy procedures under general anesthesia in the lithotomy position and did not experience these symptoms.

Conclusions.—This patient had repeated pain associated with the use of spinal lidocaine. All patients who have had spinal anesthesia in the past should be specifically asked about this complication, which many may not report.

▶ Here are two more articles (Abstract 1–11 and 1–12) emphasizing the occurrence of "transient neurologic symptoms" after lidocaine spinal anesthesia. This is a difficult problem, because in these days of ambulatory and fast-track anesthesia, we need a short-acting, safe local anesthetic. Dilution of 5.0% lidocaine does not appear to reduce the incidence of symptoms.

M. Wood, MD

Diaphragmatic Activity After Laparoscopic Cholecystectomy
Sharma RR, Axelsson H, Öberg Å, et al (Umeå Univ, Sweden; Hôpitaux Universitaires de Genéve; Centre Hospitalier Universitaire Vandois, Lausanne, Switzerland)
Anesthesiology 91:406-413, 1999   1–13

Introduction.—Diaphragmatic activity is reported to be reduced in patients undergoing laparoscopic cholecystectomy. Previous studies, however, used indirect indices to measure diaphragmatic contribution to ventilation. The authors of this study evaluated diaphragmatic activity by directly recording diaphragmatic electromyogram (EMG_{dia}) data, along with the indirect indices of pressure and volume-motion changes.

Methods.—The 13 adult patients included in the study were scheduled for elective laparoscopic cholecystectomy. All were classified as American Society of Anesthesiologists physical status 1 or 2. The patients were examined preoperatively for inspiratory tidal changes in gastric ($P_{gas-insp}$) and esophageal ($P_{eso-insp}$) pressures and for tidal changes in rib cage (V_{thor}) and abdominal (V_{abd}) cross-section areas. These values were also obtained 1, 6, and 24 hours postoperatively, together with EMG_{dia} recordings. Data were then used to derive variations in inspiratory gastric ($\Delta P_{gas-insp}$) and inspiratory transdiaphragmatic ($\Delta P_{di-insp}$) pressures.

Results.—Data obtained during the 1- and 6-hour postoperative period showed a significant reduction in the abdominal component of tidal volume (V_{abd} and $V_{abd\%}$) and an increase in the V_{thor} to V_{abd} ratio. Both of these findings indicate a shift toward a thoracic pattern of breathing. Mean $\Delta P_{di-insp}$ decreased from 11.8 cm H_2O preoperatively to 5.7 cm H_2O at 1 hour and 6.6 cm H_2O at 6 hours postoperatively. Twelve of 13 patients had reduced $\Delta P_{gas-insp}$ values at 1 and 6 hours postoperatively. There was a decrease in mean V_{abd} from 327.0 mL preoperatively to 174.0 mL at 1 hour and 175.0 mL at 6 hours. A partial recovery of these values was noted at 24 hours.

Conclusion.—Both direct and indirect indices of diaphragmatic activity showed this activity to be reduced in the immediate postoperative period in patients who have undergone laparoscopic cholecystectomy. Signs of recovery are seen on the first postoperative day.

▶ Diaphragmatic activity is affected by laparoscopic cholecystectomy—an important finding of clinical application for ambulatory patients in the post-operative period.

M. Wood, MD

Laparoscopic Renal and Adrenal Surgery in Obese Patients: Comparison to Open Surgery
Fazeli-Matin S, Gill IS, Hsu THS, et al (Cleveland Clinic Found, Ohio)
J Urol 162:665-669, 1999   1–14

Background.—The efficacy and morbidity of laparoscopic renal and adrenal surgery in obese patients have not been compared with those of open surgery. The outcomes of laparoscopic and open renal and adrenal surgery were compared in markedly and morbidly obese patients.

Methods.—Twenty-one obese persons undergoing laparoscopic renal and adrenal surgery between August 1997 and February 1998 at 1 center were compared with 21 obese patients undergoing open renal and adrenal surgery at the same center between 1994 and 1998. Most of the laparoscopic procedures were performed by the retroperitoneoscopic approach through the flank.

Findings.—Baseline parameters were comparable between groups. Median body mass indexes in the laparoscopic and open surgery groups were 34 and 31, respectively. Median operative times were 210 and 185 minutes, respectively, which were not significantly different. However, blood loss was only 100 mL in the laparoscopic group, compared with 350 mL in the open surgery group. Also, resumption of oral intake and ambulation in the 2 groups was less than 1 day and 5 days, respectively; narcotic analgesic requirements were 12 and 279 mg; median hospital stays were less than 1 day and 5 days; and convalescence was 3 weeks and 9 weeks. Six complications occurred in 4 patients undergoing laparoscopy, and 14 occurred in 9 patients undergoing open surgery.

Conclusions.—Regardless of the surgical approach, markedly obese patients are at increased risk of operative complications. Laparoscopic renal and adrenal surgery is technically feasible in markedly and morbidly obese patients. Compared with open surgery, laparoscopy results in significantly reduced blood loss, quicker return of bowel function, less analgesic requirement, shorter convalescence, and decreased length of hospital stay.

▶ Many anesthesiologists debate the use of laparoscopic surgery as opposed to open surgery in very obese patients and often believe that open surgery would have been not only faster but safer. This article suggests that the procedure is technically feasible and that there may be fewer complications with closed surgery than with open surgery; however, there were only 21 patients in each group and, as always, it is the outliers that are important.

M. Wood, MD

Cognition After Major Surgery in the Elderly: Test Performance and Complaints
Dijkstra JB, Houx PJ, Jolles J (Univ of Maastricht, The Netherlands; Academic Hosp Maastricht, The Netherlands)
Br J Anaesth 82:867-874, 1999   1–15

Objective.—Some elderly patients experience serious and permanent cognitive function after receiving general anesthesia for major surgery. There is a discrepancy between cognitive complaints and cognitive test performance. Short- and long-term postoperative cognitive dysfunction were evaluated, and the correlation between objective cognitive performance and self-reported cognitive dysfunction was investigated.

Methods.—Cognitive memory and attention tests were administered to 48 patients (35 women), aged 60 to 85 years, the day before cardiac surgery, and 7 days and 3 months after surgery, and to 50 healthy nonsurgery volunteers (23 women), aged 57 to 78 years. Scores and changes in scores were compared.

Results.—At 1 week after surgery, patients scored significantly lower than control subjects on sensorimotor speed, memory, interference susceptibility, and information processing. Patients' performance declined while control subjects' performance improved or stayed the same. At 3 months, both groups had improved, but patients improved more than control subjects. At 6 months, 14 (29%) patients said their cognitive function had worsened since they were discharged from the hospital, and 8 (17%) reported that they still had cognitive dysfunction.

Conclusion.—A subgroup of elderly patients experiences prolonged cognitive function after having general anesthesia for major surgery.

▶ I didn't need this study to tell me that as I grow old (and that is rapidly becoming the case) as opposed to "older," it is increasingly difficult to recover from any insult. It is encouraging that these seniors did indeed recover their cognition, indeed some even got better! Maybe we can tout major anesthesia and surgery as a sort of "brain tonic."

J. H. Tinker, MD

Derivation and Prospective Validation of a Simple Index for Prediction of Cardiac Risk of Major Noncardiac Surgery

Lee TH, Marcantonio ER, Mangione CM, et al (Harvard Med School, Boston; Univ of California, San Francisco)
Circulation 100:1043-1049, 1999   1–16

Objective.—There are no good overall tests for assessing the risk of cardiovascular complications during major noncardiac procedures. A simple index for the prediction of the risk of cardiac complications in major elective noncardiac surgery was prospectively derived and validated.

Methods.—Data about major cardiac complications were obtained on 4315 patients, aged 50 years or older, who underwent major elective noncardiac procedures between July 18, 1989 and February 28, 1994, requiring a hospital stay of at least 2 days at a tertiary-care teaching hospital. A reviewer blinded to preoperative and postoperative information classified cardiac complications. A Revised Cardiac Risk Index was developed using data from 2893 patients in the derivation cohort and validated in 1422 patients.

Results.—Major cardiac complications occurred in 56 (2%) patients in the derivation cohort and in 36 (2.5%) patients in the validation cohort. Total deaths in the respective cohorts were 22 (0.8%) and 21 (1.5%). Predictors of complications identified by a logistic regression model included high-risk type of surgery (odds ratio [OR], 2.8), ischemic heart disease (OR, 2.4), history of congestive heart failure (OR, 1.9), history of cerebrovascular disease (OR, 3.2), insulin-dependent diabetes (OR, 3.0), preoperative serum creatinine greater than 2.0 mg/dL (OR, 3.0). In patients with 0, 1, 2, or more factors, cardiac complication rates were 0.5%, 1.3%, 4%, and 9%, respectively for the derivation cohort and 0.4%, 0.9%, 7%, and 11%, respectively for the validation cohort.

Conclusion.—The Revised Cardiac Risk Index can identify patients at high risk and stratify patients at risk for cardiac complications during major noncardiac procedures.

▶ Dr Goldman gave us the "Cardiac Risk Index" in 1977, which proved long lived if controversial. Many attempts to validate it proved elusive, and it has largely been abandoned. Here the same "boss," who really is a "boss" now, has tackled the same problem again. The problem remains the assumption, namely, preoperative risk factor analysis can predict bad cardiovascular outcomes. I fervently wish that was true, but it ignores a major determinant of bad outcomes from anesthesia, namely US. Unfortunately, our errors and lapses, our lack of vigilance, wrong drugs, and other foul-ups are major factors that cannot be predicted by anything with any mathematical certainty. You can assume the risk of this will be higher at 3 AM, but that is about as far as you can go. I wish Dr Goldman luck, and I admire the fact that he is attempting this again. But I am much more appreciative of our roles in all this than apparently he is.

J. H. Tinker, MD

Pre-existing Medical Conditions as Predictors of Adverse Events in Day-Case Surgery

Chung F, Mezei G, Tong D (Univ of Toronto)

Br J Anaesth 83:262-270, 1999   1–17

Objective.—The predictors of perioperative adverse events after outpatient surgery have not been validated. The association of pre-existing medical conditions with perioperative adverse events was examined in a prospective observational study to establish multivariable statistical models for accurate risk assessment.

Methods.—During a 3-year period, data were collected on 17,638 consecutive surgical outpatients (two thirds female), aged 11 to 98 years, in Toronto Hospital. Eighteen pre-existing conditions and intraoperative and postoperative adverse events were entered into the backward stepwise multiple logistic regression model. Variables were stratified by age, sex, and duration and type of surgery.

Results.—The frequency of intraoperative adverse events increased with age, whereas the frequency of postoperative adverse events tended to decrease with age older than 40 years. The highest frequency of intraoperative events occurred in ophthalmic (5.4%), urologic (5.2%), and ENT-dental (4.7%) procedures. The lowest frequency occurred in gynecologic (1.4%) and chronic pain block (1.3%) procedures. The highest frequencies of adverse events in the post-anesthesia care and ambulatory care units occurred in orthopedic (20% and 10%) and ENT-dental (14% and 20%) patients, and the lowest frequencies occurred in ophthalmic (2.6% and 4.2%) and chronic pain block (4.5% and 3.2%) patients. Pre-existing conditions were present in 54% of patients. According to the model, hypertension increased the risk for intraoperative (odds ratio [OR], 2.2) and cardiovascular intraoperative (OR, 2.5) events. Obesity increased the risk of intraoperative respiratory events (OR, 3.9). Gastroesophageal reflux increased the risk of intubation-related events (OR, 8.0). Asthma (OR, 4.6), obesity (OR, 3.9), and smoking (OR, 3.8) increased the risk of postoperative respiratory events. The accuracy of the 5 models varied from 0.69 to 0.78.

Conclusion.—Hypertension was the most significant predictor of perioperative adverse events in surgical outpatients.

▶ Hypertension, obesity, asthma, reflux, smoking, etc—they found 7 predictors of post-op trouble. That's nothing surprising, but this study is a model for the kind of meticulous well-researched, concisely written studies that we have come to expect from Dr Chung and her excellent Toronto group.

J. H. Tinker, MD

A Cost Comparison of Methohexital and Propofol for Ambulatory Anesthesia

Sun R, Watcha MF, White PF, et al (Univ of Texas Southwestern Med Ctr, Dallas; Children's Hosp of Philadelphia)
Anesth Analg 89:311-316, 1999   1–18

Objective.—Newer anesthetic drugs are eliminated from patients' systems more quickly, resulting in earlier awakening, but they are also more expensive. The costs of propofol and methohexital for induction of anesthesia and of sevoflurane and desflurane for maintenance of anesthesia during ambulatory surgery were compared.

Methods.—Ambulatory surgery patients (n = 120) were randomly allocated to receive methohexital-desflurane, methohexital-sevoflurane, propofol-desflurane, or propofol-sevoflurane. Anesthesia and surgery times, adverse events, and costs were recorded.

Results.—Early recovery times, need for postoperative analgesia, incidence or severity of postoperative nausea and vomiting, and need for antiemetic medication were similar for all groups. Costs were significantly lower for patients who received methohexital and either sevoflurane or desflurane primarily because of the lower cost of induction drugs.

Conclusion.—Using methohexital rather than propofol for induction of anesthesia is less expensive. The most cost-effective combination was methohexital-desflurane.

▶ I doubt that many anesthesiologists will agree that the incidences of nausea and vomiting would be anywhere near this high in their practices. Could it be that the reason there were no differences in the incidences of these problems, between the 2 anesthetic regimens, is really because the basal incidences were so high in the first place? Most will likely stick to their propofol after reading and evaluating this study.

J. H. Tinker, MD

Relation of Surgical Volume to Outcome in Eight Common Operations: Results From the VA National Surgical Quality Improvement Program

Khuri SF, and the Participants in the VA National Surgical Quality Improvement Program (Harvard Med School, Boston; et al)
Ann Surg 230:414-432, 1999   1–19

Objective.—Most studies of surgical volume vs outcome are limited because: they are retrospective, they glean data from administrative databases, they are biased in their institutional selections, and they do not make preoperative risk adjustments. The relation between surgical volume and outcome in 8 common operations in the Veterans Health Administration data from the FY91-FY97 VA National Surgical Quality Improvement Program, which contains preoperative patient risk factors, operative data, and 30-day outcome information, were prospectively reviewed.

Methods.—There were 123 Veteran Affairs Medical Centers that contributed data on lung lobectomy/pneumonectomy, open and partial colectomy, vascular infrainguinal reconstruction, ruptured abdominal aortic aneurysmectomy, carotid endarterectomy, laparoscopic cholecystectomy, and total hip arthroplasty.

Results.—When 68,631 surgeries were analyzed, 68.4% to 81.0% were primarily performed by a resident in the presence of, or with the assistance of, a staff attending physician. Hospital volume and risk-adjusted 30-day mortality rate were not correlated in any of the procedures studied. The ratio of observed vs expected number of deaths between low-volume and high-volume hospitals varied widely, because the O/E estimate is less stable when sample sizes are small. Risk-adjusted mortality was not significant for an O/E ratio for any operation, because hospitals in lower volume quartiles had larger standard deviations than hospitals in larger volume quartiles. None of the models were able to identify a volume that specifically predicted risk-adjusted 30-day outcomes.

Conclusion.—There was no relationship between surgical volume of a particular specialty and risk-adjusted 30-day mortality. Expected mortality rates were calculated based on preoperative risk factors.

▶ This massive VA effort concludes that currently cherished dogma, namely that surgical volume is associated with outcome, is simply not true. It is a good example of a conundrum that we often see in medicine, namely that ideas that seem logical and sound do not necessarily prove to be true when rigorously examined.

J. H. Tinker, MD

A Multicentre Comparison of the Costs of Anaesthesia With Sevoflurane or Propofol
Smith I, Terhoeve PA, Hennart D, et al (Keele Univ, Stoke-on-Trent, Staffordshire, England; Academic Hosp, Utrecht, The Netherlands; Univ Hosp Erasme, Belgium; et al)
Br J Anaesth 83:564-570, 1999   1–20

Objective.—Sevoflurane is less expensive than propofol for out-patient anesthesia, but indirect costs and anesthesia maintenance costs have not been evaluated. The relative costs of propofol and sevoflurane anesthesias were assessed in a multinational, multicenter, prospective, open-label, randomized European study.

Methods.—Anesthesia was induced and maintained with propofol (group 1, n = 72), with propofol and sevoflurane (group 2, n = 70), and with sevoflurane (group 3, n = 69) in a random fashion to out-patients, aged 17 to 71 years, undergoing 15- to 90-minute procedures. Costs of anesthesia, anesthesia maintenance, analgesic medications, and disposables were tallied for all procedures.

Results.—Compared with the sevoflurane group, induction of anesthesia was significantly faster in propofol groups. Although induction times with propofol were fairly consistent, inductions times for sevoflurane were quite variable. Time to re-start of spontaneous ventilation was significantly shorter for the sevoflurane group than for the propofol groups. Although emergence and recovery times were not significantly different between propofol and sevoflurane groups, time to walk unaided was significantly longer in the sevoflurane group and incidence of postoperative nausea and vomiting (PONV) was significantly higher. Drug costs were $18.70 for group 1, $14.20 for group 2, and $17.30 for group 3. Total costs, including anesthetic drug waste and disposables costs, were $31.90 for group 1, $19.70 for group 2, and $18.80 for group 3.

Conclusion.—Propofol was more expensive than sevoflurane regimens, but sevoflurane regimens produced more PONV.

▶ The last line of the abstract originally published with this study caught my eye and engendered this comment to wit; "Although we observed increased nausea and vomiting in groups 2 and 3 and reduced patient satisfaction in group 3, *these differences should be balanced against the greater cost of propofol anaesthesia*" [italics mine]. Are we really coming to this? Would these authors choose the anesthetic for their child based on cost if the cheaper one would subject their loved one to more nausea and vomiting? I hope not. Shame on these authors! I am disgusted.

J. H. Tinker, MD

Cost Analysis of Xenon Anesthesia: A Comparison With Nitrous Oxide–Isoflurane and Nitrous Oxide–Sevoflurane Anesthesia
Nakata Y, Goto T, Niimi Y, et al (Teikyo Univ, Chiba, Japan; Ichihara Hosp, Chiba, Japan)
J Clin Anesth 11:477-481, 1999   1–21

Objective.—Costs of xenon anesthesia were compared with costs of nitrous oxide–isoflurane and nitrous oxide–sevoflurane.

Methods.—The costs of 4 anesthesia management techniques were evaluated in a hypothetical 40-year-old patient, ASA physical status 1, weighing 70 kg and undergoing minor surgery with tracheal intubation and mechanical ventilation. The 4 techniques included 240 minutes of closed-circuit anesthesia with xenon, closed-circuit anesthesia with nitrous oxide–isoflurane, semiclosed-circuit anesthesia with nitrous oxide–isoflurane, and semiclosed-circuit anesthesia with nitrous oxide–sevoflurane.

Results.—The respective costs of the 4 techniques were $356, $52, $94, and $84. Although the cost of xenon was comparable to the costs for the other anesthetics, the cost of xenon priming and flushing was significantly higher than priming and flushing costs for the other anesthetic gases.

Conclusion.—Xenon anesthesia is significantly more expensive than nitrous oxide–isoflurane or nitrous oxide–sevoflurane, primarily because of the expenses associated with xenon priming and flushing.

▶ Anesthesia with xenon is somebody's quest. It just doesn't seem to die. I have included an article or 2 on anesthesia with this noble gas in each YEAR BOOK for the past several years now. I think this study is important for one thing only, namely, that the authors have begun to think about salvaging anesthetics. The next logical step will be recycling. I can imagine a volatile agent "trap" device on the roof of the hospital, where the output of the OR scavenging system is filtered and the agents are trapped, separated, and purified for re-use. Of course, just about the time I spent the money to get the system up and running, the pharmaceutical companies would lower the price of the volatiles below my cost. Isn't capitalism wonderful?

J. H. Tinker, MD

2 Obstetric Anesthesia

Labor

Combination of Intrathecal Sufentanil 10 μg Plus Bupivacaine 2.5 mg for Labor Analgesia: Is Half the Dose Enough?

Sia ATH, Chong JL, Chiu JW (KK Women and Children's Hosp, Singapore)
Anesth Analg 88:362-366, 1999   2–1

Objective.—Intrathecal (IT) sufentanil during labor sometimes results in hypotension. Whether halving the total amount of IT sufentanil and bupivacaine would provide adequate analgesia with a concomitant reduction in incidence of hypotension was tested in a controlled, double-blind, prospective trial.

Methods.—After administration of combined spinal-epidural (CSE) analgesia, either 10 μg of sufentanil and 2.5 mg bupivacaine (group A, n = 21) or half that dose (group B, n = 21) was administered to 42 women in early labor. Baseline pain scores at 5, 15, and 30 minutes after CSE; systolic blood pressure every 5 minutes; highest sensory block to cold 5, 15, and 30 minutes after CSE; maximal degree of motor block in lower limbs at 5, 15, and 30 minutes; shivering; pruritus; nausea; vomiting; sedation; and fetal heart rate were recorded.

TABLE 3.—Incidence of Side Effects

	Group A	Group B
SBP reduced by ≥20% within 30 min of CSE	9/21	2/21*
Motor block (Bromage score >0)		
5 min after CSE	2/21	0/21
15 min after CSE	5/21	0/21*
30 min after CSE	4/21	0/21
Sedation	9	1*
Pruritus	9	8
Nausea and vomiting	1	1
Respiratory depression	0	0
Shivering	1	0
Postdural puncture headache	1	0

*Significant difference between the two groups (P < .05).
Abbreviations: CSE, Combined spinal-epidural anesthesia; SBP, systolic blood pressure.
(Courtesy of Sia ATH, Chong JL, Chiu JW: Combination of intrathecal sufentanil 10 μg plus bupivacaine 2.5 mg for labor analgesia: Is half the dose enough? *Anesth Analg* 88[2]:362-366, 1999.)

Results.—Group A patients had a significantly higher incidence of hypotension (9 vs 2), a higher incidence of lower limb motor block, and a higher incidence of sedation than did group B patients (9 vs 1). Group B patients had higher pain scores than did group A patients 5 minutes after CSE. Total amount of bupivacaine, duration of second-stage labor, mode of delivery, changes in fetal heart rate, Apgar scores, neonatal birth weight, and overall satisfaction scores were similar for the 2 groups. The incidence of side effects was similar for the 2 groups (Table 3).

Conclusion.—Half the dose of IT sufentanil and bupivacaine provided a comparable degree of analgesia. Onset of action was slower and duration of analgesia was shorter with the halved dose. The incidence of side effects was similar for the 2 groups.

▶ Early reports of IT sufentanil administration in laboring women described the administration of 10 to 15 µg of sufentanil. A growing number of anesthesiologists currently administer a smaller dose (ie, 5-7.5 µg) of IT sufentanil in laboring women. Some anesthesiologists add a small dose (ie, 1.25-2.5 mg) of bupivacaine to the sufentanil. In this study, the smaller dose of sufentanil did not result in a decreased incidence of pruritus. However, the reduced dose should reduce the incidence of other maternal side effects and complications (eg, sedation, respiratory depression).

D. H. Chestnut, MD

Bupivacaine Augments Intrathecal Fentanyl for Labor Analgesia
Palmer CM, Van Maren G, Nogami WM, et al (Arizona Health Sciences Ctr, Tucson)
Anesthesiology 91:84-89, 1999   2–2

Introduction.—Intrathecal fentanyl is an effective analgesic for labor and is frequently used as part of a combined spinal-epidural technique. Its use is limited by a short duration of action and side effects, particularly pruritus. The effect on duration and quality of analgesia of the addition of low-dose bupivacaine to intrathecal fentanyl was examined in 90 parturients in active labor who requested regional analgesia.

Methods.—Patients were randomly assigned to receive intrathecal injection of either fentanyl, 25 µg; bupivacaine, 1.25 mg, with fentanyl, 25 µg; or bupivacaine, 2.5 mg, with fentanyl, 25 µg, as part of a combined spinal-epidural technique. Visual analogue pain scores were assessed before and at intervals after injection until patient request for further analgesia. Lower extremity muscle strength was assessed before and 30 minutes after injection. Anesthetic level to cold sensation and the presence and severity of pruritus were noted.

Results.—The duration of analgesia was longer in patients who received bupivacaine, 2.5 mg, and fentanyl, 25 µg, compared with those who received fentanyl alone. The onset of analgesia was longer for both groups of patients who received bupivacaine, compared with fentanyl alone.

There were no between-group differences in muscle strength after injection. Anesthetic levels to cold were observed in all patients in the bupivacaine groups and 21 of 30 patients in the fentanyl group alone. Baseline fetal heart rates and maternal blood pressure did not change after injection in any group.

Conclusion.—The combination of fentanyl, 25 µg, with bupivacaine, 2.5 mg, lengthened the duration and accelerated onset of analgesia, compared with fentanyl, 25 µg, alone. Motor strength was similarly affected in all patient groups. Sensory changes that could alter propioception were observed in all groups.

▶ Many advocates of combined spinal-epidural analgesia now recommend the addition of a small dose (1.0-2.5 mg) of bupivacaine to the lipid-soluble opioid (fentanyl or sufentanil). This should allow the anesthesiologist to give a smaller dose of opioid, which may reduce the incidence or severity of pruritus and respiratory depression.

D. H. Chestnut, MD

Comparison of Midwife Top-ups, Continuous Infusion and Patient-controlled Epidural Analgesia for Maintaining Mobility After a Low-dose Combined Spinal-Epidural

Collis RE, Plaat FS, Morgan BM (Queens Charlotte's Hosp, London)
Br J Anaesth 82:233-236, 1999   2–3

Objective.—Motor block and the ability to ambulate safely, quality of combined spinal-epidural analgesia, and the mother's satisfaction with analgesia were compared for 3 methods of continuing analgesia during labor.

Methods.—One mL 0.25% bupivacaine (2.5 mg) and 0.5 mL fentanyl (25 µg) were injected into the cerebrospinal fluid of 133 primigravid women who were then randomly allocated to receive continuous infusion (CI, n = 46), midwife top-ups with a 10-mL bolus every 30 minutes, if requested (MW, n = 43), or patient-controlled epidural analgesia (PCEA,

TABLE 3.—Mean Bupivacaine and Fentanyl Use (Mean (SD)) in the
Continuous Infusion (Group CI), Midwife Top-up (Group MW) and
Patient-Controlled Epidural Analgesia (Group PCEA) Groups

	MW (*n* = 43)	CI (*n* = 46)	PCEA (*n* = 44)	*P* (ANOVA)
Bupivacaine (mg h⁻¹)	7.5 (3.1)	11.5 (3.3)	9.1 (2.1)	<0.001*
Fentanyl (µg h⁻¹)	18.8 (7.7)	29.9 (12.7)	21.8 (7.5)	<0.001†

*Groups MW *vs* PCEA (*P* = .02); group PCEA *vs* CI(*P* < .001)(*t* test).
†Group MW *vs* group PCEA (*P* = .07); group PCEA *vs* group CI (*P* < .001) (*t* test).
(Courtesy of Collis RE, Plaat FS, Morgan BM: Comparison of midwife top-ups, continuous infusion and patient-controlled epidural analgesia for maintaining mobility after a low-dose combined spinal-epidural. *Br J Anaesth* 82:233-236, 1999. Reprinted by permission of Oxford University Press.)

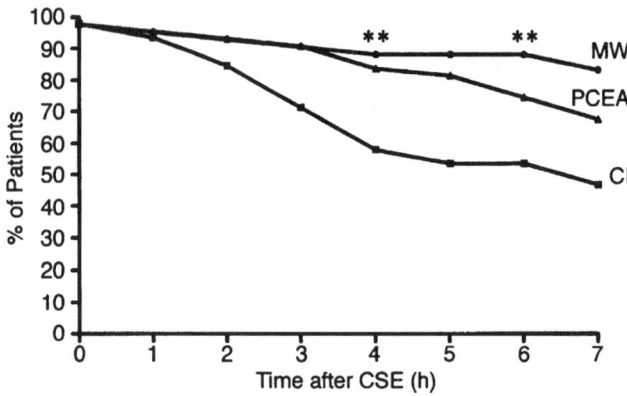

FIGURE 1.—Percentage of patients able to straight leg raise after combined spinal-epidural analgesia in the continuous infusion (group *CI*), midwife top-up (group *MW*) and patient-controlled epidural analgesia (group *PCEA*) groups. Differences among groups were significant (3 × 2 chi-square on number of patients) at 4 hours and were still significant at 6 hours (*******P* < .01). (Courtesy of Collis RE, Plaat FS, Morgan BM: Comparison of midwife top-ups, continuous infusion and patient-controlled epidural analgesia for maintaining mobility after a low-dose combined spinal-epidural. *Br J Anaesth* 82:233-236, 1999. Reprinted by permission of Oxford University Press.)

n = 44). All epidural solutions contained 0.1% bupivacaine with fentanyl 2 µg/mL. Patients assessed pain on a verbal analogue scale hourly. Motor power was assessed hourly by ability to perform a straight leg raise.

Results.—Bupivacaine use was lowest in the MW group and highest in the CI group (Table 3). Median pain scores were similar among groups. Motor block developed in 20 of 23 patients in group CI, 7 of 9 in group MW, and 9 of 15 in group PCEA (Fig 1). Analgesia and satisfaction were very high in all groups.

Conclusion.—Bupivacaine use was highest in the CI group. Analgesia and patient satisfaction were high in all groups.

▶ This study confirms the results of other studies, which have demonstrated that a continuous-epidural infusion technique results in administration of a higher total dose of bupivacaine than an intermittent bolus dose or PCEA technique in laboring women. Of interest, women in this study in the MW group received a lower total dose of bupivacaine than women in either the CI or the PCEA group. The role of PCEA in laboring women remains a matter of debate. Recently, we have gained some experience with this technique in our practice, and overall, we are pleased with the results.

D. H. Chestnut, MD

Effect of Maternal Ambulation on Labour With Low-dose Combined Spinal-Epidural Analgesia

Collis RE, Harding SA, Morgan BM (Queen Charlotte's Hosp, London)
Anaesthesia 54:535-539, 1999   2–4

Background.—Some authorities have suggested that confining women to bed during labor can prolong and worsen the pain of labor, as well as increase abnormal presentations, instrumental deliveries, and fetal distress. The effects of ambulation on labor duration, need for epidural top-ups, delivery mode, and neonatal condition were investigated.

Methods and Findings.—Two hundred twenty-nine nulliparous women requesting regional analgesia during labor were given a combined spinal-epidural (CSE) block, then randomly assigned to stay in bed or to spend 20 minutes or more of every hour out of bed. The 2 groups did not differ significantly in labor duration, analgesia requirement, delivery mode, or neonatal condition. Ambulation appeared to be safe. In both groups, women were highly satisfied with the low-dose CSE analgesia.

Conclusions.—Although ambulation duing labor does not appear to have definitive advantages over confinement to bed, ambulation has no disadvantages. Laboring women generally have a positive view of ambulation.

▶ Some anesthesiologists have expressed great enthusiasm for maternal ambulation in laboring women who receive CSE analgesia. Supervised ambulation seems safe for both the mother and the fetus, provided that the mother retains adequate motor function, proprioception, and balance. However, the benefits—if any—of maternal ambulation remain unclear.

D. H. Chestnut, MD

Effect of Combined Spinal-Epidural Ambulatory Labor Analgesia on Balance

Pickering AE, Parry MG, Ousta B, et al (Royal Free Hosp, London)
Anesthesiology 91:436-441, 1999   2–5

Background.—Because low-dose combined spinal-epidural (CSE) analgesia preserves lower limb motor power and allows ambulation during labor, this form of analgesia is popular with women. However, the safety of allowing women to walk after the analgesia is debated because of somatosensory impairment. Balance function in pregnant women after CSE analgesia was investigated in a prospective, controlled, observational study.

Methods.—After regional analgesia was instituted, 44 women underwent posturographic assessment (Fig 2). Findings were compared with those in a control group of 44 women. Another group of 6 women was tested before and after CSE analgesia.

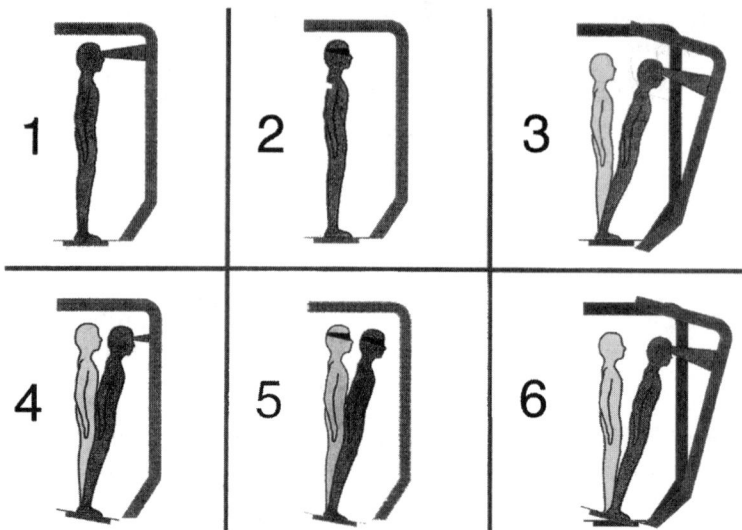

FIGURE 2.—Schematic of the sensory organization tests. For the first 3 tests, the forceplate remains fixed while the visual conditions are varied (eyes open, eyes closed, and sway-referenced visual surround) to examine the effect of loss of accurate visual orientation clues. In tests 4–6, the forceplate is sway-referenced, providing misleading somatosensory feedback, while the visual conditions are varied. In tests 3 and 6, the visual surround is sway-referenced. (Courtesy of Pickering AE, Parry MG, Ousta B, et al: Effect of combined spinal-epidural ambulatory labor analgesia on balance. *Anesthesiology* 91:436-441, 1999. Copyright American Society of Anesthesiologists, Inc. Used with permission of Lippincott-Raven Publishers.)

Findings.—After regional analgesia, 4% of the parturients had motor weakness, and 9% had clinical dorsal column sensory loss. Women given CSE analgesia had a small but significant decrease in 1 of 6 posturographic sensory-organization tests, though the difference was functionally minor. No other differences in posturography were noted between the control and CSE groups. Results in the paired study were similar, showing minimal change in balance function after CSE analgesia.

Conclusions.—Computerized dynamic posturography showed no functional impairment in balance function after CSE ambulatory analgesia in this series of women in labor, with no clinical evidence of motor block. This is the first study to objectively assess the effect of CSE analgesia on balance function.

► Supervised ambulation seems safe during administration of CSE analgesia, *provided* the mother retains adequate motor function, proprioception, and balance, and *provided* there is no evidence of postural hypotension. However, the benefits of ambulation remain unclear.

D. H. Chestnut, MD

The Safety and Efficacy of Combined Spinal and Epidural Analgesia/Anesthesia (6,002 Blocks) in a Community Hospital

Albright GA, Forster RM (Bellevue Woman's Hosp, Niskayuna, NY)

Reg Anesth Pain Med 24:117-125, 1999   2–6

Objective.—The safety and efficacy of combined spinal and epidural (CSE) analgesia for cesarean delivery was retrospectively reviewed.

Methods.—Outcomes, side effects, complications, and failure rates for 6002 CSE blocks administered between January 1, 1994 and December 31, 1997 were compared with those of spinal and epidural anesthesia. The respiratory rate was recorded every 30 minutes for 4 hours and then hourly for 12 to 24 hours. Patients were monitored with a pulse oximeter for at least 12 hours.

Results.—Intrathecal administration of sufentanil rarely induced nausea and vomiting requiring treatment unless epinephrine was also given. Hypotension developed in 2.2% of patients. The corrected failure rate for anesthesia via an epidural catheter was 3.8%. Twelve patients required general anesthesia. The initial regional anesthesia failure rate in patients not having a CSE labor block was 0.9%. Side effects of intrathecal sufentanil requiring IV treatment included pruritus (n = 8), dysphagia (n = 71), and low partial pressure of oxygen in alveoli/drowsiness (n = 24). One percent of non–cesarean delivery patients required general anesthesia. For cesarean deliveries, 1.5% of patients required general anesthesia. The corrected prevalence of no CSF in the spinal epidural needle was 0.6%. The prevalence of pruritus, dysphagia, low partial pressure of oxygen in alveoli, or any side effect increased with the intrathecal dose of sufentanil.

Conclusion.—The anesthesia complication rate for CSE is similar to the complication rates found in the literature for CSE and epidural anesthesia. CSE is effective for labor analgesia and surgical anesthesia in cesarean and non-cesarean deliveries. Monitoring patients with a pulse oximeter lowers the risk of acute respiratory depression.

▶ These authors have called attention to the increased risk for maternal sedation and respiratory depression in laboring women who receive intrathecal opioid analgesia *after* systemic opioid administration. They recommend careful patient observation—including the use of continuous pulse oximetry—for 1 to 2 hours after intrathecal administration of a lipid-soluble opioid such as sufentanil.

D. H. Chestnut, MD

Analgesia, Pruritus, and Ventilation Exhibit a Dose-Response Relationship in Parturients Receiving Intrathecal Fentanyl During Labor

Herman NL, Choi KC, Affleck PJ, et al (Cornel Univ, New York; Wilford Hall Med Ctr, Lackland Air Force Base, Tex; 48th Med Operations Squadron, Royal Air Force Lakenheath, England)

Anesth Analg 89:378-383, 1999   2–7

Background.—Although several studies have reported on the 50% and 95% effective doses of intrathecal (IT) sufentanil for labor analgesia, few have investigated these criteria for fentanyl, a less expensive alternative. Also, the ventilatory effects of IT fentanyl at clinically relevant doses have not been established. The dose-response relationship of IT fentanyl for both analgesia and ventilatory depression was investigated.

Methods.—By random assignment, 90 parturients in active early labor were given IT fentanyl in doses of 5, 7.5, 10, 15, 20, or 25 µg. The percentage of women attaining analgesic success was used to construct quantal dose-response curves, from which the ED_{50} and ED_{95} values were derived for the total population, nulliparous subgroup, and multiparous subgroup.

Findings.—The overall 50% value was 5.5 µg, and the overall 95% value was 17.4 µg. Nulliparous values were 5.3 and 15.9 µg, respectively, compared with 6.9 and 26 µg, respectively, for multiparous women. How-

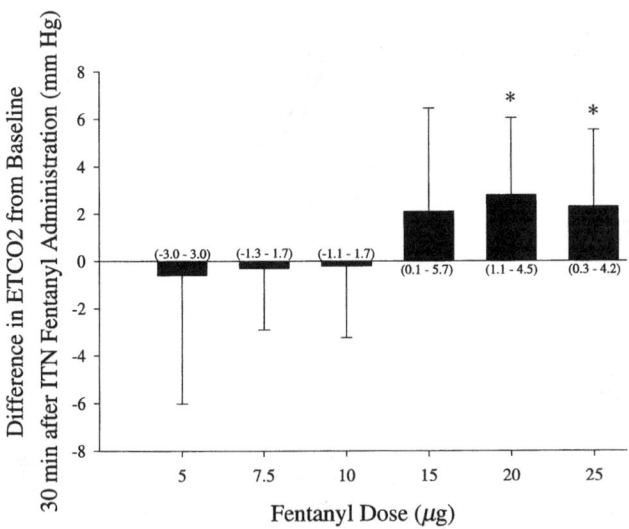

FIGURE 2.—Mean of the differences in end-tidal carbon dioxide concentration (ET_{CO_2}) in parturients with analgesic success for the 6 IT fentanyl groups (5 µg, n = 5; 7.5 µg, n = 11; 10 µg, n = 11; 15 µg, n = 9; 20 µg, n = 15; and 25 µg, n = 11) at the 30-minute sampling point when the ET_{CO_2} response was maximal. *Asterisk* indicates significant differences from baseline ($P \leq .05$, Bonferroni adjustment). The *error bars* represent the standard deviation. The values within the parentheses are the 95% CIs for each group. *Abbreviation: ITN*, intrathecal narcotics. (Courtesy of Herman NL, Choi KC, Affleck PJ, et al: Analgesia, pruritus, and ventilation exhibit a dose-response relationship in parturients receiving intrathecal fentanyl during labor. *Anesth Analg* 89[2]:378-383, 1999.)

ever, the former values were within the 95% CIs of the total population. The incidence of pruritus in women attaining analgesic success showed a dose-response relationship identical to that for analgesia. A dose-related increase occurred in end-tidal carbon dioxide concentration, especially at doses of 15 µg or more, with no concomitant changes in respiratory rate of arterial oxygen percent saturation, suggesting a reduction in tidal volume (Fig 2). Even without overt signs or symptoms of somnolence, IT fentanyl at doses within the effective analgesic range produced ventilation changes that may have lasted longer than the 30 minutes of observation.

Conclusion.—IT fentanyl induces rapid, effective, dose-dependent analgesia in early labor. However, it also results in dose-related reductions in ventilation in the absence of overt somnolence.

▶ The authors of this study observed "dose-related decreases in ventilation in the absence of overt somnolence." They observed no change in respiratory rate, which suggests that the increased end-tidal carbon dioxide concentration occurred as a result of decreased tidal volume. Further, oxygen saturation decreased significantly only in those patients who received 25 µg of fentanyl. This study highlights the importance of adequate monitoring of patients who receive an intrathecal opioid during labor. Further, anesthesiologists should exercise caution when giving an IT opioid to a patient who has received systemic opioids earlier in labor.

D. H. Chestnut, MD

Respiratory Arrest Following Intrathecal Injection of Sufentanil and Bupivacaine in a Parturient
Katsiris S, Williams S, Leighton BL, et al (Univ of Toronto)
Can J Anaesth 45:880-883, 1998   2–8

Introduction.—The combined spinal-epidural (CSE) has become increasingly popular as a means of relieving pain in laboring parturients. Lower drug dosage, minimal motor and sympathetic blockage with highly selective sensory blockade, and rapid onset of analgesia make CSE an attractive alternative to epidural in the obstetric patient. Described was a healthy parturient in labor who experienced respiratory arrest after initiation of CSE.

Case Report.—Woman, 20, was admitted to the hospital in active labor. She had no drug allergies and was taking no regular medication. She reported that she had not taken any drugs before admission. The patient had never been exposed to opioids. She requested analgesia within 30 minutes of admission and received 10 µg sufentanil and 2.5 mg bupivacaine intrathecally as part of a CSE. About 15 minutes after the intrathecal injection, she complained of mild pruritus. Five minutes later, she complained of sleepiness, although she was alert and responsive. At 23 minutes after intrathecal injection, the patient was unresponsive and experienced a respiratory arrest. Naloxone, 0.4 mg, was administered IV 3 minutes after respiratory arrest, with immediate return of consciousness and respiratory efforts. She remained awake and was drowsy, so additional doses of naloxone, 0.4 mg, were administered IV at 7 and 13 minutes from initiation of resuscitation. At 105 minutes after the intrathecal injection, the patient experienced pain with contractions. Bupivacaine 0.125% with epinephrine, 1:600,000, was administered at 8 mL/h for 115 minutes. One hour later, vacuum delivery was performed and the patient delivered a healthy male infant. The remaining 8 mL of diluted sufentanil were tested; an overdose did not occur.

Conclusion.—Respiratory arrest is an unusual, yet potentially life-threatening, complication associated with the use of intrathecal opioids for labor analgesia. Patients must be carefully monitored after administration of these drugs.

▶ Most cases of intrapartum respiratory depression after intrathecal opioid administration have occurred in parturients who received 10 to 15 µg of sufentanil intrathecally. For this reason, I prefer to give a smaller dose (5-7.5 µg) of sufentanil, with or without a small dose (1-2.5 mg) of bupivacaine. Regardless of the dose, vigilance is essential.

D. H. Chestnut, MD

Intrathecal Bupivacaine Reduces Pruritus and Prolongs Duration of Fentanyl Analgesia During Labor: A Prospective, Randomized Controlled Trial
Asokumar B, Newman LM, McCarthy RJ, et al (Rush-Presbyterian-St Luke's Med Ctr, Chicago)
Anesth Analg 87:1309-1315, 1998   2–9

Introduction.—Pruritus is a common complication (40%-100%) of intrathecal (IT) administration of fentanyl (F) at 25 µg in laboring parturients. It frequently requires antipruritic therapy. The frequency of pruritus when using combined F and bupivacaine (B) 2.5 mg has been reported to be 17.3% in a nonrandomized trial of 300 consecutive parturients. The effect of IT B and F on the incidence and distribution of pruritus was examined in 65 laboring parturients. Analgesic duration was also assessed.

Methods.—Patients were randomly assigned to either IT F, B, or F + B as part of a combined spinal-epidural technique. Visual Analogue Scores, sensory level, motor strength, and pruritus were recorded at baseline before injection and at intervals thereafter. Distribution of pruritus was examined, when present. The duration of analgesia was considered as the time from IT drug administration until the patient requested supplemental analgesia.

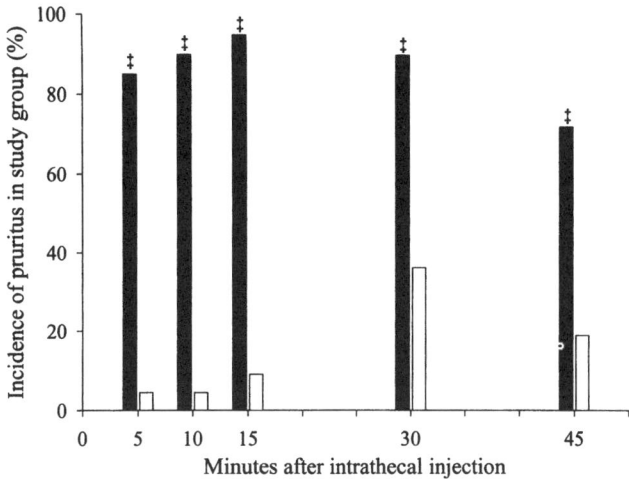

FIGURE 2.—The incidence of pruritus in the fentanyl (*black bars*) and the fentanyl + bupivacaine (*white bars*) study groups as a function of time after intrathecal drug administration. *Double dagger* indicates significantly different from fentanyl + bupivacaine at a specified time ($P < .05$). (Courtesy of Asokumar B, Newman LM, McCarthy RJ, et al: Intrathecal bupivacaine reduces pruritus and prolongs duration of fentanyl analgesia during labor: A prospective, randomized controlled trial. *Anesth Analg* 87[6]:1309-1315, 1998.)

Results.—The median duration of analgesia was 94.5 minutes for the F + B group. For the F and B groups, these times were 62.5 minutes and 55.0 minutes, respectively. The frequency of pruritus was 95% in the F group and 36.4% in the F + B group (Fig 2). Facial pruritus was 25% in both the F and F + B group. The occurrence of pruritus distributed over the rest of the body was significantly higher in the F group, compared with the F + B group.

Conclusion.—The duration of labor analgesia is prolonged with IT administration of F + B, compared with F alone or B alone. The combined therapy also diminishes the incidence of pruritus, except in the facial region.

▶ The addition of a small dose of local anesthetic (eg, bupivacaine) to a lipid-soluble opioid allows a reduction in the dose of IT opioid in laboring women. For example, the addition of bupivacaine (1-2.5 mg) allows administration of smaller IT doses of fentanyl (15-20 µg) or sufentanil (5 to 7.5 µg). Administration of a smaller dose of opioid should reduce the risk of respiratory depression. In this study, the authors identified an additional (albeit unexplained) benefit: a reduced incidence of truncal pruritus. It will be interesting to see whether other studies confirm this observation.

D. H. Chestnut, MD

The Incidence of Fetal Heart Rate Changes After Intrathecal Fentanyl Labor Analgesia

Palmer CM, Maciulla JE, Cork RC, et al (Univ of Arizona, Tucson; Louisiana State Univ, Shreveport; Southern Arizona Anesthesia, Tucson)
Anesth Analg 88:577–581, 1999   2–10

Background.—Although intrathecal (IT) fentanyl is effective for analgesia in laboring parturients, concerns have been raised that it may adversely affect fetal heart rate (FHR). The current study compared the incidence of new FHR abnormalities after IT fentanyl and conventional epidural labor analgesia.

Methods.—The first 100 parturients in active labor receiving epidural analgesic, and with FHR recorded for 30 minutes before and after injection, were compared with the first 100 parturients given IT fentanyl analgesic. A perinatologist unaware of the anesthetic method used assessed each recording and identified FHR changes.

Findings.—The incidence of new "negative" changes, indicating worsened fetal status, was 6% in the epidural group and 12% in the IT group. No differences occurred in the incidence or degree of blood pressure change, need for cesarean delivery, neonatal outcome, parity, or oxytocin use. No urgent or emergent cesarean deliveries were performed. All FHR changes resolved within the 30-minute observation period (Table 2).

Conclusions.—With both analgesic techniques evaluated, the incidence of FHR changes was low. Neonatal outcomes in the 2 groups did not differ. However, a much larger study is needed to verify and determine the clinical implications of these findings.

▶ This study is subject to the potential for a type II statistical error. That is, the authors may not have reviewed a sufficient number of cases to exclude the possibility that FHR abnormalities are more common after IT opioid analgesia than after epidural analgesia. For example, the authors observed five cases of fetal bradycardia in the IT group versus only one case in the epidural group. The authors correctly acknowledged that "a much larger series would be necessary to determine whether there. . .is a difference in

TABLE 2.—Type of Negative FHR Changes

	Intrathecal	Epidural
Decelerations		
Early	2	
Variable	3	3
Late	2	2
Isolated bradycardia(s)	5	1

Abbreviation: FHR, Fetal heart rate.
(Courtesy of Palmer CM, Maciulla JE, Cork RC, et al: The incidence of fetal heart rate changes after intrathecal fentanyl labor analgesia. *Anesth Analg* 88:[3]:577-581, 1999.)

the incidence of FHR changes between these techniques, and further study of the clinical significance of such FHR changes is necessary."

D. H. Chestnut, MD

A Randomized Study of Combined Spinal-Epidural Analgesia Versus Intravenous Meperidine During Labor: Impact on Cesarean Delivery Rate
Gambling DR, Sharma SK, Ramin SM, et al (Univ of Texas, Dallas)
Anesthesiology 89:1336-1344, 1998   2–11

Introduction.—Combined spinal-epidural (CSE) analgesia offers rapid-onset pain relief and allows ambulation in early labor. Epidural local anesthetics may add to operative deliveries by reducing perineal sensation and producing motor weakness. It is possible that CSE may reduce operative delivery rates by avoiding or delaying administration of local anesthetics. The effects of CSE were compared with those of IV meperidine on the rate of cesarean delivery in laboring parturients with normal full-term pregnancies.

Methods.—Patients were randomized to receive either CSE or IV meperidine analgesia. Patients in the CSE group received 10 µg intrathecal sufentanil. This was followed by epidural bupivacaine and fentanyl for subsequent requests for analgesia. Patients in the meperidine group received 50 mg of IV meperidine on demand. The maximum was 200 mg in 4 hours. Labor and delivery outcomes were recorded and compared.

Results.—An intent-to-treat analysis of 1223 women showed that CSE did not raise the rate of cesarean delivery for dystocia in nulliparous and parous women or in nulliparous women alone. Profound fetal bradycardia

---

TABLE 3.—Mode of Delivery Analyzed by Intent to Treat

Delivery	CSE (n = 616) (%)	Meperidine (n = 607) (%)	Significance
Spontaneous	526 (86)	539 (89)	NS
Outlet forceps	10 (1.5)	10 (1.5)	NS
Low forceps	41 (6.5)	24 (4)	0.036
Forceps indication			
Failure to progress	16 (2.5)	14 (2.2)	NS
Nonreassuring FHR	35 (5.5)	20 (3.3)	0.045
Cesarean delivery	39 (6)	34 (5.5)	NS
Dystocia	23 (3.5)	25 (4.0)	NS
Nonreassuring FHR strip	16 (2.5)	9 (1.5)	NS
Profound fetal bradycardia within 60 min of initial administration of analgesic	9 (1.5)	0	<0.005

Abbreviations: CSE, combined spinal-epidural; *FHR*, fetal heart rate; *NS*, not significant.
(Courtesy of Gambling DR, Sharma SK, Ramin SM, et al: A randomized study of combined spinal-epidural analgesia versus intravenous meperidine during labor: Impact on cesarean delivery rate. *Anesthesiology* 89:1336-1344, 1998. Copyright American Society of Anesthesiologists, Inc. Used with permission of Lippincott-Raven Publishers.)

that required emergency cesarean delivery within 1 hour of the time the mother received sufentanil occurred in 8 of 400 women, compared with 0 of 352 who received meperidine (the difference was significant) (Table 3). The method of fetal monitoring varied between groups. Overall neonatal outcomes were similar between groups, despite differences in monitoring.

Conclusion.—The cesarean delivery rate for dystocia in healthy parturients at full term does not increase with administration of CSE analgesia during labor. An unexpected rise in the number of cesarean deliveries for profound fetal bradycardia after administration of intrathecal sufentanil was seen in this patient series. Further investigation is needed.

▶ This study represents this group's third prospective, randomized study of CSE versus IV meperidine analgesia during labor. In this study, the most important observation was a significant increase in the incidence of emergency cesarean section for fetal bradycardia in the CSE group. Other anesthesiologists have observed anecdotal cases of fetal bradycardia after intrathecal opioid administration, but most studies have not demonstrated a significant increase in the requirement for emergency cesarean section in patients who received intrathecal opioid analgesia.

Some anesthesiologists have hypothesized that fetal bradycardia may follow intrathecal opioid administration because of increased uterine tone resulting from an abrupt decline in maternal plasma concentrations of epinephrine. Additional studies are needed to determine whether intrathecal administration results in an increased incidence of fetal bradycardia and, if so, whether the bradycardia can be treated conservatively (for example, with nitroglycerin) or requires emergency cesarean section.

D. H. Chestnut, MD

Is Combined Spinal-Epidural Analgesia Associated With More Rapid Cervical Dilation in Nulliparous Patients When Compared With Conventional Epidural Analgesia?
Tsen LC, Thue B, Datta S, et al (Harvard Med School, Boston)
Anesthesiology 91:920-925, 1999   2–12

Background.—The combined spinal-epidural (CSE) technique is reportedly associated with rapid onset of labor analgesia and shorter labor duration. By contrast, epidural analgesia appears to modestly prolong labor. However, whether more rapid cervical dilation in patients undergoing CSE analgesia is a physiologic effect of the method or an artifact of patient selection is not clear. The effects of CSE analgesia were compared with those of epidural analgesia on cervical dilation rate.

Methods.—One hundred healthy nulliparous parturients in spontaneous labor were enrolled in the double-blind trial. All were delivering singleton, vertex, full-term fetuses. Before cervical dilation reached 5 cm, the women were assigned randomly to combined CSE analgesia or the

TABLE 1.—Progress of Labor

	Combined Spinal-Epidural	Epidural
Onset of labor to analgesia (h)	10.0 ± 5.2	11.6 ± 8.9
Analgesia to full cervical dilation (h)	3.8 ± 2.6	5.1 ± 2.6*
Full cervical dilation to delivery (h)	1.8 ± 1.2	2.2 ± 1.5
Initial cervical dilation rate (cm/h)†	2.1 ± 2.1	1.0 ± 1.0*
Mean cervical dilation rate‡	2.3 ± 2.6	1.3 ± 0.7*
Mode of delivery (%)		
Spontaneous vaginal	68	66
Instrumental vaginal	16	16
Cesarean section	16	18

Note: Times and cervical dilation rates are shown as mean ± SD.
*$P < .05$ for difference between analgesic groups.
†Initial cervical dilation rate = (first cervical examination after analgesia − last cervical examination before analgesia)/time between examinations.
‡Mean cervical dilation rate = (10 − last cervical examination before analgesia)/time between examinations.
(Courtesy of Tsen LC, Thue B, Datta S, et al: Is combined spinal-epidural analgesia associated with more rapid cervical dilation in nulliparous patients when compared with conventional epidural analgesia? *Anesthesiology* 91:920-925, 1999. Copyright American Society of Anesthesiologists, Inc. Used with permission of Lippincott-Raven Publishers.)

epidural technique. Data on cervical dilation, pain, sensory level, and motor blockade were analyzed.

Findings.—After the induction of regional analgesia in comparable groups at 3 cm of cervical dilation, the mean initial cervical dilation rates were significantly more rapid in the CSE group. Five women in the CSE group and none in the epidural group had a very rapid rate of mean initial cervical dilation, exceeding 5 cm/h (Table 1). Overall mean cervical dilation rates in women achieving full cervical dilation were 2.3 cm/h with CSE and 1.3 cm/h after epidural analgesia.

Conclusions.—CSE analgesia provides more rapid cervical dilation than epidural analgesia in healthy nulliparous parturients in early labor. More research is needed to determine the cause and overall effect of this difference.

▶ In this study, women who received CSE analgesia had more rapid cervical dilation than women who received epidural analgesia alone. Similarly, Leighton et al[1] observed that women who received lumbar sympathetic block had more rapid cervical dilation than women who received epidural analgesia. However, there was no difference between the 2 groups in obstetric outcome (ie, method of delivery) in either study.

D. H. Chestnut, MD

Reference

1. Leighton BL, Halpern SH, Wilson DB: Lumbar sympathetic blocks speed early and second stage induced labor in nulliparous women. *Anesthesiology* 90:1039-1046, 1999.

Observations on Labor Epidural Analgesia and Operative Delivery Rates
Yancey MK, Pierce B, Schweitzer D, et al (Tripler Army Med Ctr, Honolulu, Hawaii)
Am J Obstet Gynecol 180:353-359, 1999   2–13

Objective.—The operative delivery rates in a large population of women who gave birth at military medical centers when the use of epidural analgesia was highly restricted were retrospectively compared with the operative delivery rates in a group of women who gave birth when epidural analgesia was available on request.

Methods.—Before October 1993, epidural analgesia was available only to patients who were determined to have a medical need. After October 1993, the US Department of Defense mandated that epidural analgesia be available on demand to laboring women. Two cohorts of women who gave birth either 20 months immediately before the mandate or 20 months immediately after the mandate were compared. Epidural demand stabilized at about 60%. The proportions of vaginal and cesarean births were compared.

Results.—There were 4778 women with singleton pregnancies in the "before" group and 4859 women in the "after" group. The percentages of women requiring operative delivery before and after the mandate were not significantly different (13.8% and 14.9%, respectively). The modes of delivery before and after the mandate were spontaneous vaginal delivery (68.3% vs 69.5%), forceps delivery (5.5% vs 5.9%), vacuum (6.4% vs 5.2%), vaginal breech delivery (0.4% vs 0.4%), primary cesarean (13.4% vs 13.2%), and repeated cesarean (6.0% vs 5.8%). Nulliparous women who requested and received epidural analgesia were almost twice as likely to require a cesarean section or operative delivery as women who did not receive epidural analgesia. The effect of epidural analgesia on labor and delivery could not be explained.

Conclusion.—Although epidural analgesia does not appear to increase a laboring woman's risk for cesarean or operative delivery, a subset of nulliparous laboring women who requested and received epidural analgesia had almost twice the risk of a cesarean or operative delivery.

▶ This article presents yet another study that has demonstrated that the introduction of an epidural analgesia service did not result in an increased incidence of cesarean section. Of interest, the epidural analgesia rate was 59% during the "after" period. These results are similar to the observations made in other "sentinel event" studies. Maternal-fetal factors and obstetric management—not epidural analgesia—are the major determinants of the cesarean section rate.

D. H. Chestnut, MD

Epidural Analgesia and Active Management of Labor: Effects on Length of Labor and Mode of Delivery
Rogers R, Gilson G, Kammerer-Doak D (Univ of New Mexico, Albuquerque)
Obstet Gynecol 93:995-998, 1999   2–14

Introduction.—Controversy continues regarding use of epidural analgesia in early labor versus at a time when cervical dilatation is more advanced. Medical records of 255 women who requested epidural analgesia and were randomly assigned to active management of labor or a control protocol were examined retrospectively to determine whether cervical dilatation at the time of placement of patient-requested epidural affects incidence of cesarean deliveries or duration of labor.

Methods.—Of 255 women evaluated, 125 were randomly assigned to active management of labor and 130 to control protocols. Active management of labor included amniotomy within 2 hours of admission; augmentation of labor with oxytocin if there was not 1 cm dilatation per hour in the first stage of labor or 1 cm of descent per hour in the second stage; use of uterine pressure transducers if clinically indicated; and electronic fetal heart rate monitoring. Control protocol included admission to the labor suite based on cervical dilatation of 3 to 4 cm with regular, painful uterine contractions; or oxytocin augmentation if labor did not progress adequately. Patients were stratified according to early epidural placement (up to 4 cm cervical dilatation) versus late placement (more than 4 cm).

Results.—Women with early epidural placement had significantly shorter labors, compared with those with late placement. Duration of labor was significantly shorter in women randomized to active management, compared with controls (10.9 vs 12.3 hours). Women with early epidurals had a nonsignificantly higher cesarean rate, compared with those with late epidurals. Women who had actively managed labors had a nonsignificantly lower cesarean rate, compared with control subjects; this was not affected by timing of epidural placement. Early epidural placement did not lengthen the second stage of labor, nor did it raise the rates of operative vaginal deliveries.

Conclusion.—Early epidural placement did not affect the duration of labor or cesarean rate and was associated with shorter labor than was late placement. Regardless of timing of epidural placement, women whose labors were managed actively had shorter labors than control subjects did.

The Influence of the Obstetrician in the Relationship Between Epidural Analgesia and Cesarean Section for Dystocia
Segal S, Blatman R, Doble M, et al (Brigham and Women's Hosp, Boston)
Anesthesiology 91:90-96, 1999   2–15

Introduction.—Retrospective and prospective randomized trials evaluating the effect of epidural analgesia on the progress and outcome of labor have been plagued with methodologic difficulties. It seemed likely that if epidural analgesia affected the rate of cesarean sections, then obstetricians with higher utilization rates of epidural analgesia for labor would have higher rates of cesarean section because of dystocia. The frequency of use of epidural analgesia and the frequency of occurrence of various patient risk factors for cesarean section were analyzed for 110 obstetricians caring for 50 or more low-risk parturients.

Methods.—Summaries of deliveries for each obstetrician were obtained and were analyzed according to type of delivery and primary type of anesthesia. Additional data were abstracted regarding maternal and fetal characteristics. Stepwise regression using 3 variables (gestational age, provider volume, and frequency of induction of labor) was performed to help predict obstetricians' cesarean rates in relation to the incidence of various patient and provider risk factors.

Results.—There was no significant relationship between the frequency of epidural analgesia use and the rate of cesarean section because of dystocia across practitioners. These findings were not changed when weighting each obstetrician's data for the number of patients cared for during the evaluation period. Stepwise linear regression modestly predicted obstetricians' cesarean section rates because of dystocia and provided a model containing 12 variables not including epidural analgesia: gestational age, induction of labor, maternal age, provider volume, nulliparity, and 7 interactions.

Conclusion.—Frequency of use of epidural analgesia was not predictive of obstetricians' rates of cesarean section because of dystocia. After accounting for several known patient risk factors, individual obstetrician practice style seemed to be a primary determinant of rates of cesarean section.

▶ Several randomized clinical trials have demonstrated that the contemporary use of epidural analgesia does *not* increase the overall incidence of cesarean section. These 2 studies support my long-standing belief that maternal-fetal factors and obstetric management—not epidural analgesia—are the most important determinants of the cesarean section rate.

D. H. Chestnut, MD

Effects of Providing Hospital-based Doulas in Health Maintenance Organization Hospitals
Gordon NP, Walton D, McAdam E, et al (Kaiser Permanente Medical Care Program of Northern California, Oakland; Kaiser Permanente Med Ctr, Oakland, Calif; Kaiser Permanente Medical Care Program, Oakland, Calif)
Obstet Gynecol 93:422-426, 1999   2–16

Background.—There are reports that some women in labor who receive doula support have decreased odds of cesarean delivery; use of forceps, oxytocin, epidural anesthesia, and analgesia; and long labor. It has also been reported that women who have doula support during labor report better coping, lower perception of labor pain, quicker bonding with the baby, and less postpartum anxiety and depression. It is unclear whether the results of these studies apply to current labor and delivery conditions in the United States, or to populations of privately insured women giving birth in private hospitals.

Methods.—In a randomized study, 314 nulliparous women enrolled in a health maintenance organization were studied. The women gave birth in 1 of 3 hospitals managed by a health maintenance organization. Of the 314 women, 149 had doulas and 165 did not. Data were obtained from medical charts, study intake forms, and phone interviews.

Results.—Compared with women who did not have doula support during labor, women who had doulas had significantly less use of epidural anesthesia and were also significantly more likely to rate the birth experience as good, to feel that they coped well with labor, and to feel that labor had a positive effect on their feelings as a woman and on their perception of their bodies' strength and performance. Rates of cesarean, vaginal, forceps, and vacuum delivery; oxytocin use; breast-feeding; postpartum depression; and measures of self-esteem were similar in the 2 groups.

Discussion.—In these patients in this labor and delivery setting, labor support from doulas had a positive effect on the use of epidural anesthesia and on women's feelings about the birth experience. The need for operative deliveries was not affected by use of doulas. Although technology has replaced the human aspect of patient care in some areas, outcome has not improved. The effect of experienced woman labor companions on the outcome of labor and delivery deserves reevaluation.

▶ This study did not confirm the results of earlier studies, which suggested that maternal support from doulas results in a decreased requirement for operative delivery. In this study, there was a modest decrease in the use of epidural analgesia among women in the doula group. It is arguable whether this is a desirable outcome.

D. H. Chestnut, MD

Lumbar Sympathetic Blocks Speed Early and Second Stage Induced Labor in Nulliparous Women

Leighton BL, Halpern SH, Wilson DB (MCP Hahnemann Univ, Philadelphia; Univ of Toronto; Women's College Hosp)
Anesthesiology 90:1039-1046, 1999   2–17

Objective.—Epidural analgesia prolongs the first and second stages of labor. Results of a single-blind pilot study to compare the effects of lumbar sympathetic block (LSB) with those of epidural analgesia on labor speed and delivery route in nulliparous women undergoing labor induction were presented.

Methods.—The rate of cervical dilation in the first 2 hours after block placement, the rate of cervical dilation in active first-stage labor (4- to 10-cm cervical dilation), the length of the second labor stage, the rate of cesarean delivery for dystocia, block complications, and maternal satisfaction were assessed in full-term, nulliparous women, average age 32. Women were randomly allocated to receive initial labor analgesia with either epidural analgesia (10 mL 0.125% bupivacaine, 50 µg fentanyl, and 100 µg epinephrine and sham LSB) (n = 19) or LSB analgesia (10 mL 0.5% bupivacaine, 25 µg fentanyl, and 50 µg epinephrine bilateral and epidural catheters) (n = 17).

Results.—The rate of cervical dilation (57 vs 120 min/cm) and speed of second-stage labor was significantly faster in the LSB group than in the epidural group (105 vs 270 minutes). The speed of first-stage labor was rapid and similar for both groups. The rate of cesarean delivery was 26% in the epidural group and 6% in the LSB group. After 30 minutes, the epidural group had significantly more dermatomes blocked than did the LSB group (13 vs 4). Whereas fright inhibits uterine contractions, alpha-adrenergic blockage abolishes the tocolytic effects of fright.

Conclusion.—Patients receiving LSB had more rapid cervical dilation during the first 2 hours, a shorter second stage of labor, and a lower cesarean delivery rate.

▶ LSB remains a useful technique in selected parturients with abnormal spinal anatomy (eg, Harrington rod instrumentation). The results of this study support earlier, uncontrolled observations that LSB may accelerate the first stage of labor, and this technique may have a role in a larger population of patients. The authors' hypothesis (see Fig 3) deserves further investigation.

D. H. Chestnut, MD

Labor Analgesia With Paravertebral Lumbar Sympathetic Block
Suelto MD, Shaw DB (Univ of Alabama, Birmingham)
Reg Anesth Pain Med 24:179-181, 1999   2–18

Objective.—The use of paravertebral lumbar sympathetic block (LSB) to provide first-stage labor analgesia in 2 laboring mothers with spine pathology was discussed.

> *Case 1.*—Woman, 27, with spina bifida, had premature membrane rupture at 24 weeks' gestation. Bupivacaine LSB was placed with the patient in the sitting position. Analgesia was effective in 7 minutes, and complete cervical dilation and effacement was achieved in 155 minutes. The infant was delivered and had Apgar scores of 2 and 6 at 1 and 5 minutes, respectively.
>
> *Case 2.*—Woman, 33, who had had Harrington rod placement for scoliosis 18 years earlier, went into labor at 39 weeks' gestation.

Bupivacaine right-sided LSB was placed with the patient in the sitting position. The infant was delivered 108 minutes later and had Apgar scores of 8 and 9 at 1 and 5 minutes, respectively.

Conclusion.—Paravertebral LSB provides effective and lasting analgesia for patients with spine pathology.

▶ LSB remains a useful technique for selected parturients with previous back surgery (eg, Harrington rod instrumentation). In a recent study, Leighton et al[1] observed that nulliparous women who received LSB had faster cervical dilation during the first 2 hours of analgesia, as well as a shorter second stage of labor, compared with similar women who received epidural analgesia.

D. H. Chestnut, MD

Reference

1. Leighton BL, Halpern SH, Wilson DB: Lumbar sympathetic blocks speed early and second stage induced labor in nulliparous women. *Anesthesiology* 90:1039-1046, 1999.

The Effects of Needle Bevel Orientation During Epidural Catheter Insertion in Laboring Parturients
Richardson MG, Wissler RN (Univ of Rochester, NY; Strong Mem Hosp, Rochester, NY)
Anesth Analg 88:352-356, 1999   2–19

Objective.—Inadvertent dural puncture with an epidural needle bevel orifice oriented laterally may result in reduced incidence of postdural puncture headache. The analgesia success, side effects, and complications associated with catheter insertion through lateral- and cephalad-oriented Tuohy needle bevels in women in labor were prospectively investigated.

Methods.—Anesthesia residents were randomly selected to identify the epidural space with the needle bevel oriented either cephalad or lateral for the first half of the month and the other way for the second half of the month using an 18-gauge Tuohy needle followed by a 20-gauge open-ended, nonstyletted, single-orifice polyamide catheter. Patients rated labor pain before and 20 minutes after administration of analgesia. Pain scores on a Visual Analogue Scale were compared between the lateral (n = 240) and cephalad (n = 294) patients.

Results.—Outcomes of 475 catheter insertions in 445 patients were reported. First attempts resulted in successful analgesia in significantly more patients in the cephalad group than in the lateral group (91.1% vs 80.2%, respectively). Initial unsuccessful catheter insertion was subsequently successful in 1.9% and 12.4%, respectively. Paresthesias during catheter insertion occurred with greater frequency in the lateral group than in the cephalad group (31% vs 23%, respectively), but IV cannulation (5.8% vs 5.1%), dural puncture (3.8% vs 2.0%), postdural puncture headache (0.4% vs 0.7%), and asymmetric block (31% vs 27%) rates were similar. Patients in the lateral group who experienced paresthesias were significantly more likely to report them on the same rather than the opposite side (78% vs 22%), and the greatest block was more often on the same side as the paresthesia (78% vs 22%). There were no differences in pain scores between groups.

Conclusion.—Whereas the lateral approach reduces the incidence of postdural puncture headache, it increases the risk of dural puncture, resulting in a greater incidence of paresthesias.

▶ The results of this study seem intuitive, namely that insertion of the epidural catheter with the epidural needle orifice oriented in a cephalad direction results in a greater likelihood of satisfactory epidural analgesia in laboring women.

D. H. Chestnut, MD

Increased Risk of Unintentional Dural Puncture in Night-time Obstetric Epidural Anesthesia
Aya AGM, Mangin R, Robert C, et al (CHU Gaston Doumergue, Nîmes, France)
Can J Anesth 46:665-669, 1999   2–20

Background.—Operator experience and training are generally considered to be the main factors affecting the incidence of unintentional dural puncture (UDP). Operator experience and the time of epidural anesthesia as factors contributing to UDP were investigated.

Methods and Findings.—Data on 1489 consecutive epidural procedures were analyzed. Twelve women had UDP, for an incidence of 0.8%. The relative risk of UDP was greater at night than during the day, with a risk ratio of 6.33. Seven punctures were caused by 3 operators with little expertise. Five were caused by 2 skilled obstetric anesthesiologists.

Conclusion.—Operator experience and the hour of the procedure are important risk factors for UDP. The increase in UDP risk at night may be the result of human factors, such as fatigue.

▶ The authors of the present study noted that other studies performed in nonmedical settings have demonstrated a "circadian variation in accident frequency." Likewise, Bromage[1] noted that "most medical and nonmedical accidents occur on the night shift, with a peak incidence in the early morning between 3 AM and 7 AM, when the human circadian rhythm sets the biologic clock for its nadir of wakefulness."[1,2]

D. H. Chestnut, MD

References

1. Bromage PR: Neurologic complications of labor, delivery, and regional anesthesia, in Chestnut DH (ed): *Obstetric Anesthesia: Principles and Practice*, ed 2. St Louis, Mosby, 1999, pp 639-661.
2. Moore-Ede MC: Medical care whenever you need it: Human fatigue and the law, in *The Twenty-Four Hour Society*. Reading, Mass, Addison-Wesley, 1993, pp 97-107, 137-147.

Does Epinephrine Improve the Diagnostic Accuracy of Aspiration During Labor Epidural Analgesia?

Norris MC, Ferrenbach D, Dalman H, et al (Washington Univ, St Louis)
Anesth Analg 88:1073-1076, 1999   2–21

Objective.—False-positive epinephrine tests can cause laboring women to undergo unnecessary repeat epidural catheter insertion. Because aspiration detects most intravascular catheters, a supplemental epinephrine 15-µg test dose may be unnecessary. This hypothesis was tested in 532 consecutive patients requesting neuraxial labor analgesia.

Methods.—Multiorifice catheters (n = 575) were inserted epidurally in 532 laboring women as part of an epidural (n = 305) or combined spinal-epidural (n = 270) technique. Aspiration followed by administration of 3 mL of 1.5% lidocaine with 5 µg/mL epinephrine, followed by bolus injection or infusion of 10 to 20 mL of 0.125% bupivacaine and 10 µg of sufentanil in 5-mL increments was used to detect catheter position.

Results.—Aspiration detected 47 of 48 misplaced catheters. The epinephrine generated 10 positive responses of which 7 were false positive, 2 were true positive, and 1 was inadequately tested. The sensitivity, specificity, positive predictive value, and negative predictive value of aspiration and epinephrine were 97.9% and 100%, 100% and 98.7%, 100% and 12.5%, and 99.8% and 100%, respectively.

Conclusion.—Aspiration detects more than 99.5% of all misplaced multiorifice intravascular catheters in laboring women. The use of epinephrine provides no useful additional information.

▶ David Birnbach and I summarized our review of this manuscript in a recently published editorial.[1] We concluded that editorial with the following statement: "There is no substitute for careful observation, vigilance, and sound clinical judgment. Careful aspiration, followed by an appropriate test dose, increases the likelihood that an intravascular catheter will be detected and that a systemic reaction to local anesthetic will be avoided."[1]

I continue to use an epinephrine-containing test dose during administration of epidural analgesia in laboring women.

D. H. Chestnut, MD

Reference

1. Birnbach DJ, Chestnut DH: The epidural test dose in obstetric patients: Has it outlived its usefulness? *Anesth Analg* 88:971-972, 1999.

Comparative Evaluation of Four Different Infusion Rates of Ropivacaine (2 mg/mL) for Epidural Labor Analgesia
Cascio MG, Gaiser RR, Camann WR, et al (Magee-Womens Hosp, Pittsburgh, Pa; Univ of Pennsylvania, Philadelphia; Brigham & Women's Hosp, Boston; et al)
Reg Anesth Pain Med 23:548-553, 1998   2–22

Introduction.—Earlier trials have reported comparable efficacy for ropivacaine and bupivacaine when used for labor analgesia in concentrations of 2.5 mg/mL. The current trend is to minimize motor blocks during labor and delivery. Lower doses of bupivacaine have been used to achieve minimal motor block. No trials have examined the use of 2 mg/mL of ropivacaine in an obstetric population. The efficacy and safety of 4 different epidural infusion rates of 2 mg/mL ropivacaine were examined during labor for pain management in 128 women at term in a prospective, open, randomized, multicenter trial.

Methods.—Analgesia was initiated with a 5-mL test dose, then 5 to 15 mL of 2 mg/mL ropivacaine. Patients were then randomly assigned to receive ropivacaine, 2 mg/mL, at a fixed rate of either 4, 6, 8, or 10 mL/h administered by a lumbar epidural catheter. Rescue analgesia was administered with 5-mL "top-up" injections as needed for maternal comfort. Efficacy was measured by a visual analogue pain scale, incidence and intensity of the motor block, and number of supplemental bolus doses. Neonatal safety was assessed by neurologic adaptive capacity scores, Apgar scores, and adverse events.

Results.—Ratings on the visual analogue pain scale were effectively diminished by all 4 infusion regimens. Most patients in all 4 groups had minor or no motor block at the end of the first stage of labor. The mean total number of top-up injections needed per patient were 3, 2, 1.5, and 1.4, respectively for patients the 4-, 6-, 8-, and 10-mL/h groups ($P < .05$, 4 mL/h vs all other groups). The 4 mL/h–group had more total bolus dosages; it had less motor block in the lower extremities. All groups had similar neurologic adaptive capacity scores and Apgar scores.

Conclusion.—With the availability of supplemental analgesia at epidural infusion rates of 4, 6, 8, and 10 mL/h, 2 mg/mL of ropivacaine produces satisfactory labor analgesia. Among the 4 infusion rates, a rate of 6 mL/h may offer the lowest effective rate that provides the best combination of pain relief, motor block, and re-bolusing.

▶ It remains unclear whether epidural administration of ropivacaine offers any advantages over equipotent epidural doses of bupivacaine in laboring women.

D. H. Chestnut, MD

Relative Analgesic Potencies of Ropivacaine and Bupivacaine for Epidural Analgesia in Labor: Implications for Therapeutic Indexes
Polley LS, Columb MO, Naughton NN, et al (South Manchester Univ Hosp, Withington, England)
Anesthesiology 90:944-950, 1999   2–23

Objective.—Epidural bupivacaine has the potential for motor blockade and cardiovascular toxicity. Whereas ropivacaine has a lower side effects profile, its analgesic efficacy and side effects profile relative to bupivacaine has not been tested. The relative analgesic potencies of bupivacaine and ropivacaine were evaluated by determining their respective minimum local analgesic concentration values in a double-blinded, randomized, prospective study.

Methods.—Laboring women were randomly allocated to receive 20 mL ropivacaine (n = 34) or 20 mL bupivacaine (n = 39) via a lumbar epidural catheter. Efficacy was assessed with a 100-mm visual analogue pain scale (VAPS) at 5-minute intervals for the first 30 minutes. A VAPS score of 10 mm or less was considered effective. Outcome measures were the duration of effective analgesia and the number of women reporting a VAPS 10 mm or less until the first request for additional medication.

Results.—Data for 25 patients in each group were available for analysis. Ropivacaine was significantly less potent than bupivacaine (potency ratio, 0.6). There was no significant difference between groups in the number of segments blocked, in motor block, or in fetal heat rate tracings. Compared with the bupivacaine group, the ropivacaine group had a longer duration of analgesia (93.7 vs 73.2 minutes).

Conclusion.—Compared with bupivacaine, ropivacaine was significantly less potent but longer lasting.

Relative Potencies of Bupivacaine and Ropivacaine for Analgesia in Labour
Capogna G, Celleno D, Fusco P, et al (Fatebenefratelli Gen Hosp, Rome; Ospedale S Giacomo in Augusta, Rome; St James's Univ, Leeds, England; et al)
Br J Anaesth 82:371-373, 1999   2–24

Objective.—The relative analgesic potencies of bupivacaine and ropivacaine when given for pain relief in the first stage of labor were established by determining the minimum local analgesic concentration (MLAC) in a randomized, double-blind, up-down sequential allocation study.

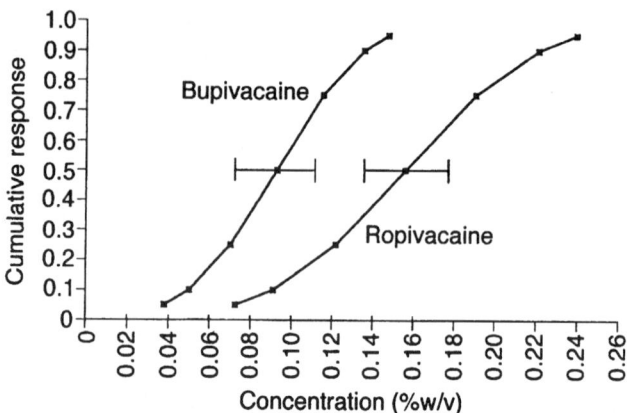

FIGURE 3.—EC$_{50}$ for ropivacaine and bupivacaine with 95% confidence intervals. Derived point estimates are plotted to demonstrate the concentration-response relationship. (Courtesy of Capogna G, Celleno D, Fusco P, et al: Relative potencies of bupivacaine and ropivacaine for analgesia in labour. *Br J Anaesth* 82:371-373, 1999. Reprinted by permission of Oxford University Press.)

Methods.—Either 20 mL of bupivacaine (n = 43) or 20 mL of ropivacaine (n = 44) was administered epidurally to women in the first stage of labor. The concentration of the dose of the next woman was determined by the response of the previous woman. Efficacy was assessed using a visual analogue pain scale (VAPS) at 0, 15, and 30 minutes. A VAPS 10 mm or less was defined as effective.

Results.—The MLAC was 0.093 for bupivacaine, significantly lower than the MLAC of 0.156 for ropivacaine. The relative potency of ropivacaine compared with bupivacaine was 0.6. The molar MLAC (EC$_{50}$) for ropivacaine and bupivacaine were 5.02 and 2.86, respectively (Fig 3).

Conclusion.—Epidural ropivacaine was significantly less potent than bupivacaine for women in the first stage of labor.

▶ Both of these studies (Abstracts 2–23 and 2–24) compared the MLAC for epidural ropivacaine versus bupivacaine, and both studies noted that epidural ropivacaine is significantly less potent than bupivacaine in laboring women. In the first study, the MLAC for bupivacaine and ropivacaine was 0.067% and 0.111%, respectively. In the second study, the MLAC for bupivacaine and ropivacaine was 0.093% and 0.156%, respectively. Although the absolute values differed between the 2 studies, the potency ratio (ie, 0.6) was identical in the 2 studies. In an editorial that accompanied the study by Polley et al, D'Angelo and James[1] correctly noted that "differences in potency [between ropivacaine and bupivacaine] could have accounted for differences in side effects and toxicity observed in all previous studies."

D. H. Chestnut, MD

Reference

1. D'Angelo R, James RL: Is ropivacaine less potent than bupivacaine? (editorial). *Anesthesiology* 90:941-943, 1999.

Epidural Analgesia and Intrapartum Fever: Placental Findings
Dashe JS, Rogers BB, McIntire DD, et al (Univ of Texas, Dallas)
Obstet Gynecol 93:341-344, 1999   2–25

Objective.—Studies have demonstrated that epidural analgesia increases the risk of fever by 4 to 14 times, but the cause is controversial. Whether placental examination for acute inflammation might permit a better understanding of the relationship between epidural analgesia and maternal fever in labor was investigated in a prospective, observational study.

Methods.—During June 1997 at Parkland Memorial Hospital in Dallas, placentas were collected within 48 hours of delivery from 80 women who received epidural analgesia and 69 women who did not. Four grades of leukocyte infiltration were used to evaluate inflammation. Maternal temperature was recorded every 15 minutes for 1 hour and then hourly for the duration of labor.

Results.—Fever (38°C or higher) was significantly more likely to occur in women receiving epidural analgesia than in women not receiving epidural analgesia (46% vs 26%, respectively). Women receiving epidural analgesia were significantly more likely to have placental inflammation (61% vs 36%), significantly more likely to have combined fever and placental inflammation (35% vs 17%), and more likely to have a longer labor (11.8 vs 9.6 hours). Women receiving epidural analgesia had a significantly longer duration of membrane rupture. Incidence of maternal fever was similar in both the epidural group and the group not having epidural analgesia in the absence of placental inflammation (11% vs 9%).

Conclusion.—Epidural analgesia is associated with fever only in the presence of placental inflammation.

▶ Women with prolonged labor are more likely to choose and receive epidural analgesia than women who labor rapidly. This is especially true in hospitals with a low utilization rate for epidural analgesia. Further, epidural analgesia itself may result in a modest prolongation of labor, although this effect is less significant than the effect of selection bias. Women with prolonged labor are more likely to show evidence of chorioamnionitis and fever. Epidural analgesia may also result in thermoregulatory changes not discussed by the authors of this study. However, many anesthesiologists would agree with the authors' conclusion that "maternal fever linked to epidural analgesia is not a side effect of the analgesia, but a consequence of longer labor that predisposes these women to intrapartum infection."

D. H. Chestnut, MD

Epidural Analgesia During Labor and Maternal Fever

Philip J, Alexander JM, Sharma SK, et al (Univ of Texas, Dallas)
Anesthesiology 90:1271-1275, 1999   2–26

Background.—Recent observational studies have reported maternal fever associated with epidural analgesia at the patient's request during labor. A secondary analysis of fever in women randomized to epidural or patient-controlled IV analgesia during labor was conducted.

Methods.—Seven hundred fifteen women at term were assigned to epidural analgesia with bupivacaine and fentanyl or to patient-controlled IV analgesia with meperidine. Maternal tympanic temperature was assessed during spontaneous labor.

Findings.—Epidural analgesia was associated with maternal fever, with an odds ratio of 4.0. Nulliparity and labor exceeding 12 hours were also associated with maternal fever, with odds ratios of 4.1 and 5.4, respectively (Fig 1). All these factors were independent variables when analyzed using a logistic regression analysis.

Conclusions.—These data indicate that epidural analgesia is associated with maternal fever, although nulliparity and dysfunctional labor are also significant covariates. In the absence of maternal fever, epidural analgesia is not correlated with neonatal sepsis evaluations. Thus, clinicians need not avoid epidural analgesia because of concerns about fever or about unnecessary neonatal evaluations for possible sepsis.

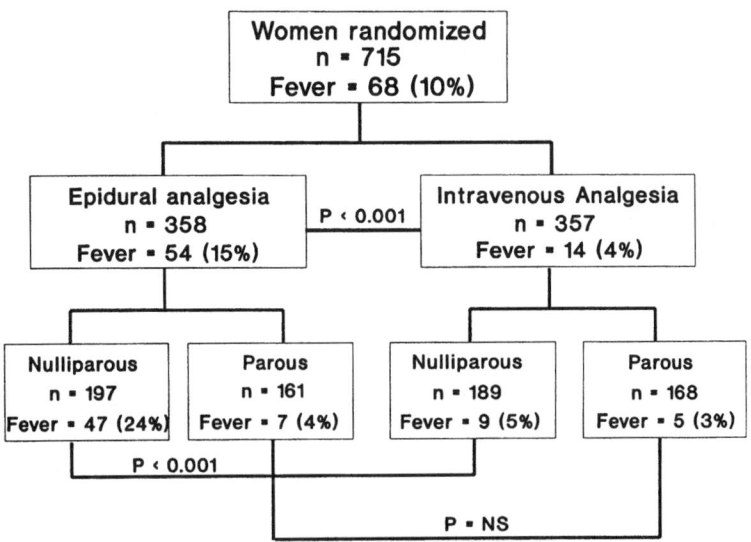

FIGURE 1.—Maternal fever in relation to type of analgesia and parity. (Courtesy of Philip J, Alexander JM, Sharma SK, et al: Epidural analgesia during labor and maternal fever. *Anesthesiology* 90:1271-1275, 1999. Copyright American Society of Anesthesiologists, Inc. Used with permission of Lippincott-Raven Publishers.)

▶ Several studies have demonstrated that epidural analgesia is associated with maternal fever during labor. It is likely that this association largely reflects the increased use of epidural analgesia in nulliparous women with prolonged labor. Epidural analgesia also may alter maternal temperature regulation, but the clinical significance is unclear. Regardless, no study has shown that the modest increase in maternal temperature associated with intrapartum epidural analgesia adversely affects the fetus.

D. H. Chestnut, MD

Cesarean Section

Obstetricians' Ability to Assess the Airway
Gaiser RR, McGonigal ET, Litts P, et al (Univ of Pennsylvania Health System, Philadelphia)
Obstet Gynecol 93:648-652, 1999   2–27

Objective.—Identifying women at risk for difficult intubation during labor and delivery is important for decreasing the risk of complications and death; however, no studies have assessed the ability of obstetricians to make this judgment. Obstetricians' ability to assess the airway and predict possible difficult intubation was assessed by comparing obstetricians' airway examinations with those of an attending anesthesiologist.

Methods.—Four physicians—an attending obstetrician and a resident obstetrician and an attending and a resident anesthesiologist—examined the airways of 80 laboring women without receiving guidance or education. They then examined the airways of another 80 laboring women after 30 minutes of airway examination instruction and after observing an airway examination by an anesthesiologist. The residents, attending obstetricians, and attending anesthesiologist completed a questionnaire. With the anesthesiologist's responses as the standard, the sensitivity, specificity, and positive and negative predictive values were calculated for responses of the other physicians.

Results.—Instruction did not affect the results of the obstetricians' airway assessment. The sensitivities and specificities of the attending obstetrician and obstetric resident before instruction were 0.59 and 0.82 and 0.41 and 0.89, respectively. After instruction, the corresponding figures were 0.60 and 0.83 and 0.50 and 0.87, respectively. Instruction did not affect the number of consultations requested by resident and attending obstetricians for possible difficult intubations. Attending obstetricians were significantly more likely to use epidural analgesia at 2-cm cervical dilatation in women with possible difficult intubations.

Conclusion.—Instruction in airway examination did not affect the obstetricians' ability to assess a difficult airway. Obstetricians were significantly more likely to use epidural analgesia in women with a possible difficult airway.

▶ Airway assessment remains subjective—even when performed by an experienced anesthesiologist. It is probably unrealistic to expect an obstetrician to perform an airway examination with the same sensitivity and specificity as that performed by an anesthesiologist. However, it remains useful for anesthesiologists to remind our obstetric colleagues that airway complications (eg, failed intubation, pulmonary aspiration) remain the leading causes of anesthesia-related maternal mortality.

D. H. Chestnut, MD

Comparison of Epidural Anaesthesia With Ropivacaine 0.5% and Bupivacaine 0.5% for Caesarean Section
Crosby E, Sandler A, Finucane B, et al (Univ of Ottawa, Ont; Univ of Toronto; Univ of Alberta; et al)
Can J Anaesth 45:1066-1071, 1998   2–28

Background.—In animal models, it has been shown that ropivacaine has a lower CNS and cardiotoxic potential than bupivacaine. In humans, ropivacaine is less likely than bupivacaine to produce mild CNS and cardiovascular changes after IV administration. The quality and nature of epidural block with ropivacaine and bupivacaine were determined in women undergoing cesarean section.

Methods.—In a randomized, double-blind, parallel-group trial, healthy pregnant women undergoing elective cesarean section were studied. Epidural block was achieved with 20 to 30 mL ropivacaine 0.5% or bupivacaine 0.5%, and surgery was started when anesthesia reached dermatome level T_6. Maternal heart rate and blood pressure and fetal heart rate were monitored at baseline and at 5-minute intervals. Sensory and motor block characteristics were also monitored at 5-minute intervals. Postpartum Apgar scores and Neurologic and Adaptive Capacity Scores were determined. Adverse effects were noted.

Results.—There were 65 women enrolled, and data from 61 women were analyzed. Of the 61 women, 30 received ropivacaine and 31 received bupivacaine. The time from the last injection to the start of surgery was 46 minutes in the ropivacaine group and 53 minutes in the bupivacaine group. The median length of analgesia was 1.7 to 4.2 hours in the ropivacaine group and 1.8 to 4.4 hours in the bupivacaine group. Bromage 4 block lasted longer in women who had bupivacaine. The quality of analgesia was satisfactory in 93% of women given ropivacaine and in 87% of women given bupivacaine, although supplemental opioid was needed in 10 women who had ropivacaine and in 7 women who had bupivacaine. In all neonates, Apgar scores were 7 at 5 minutes. The most common maternal adverse effects were hypotension and nausea.

Discussion.—Ropivacaine 0.5% and bupivacaine 0.5% are effective for epidural anesthesia in women having cesarean section, although supplemental opioid may be needed. This need for supplemental opioid is concerning. Maternal adverse effects are similar with the 2 drugs and are probably more related to technique than to drug.

▶ The role of epidural ropivacaine in obstetric anesthesia practice remains unclear. I rarely use 0.5% bupivacaine when giving epidural anesthesia for cesarean section. The anesthesia is often inadequate, and I prefer to avoid the risk of cardiotoxicity, which is associated with administration of a large dose of bupivacaine. Why use epidural ropivacaine for cesarean section? It does *not* provide analgesia superior to that provided by bupivacaine. Further, 2% lidocaine with epinephrine is an excellent local anesthetic for most patients who receive epidural anesthesia for cesarean section.

D. H. Chestnut, MD

Clinical Effects and Maternal and Fetal Plasma Concentrations of 0.5% Epidural Levobupivacaine Versus Bupivacaine for Cesarean Delivery
Bader AM, Tsen LC, Camann WR, et al (Harvard Med School, Boston; Brigham and Women's Hosp, Boston)
Anesthesiology 90:1596-1601, 1999   2–29

Objective.—Research suggests that the levo enantiometer of bupivacaine results in less CNS and cardiovascular toxicity while maintaining equal local anesthetic potency dexbupivacaine. The efficacy and safety of 0.5% levobupivacaine and 0.5% bupivacaine for epidural anesthesia were compared in patients undergoing elective cesarean section in a randomized, double-blind study.

Methods.—Either 30 mL 0.5% levobupivacaine or 30 mL 0.5% bupivacaine was administered epidurally in 60 healthy women undergoing elective cesarean section. Outcome measures were onset, offset, and quality of anesthesia. Neonatal blood gases, Apgar scores, and neurobehavior were assessed. Pharmacokinetic studies were performed on venous blood samples obtained from women in each group.

Results.—Sensory and motor block characteristics were similar for both groups. The incidence of hypotension was 84.4% in the levobupivacaine group and 100% in the bupivacaine group. Maximum drug concentrations for levobupivacaine and bupivacaine (1.017 and 1.053 µg/mL, respectively) and areas under the plasma drug concentration–time curve (4.082 and 3.765 hours per µg/mL), respectively) were similar for both groups. Patient-perceived quality of anesthesia and neonatal outcomes were similar for both groups. Incidences of nausea and postoperative pain were similar in both groups.

Conclusion.—Epidural levobupivacaine (0.5%) and bupivacaine (0.5%) were equally efficacious for cesarean section.

The Placental Transfer and Fetal Effects of Levobupivacaine, Racemic Bupivacaine, and Ropivacaine

Santos AC, Karpel B, Noble G (Albert Einstein College of Medicine, Bronx, NY; State Univ of New York, Stony Brook)
Anesthesiology 90:1698-1703, 1999   2–30

Introduction.—Levobupivacaine, the single levorotary isomer of bupivacaine, offers the beneficial blocking properties of racemic bupivacaine but with reduced cardiotoxic effects. This agent is being studied for obstetric use, although its effects on uterine blood flow and the fetus are unknown. The placental transfer and fetal tissue uptake of levobupivacaine, as well as its effects on uterine blood flow and fetal well-being, were studied in sheep.

Methods.—After instrumentation for long-term monitoring, pregnant ewes received 2-step, 1-hour IV infusion of levobupivacaine, bupivacaine, or ropivacaine. In addition to monitoring of maternal and fetal hemodynamics, maternal and fetal arterial blood was sampled to measure acid-base status and serum drug levels. Drug levels were also measured in the fetal heart, brain, liver, lungs, adrenal glands, and kidneys.

Results.—None of the anesthetic agents studied significantly altered maternal blood pressure, central venous or intra-amniotic pressure, acid-base status, or uterine blood flow. Bupivacaine decreased the maternal heart rate slightly but significantly. None of the 3 agents adversely affected fetal well-being. Maternal serum levels were similar with all 3 drugs, as were fetal serum levels, fetal tissue levels, and tissue-serum concentration ratios.

Conclusions.—Like bupivacaine and ropivacaine, levobupivacaine has no significant hemodynamic effects in pregnant and fetal sheep. Infusion of all 3 local anesthetics produces steady-state serum concentrations within the range used for epidural anesthesia for cesarean section. Fetal serum and tissue levels of the 3 drugs are similar.

▶ Levobupivacaine is the single levorotary isomer formulate of bupivacaine (Abstracts 2–29 and 2–30). Laboratory studies suggest that levobupivacaine may cause fewer arrhythmias or other ECG changes than either the dextrorotary or racemic formulation of bupivacaine. A recent clinical study suggested that levobupivacaine and racemic bupivacaine have similar potency when given epidurally in laboring women.[1] However, it is likely that levobupivacaine will be more expensive than racemic bupivacaine. Most anesthesiologists administer a dilute solution of bupivacaine, with or without an opioid, when providing epidural analgesia in laboring women. This fact, coupled with other safety precautions (eg, administration of a test dose, fractionation of the therapeutic dose of local anesthetic), have made administration of epidural analgesia a very safe procedure in laboring women. Levobupivacaine might offer a greater potential for advantage in patients receiving epidural anesthesia for cesarean section, except that lidocaine with epinephrine is a satisfactory choice for most patients. Thus the role of the single levorotary isomers of local anesthetic (eg, levobupivacaine, ropivacaine) in obstetric anesthesia practice remains unclear.

D. H. Chestnut, MD

Reference

1. Lyons G, Columb MO, Wilson RC, et al: Epidural pain relief in labour: Potencies of levobupivacaine and racemic bupivacaine. *Br J Anaesth* 81:899-901, 1998.

Spinal Block Levels and Cardiovascular Changes During Post-Cesarean Transport
Bandi E, Weeks S, Carli F (McGill Univ, Montreal)
Can J Anesth 46:736-740, 1999

2–31

Background.—Cardiovascular changes have been associated with transport after surgery with spinal anesthesia. Patients who are extensively vasodilated may be unable to compensate for postural blood flow redistribution. Preoperative and postoperative sensory levels and hemodynamic changes during the postoperative transport period were investigated.

Methods.—One hundred ninety-nine women undergoing cesarean section under spinal anesthesia were studied. All were at level 1 or 2 according to the American Society of Anesthesiologists scale. Hyperbaric bupivacaine 12 to 15 mg and morphine 0.25 mg were used. One hundred eleven patients (group A) were transferred to the recovery room on a stretcher with the upper body flexed 30°, head up. Eighty-eight patients (group B) remained supine during transport.

Findings.—At the end of surgery, 95% had upper sensory levels of T_4 and higher. The block ascended 2 to 7 dermatomes compared with preoperative levels in 17.5% of the patients. The incidence of hypotension on recovery room arrival was 10% in group A and 9% in group B, a nonsignificant difference.

Conclusions.—Extensive sympathetic block persists at the end of cesarean section. Transport to the recovery room was associated with the development of marked hypotension in about 10% of the patients. Transport position did not affect this incidence. The level of sensory block should be recorded at the end of surgery, and monitoring during transport to the recovery room should be increased.

▶ Other studies have noted that hospitalized critically ill patients are most vulnerable during transport from 1 part of the hospital to another. Some physicians have quipped that patients are near—but not actually in—a hospital during periods of transport. The authors of the present study noted that "the transfer period remains 1 of the least monitored periods during the surveillance of the surgical patient." Further, they stated that "the transfer period deserves closer scrutiny and monitoring, as this is a time when disasters can occur."

The authors also called attention to the fact that many anesthesiologists do not determine serial sensory levels in patients who receive spinal anesthesia. They recommended that anesthesiologists determine the sensory level at the conclusion of surgery in patients who have received spinal anesthesia for cesarean section.

Finally, this study calls attention to the importance of good postanesthesia care after cesarean section. Postanesthesia care standards for obstetric patients should be similar to those for nonobstetric patients who undergo surgery elsewhere in the hospital.

D. H. Chestnut, MD

Obstetric Postanesthesia Care Unit Stays: Reevaluation of Discharge Criteria After Regional Anesthesia

Cohen SE, Hamilton CL, Riley ET, et al (Stanford Univ, Calif)
Anesthesiology 89:1559-1565, 1998   2–32

Introduction.—There are few data describing the course and recovery characteristics of patients in the obstetric postanesthesia care unit (OB-PACU). Most patients in the OB-PACU have received general anesthesia for cesarean delivery or tubal ligation. They may have prolonged OB-PACU stays after surgery because of residual regional block or other conditions. Modified discharge criteria were examined to determine whether they might allow for earlier discharge without compromising patient safety.

Methods.—Data for 358 patients who underwent cesarean section or tubal ligation and recovered in the OB-PACU were prospectively collected for 6 months. Ninety-four percent of these patients received regional anesthesia. Duration of anesthesia and PACU stay, occurrence and treatment of events in the PACU, and the regression of neural blockade were recorded. Discharge from the OB-PACU necessitated a 1-hour minimum stay, stable vital signs, adequate analgesia, and ability to flex the knees. Events that occurred after a 1-hour minimum stay in the OB-PACU were documented and reevaluated by a focus group consisting of 3 obstetric anesthesiologists and 3 senior nurse managers as to whether patients needed to stay in the OB-PACU for medical reasons. The focus group defined "needed to stay" events as including bleeding, cardiorespiratory problems, sedation, dizziness, and pain. "Safe to leave" events included pruritis, nausea, and residual neural blockade.

Results.—For each time interval evaluated, residual block was responsible for most stays (34% to 47%) that were considered unnecessary. The focus group determined from using their revised discharge criteria that over 50% of patients who remained in the OB-PACU at any time could have been discharged (Fig 3). One patient had a transient bout of tachycardia 91 to 120 minutes into her PACU stay. She had no other events before or after that required a PACU stay. Had the revised criteria been used during the 6-month evaluation period, 212.5 hours (429 hours annually) of one-to-one care from a registered nurse could have been saved. This could have meant a cost savings of $20,292.

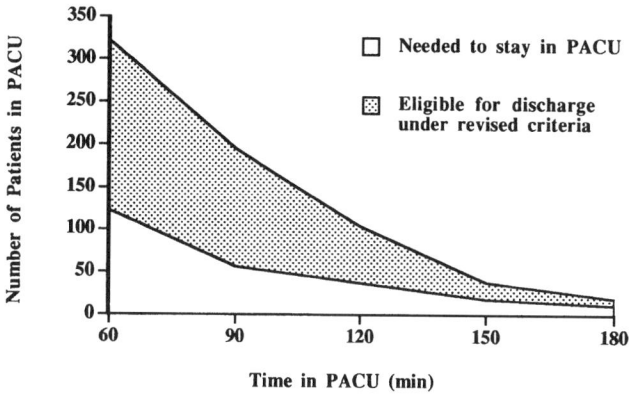

FIGURE 3.—Number of patients remaining in the obstetric postanesthesia care unit (*PACU*) who needed to stay for medical reasons or who would have been eligible to leave by the revised discharge criteria. (Courtesy of Cohen SE, Hamilton CL, Riley ET, et al: Obstetric postanesthesia care unit stays: Reevaluation of discharge criteria after regional anesthesia. *Anesthesiology* 89:1559-1565, 1998. Copyright American Society of Anesthesiologists, Inc. Used with permission of Lippincott-Raven Publishers.)

Conclusion.—The duration of the OB-PACU stay for most patients could safely be shortened by continuing observation of resolving neural blockage and treatment of opioid side effects in a lower-acuity setting. The reduced need for one-on-one care by a registered nurse should allow for increased productivity, greater flexibility in staffing, and modest direct cost savings as a result of the differences in nursing salaries needed to pay for patients on the postpartum unit versus the OB-PACU.

▶ The authors' conclusions depend on 2 assumptions: (1) the option to close the OB-PACU and reassign nursing personnel to other duties when no surgical patients are present and (2) the option to send nurses home without pay for a complete shift during times of decreased patient census. Further, the authors acknowledge that their calculations may have overestimated cost savings on those occasions when more than 1 patient was present in the OB-PACU. Nonetheless, this interesting study should prompt anesthesiologists to reevaluate OB-PACU discharge criteria.

D. H. Chestnut, MD

The Development of a Maternal Satisfaction Scale for Caesarean Section

Morgan PJ, Halpern S, Lo J (Mount Sinai Hosp, Toronto; Univ of Toronto)
Int J Obstet Anesth 8:165-170, 1999   2–33

Background.—Satisfaction has become an important health care outcome measure. This study was undertaken to develop a health measurement scale for satisfaction in women undergoing cesarean section under regional anesthesia.

Study Design.—The initial study group consisted of 25 nulliparous and multiparous women who received regional anesthesia for elective or non-emergent cesarean section. Face validity was ensured by having patients generate items before and after cesarean section. Content validity was ensured by interviewing until no new items were generated. All items were then grouped into 4 factors, and a Likert scale was generated for each item. The resulting questionnaire was then administered to 115 women who had undergone cesarean section. The questionnaire was correlated with a Visual Analogue Scale for satisfaction, which was administered at the same time. Items endorsed by less than 15% of the study group were eliminated. Reliability was measured with Cronbach's α.

Findings.—Of the initial 33 items on the draft satisfaction scale, 6 were excluded because of lack of sufficient endorsement. Five more items were excluded after principal component and factor analysis. Two more items were excluded after item-total correlations. The correlation between the scale and the visual analogue scale was 0.48. Cronbach's α was 0.82 for the overall scale. Maternal sense of control was the single item on the scale that most related to satisfaction.

Conclusion.—This study produced a 22-item satisfaction scale for women undergoing cesarean section under regional anesthesia. The scale was determined to have face, content, and construct validity as well as reliability. The results of this study indicated that maternal sense of control and good communication with staff appeared to be important in a positive cesarean delivery experience. Further work is necessary before there is widespread use of this scale for the measurement of satisfaction in women undergoing nonemergent cesarean section.

▶ Several studies have assessed maternal satisfaction during labor. In a discussion of those studies, the authors noted that "communication be-tween staff and patient, participation in the decision-making process, maternal feeling of control of the situation and personal behavior strongly correlate with [maternal] satisfaction" during labor. In the present study, the authors concluded that their observations of maternal satisfaction for women undergoing cesarean section "mirror" the findings of earlier studies of maternal satisfaction during labor.

D. H. Chestnut, MD

Post-Cesarean Analgesia

Dose-Response Relationship of Intrathecal Morphine for Postcesarean Analgesia

Palmer CM, Emerson S, Volgoropolous D, et al (Univ of Arizona, Tucson; Univ of Washington, Seattle; Southern Arizona Anesthesia, Tucson; et al)
Anesthesiology 90:437-444, 1999   2–34

Objective.—Whereas small doses of intrathecal (IT) morphine prolong analgesia in patients with chronic pain, the dose-response relationship of IT morphine for postcesarean analgesia has not been carefully evaluated.

The minimum effective dose of IT morphine for postcesarean analgesia, the relationship of side effects to morphine dose, and the analgesic failure rate at various doses were evaluated for analgesic efficacy, incidence of side effects, and need for treatment interventions.

Methods.—One hundred eight patients undergoing elective cesarean section were randomly allocated to receive 0.0, 0.025, 0.05, 0.075, 0.1, 0.2, 0.3, 0.4, or 0.5 mg IT morphine as a single dose. Patient-controlled analgesia (PCA) was provided. Patients were followed for 4 hours, and level of sensory anesthesia; occurrence of pruritus, nausea, and vomiting; and need for treatment interventions were recorded by a blinded investigator.

Results.—The 0.075-, 0.10-, 0.30-, 0.40-, and 0.50-mg morphine groups used significantly less morphine than the 0.0-mg group. Twenty-four-hour PCA morphine use was 45.7 mg lower in the 0.075-mg group than in the 0.0-mg group and 4.1 mg lower in the 0.5-mg group than in the 0.075-mg group. Whereas the incidence of nausea was similar among groups, the severity of pruritus was significantly lower in the 0.0-mg group than in the 0.5-mg group. The severity of pruritus was dose-related. Nalbuphine use was significantly higher in the 0.2- to 0.5-mg groups than in the 0.0- to 0.1-mg groups. The 0.4-mg group had a significantly higher use of nalbuphine than did the 0.0- and 0.075-mg groups. The need for treatment intervention tended to increase with increasing dose.

Conclusion.—Whereas doses of 0.1 mg or less to 0.5 mg PCA produced comparable analgesia, severity of pruritus and need for treatment interventions increased with increasing dose. The incidences of nausea and vomiting were not dose-related.

Determination of an Effective Dose of Intrathecal Morphine for Pain Relief After Cesarean Delivery
Gerancher JC, Floyd H, Eisenach J (Wake Forest Univ, Winston-Salem, NC)
Anesth Analg 88:346-351, 1999 2–35

Objective.—The dose-response curve for small doses of intrathecal (IT) morphine after cesarean delivery has not been completely documented. Results of a double-blind study to determine the effective postoperative pain dose of very small doses of IT morphine while minimizing side effects and to analyze the acquisition costs and nursing care time were presented. Data were compared with a historical cohort of patients receiving patient-controlled analgesia (PCA).

Methods.—IT morphine was administered to 40 patients undergoing elective cesarean delivery in an up-down method of dose allocation, beginning with 200 µg and decreasing by 25 µg for success or increasing by 50 µg for failure to a maximum of 500 µg and a minimum of 0 µg. Postoperative pain was treated first with 5 mg oral hydrocodone and 1 or 2 tablets of 500 mg acetaminophen every 4 hours as needed. If pain relief was ineffective, IV morphine was administered in 4-mg increments. Morphine use and pain scores were recorded. Patients were followed for 12 hours.

Results.—Whereas no IT dose-response analgesia curve was discovered, patients in this study required no more time commitment than did patients in the historical PCA cohort. Drug acquisition costs for the IT morphine group were significantly lower than for the PCA group ($15.13 vs $34.64, respectively).

Conclusion.—Small doses of IT morphine provide effective and cost-effective pain relief for patients after cesarean delivery.

▶ Both of these studies (Abstracts 2–34 and 2–35) attempted to determine the minimum effective dose of IT morphine for postcesarean analgesia. In the first study, Palmer et al concluded that there is little justification for administration of a dose of IT morphine larger than 0.1 mg for postcesarean analgesia. Larger doses of IT morphine did not result in decreased use of supplemental PCA morphine, and the severity of pruritus seemed to be dose related (ie, more severe pruritus occurred with larger doses of IT morphine). In the second study, Gerancher et al used a different methodology in an attempt to define the median effective dose for IT morphine for postcesarean analgesia. They concluded that their "best estimate" of a median effective dose for IT morphine is 0.22 mg. However, the authors defined failure as the administration of IV morphine at *any* time during the first 12 hours after IT morphine administration. If the goal is to eliminate all supplemental parenteral doses of opioid, then higher doses of IT morphine must be administered. However, I favor the approach of Palmer et al. Namely, it seems preferable to give a small dose (0.1-0.2 mg) of IT morphine and then provide supplemental analgesia as needed. Regardless, both studies clearly suggested that it is unnecessary to give a dose larger than 0.25 mg for postcesarean analgesia.

D. H. Chestnut, MD

Comparison of 0.25 mg and 0.1 mg Intrathecal Morphine for Analgesia After Cesarean Section
Yang T, Breen TW, Archer D, et al (Univ of Calgary, Alta)
Can J Anesth 46:856-860, 1999   2–36

Background.—Intrathecal (IT) morphine, 0.25 mg, widely used for analgesia after cesarean delivery under spinal anesthesia, is associated with troublesome adverse effects. IT morphine, 0.1 mg, plus nonsteroidal anti-inflammatory drugs (NSAIDs) may provide satisfactory analgesia after cesarean section with fewer side effects than 0.25 mg IT morphine.

Methods.—Sixty women scheduled for elective cesarean delivery under spinal anesthesia were assigned randomly to 0.1 or 0.25 mg IT morphine combined with 0.75% hyperbaric bupivacaine and 20 µg fentanyl. A 100-mg indomethacin suppository was given to all patients at the end of

TABLE 2.—Proportion of Women Requesting Additional Medications

	0.1 mg (Number/Total)	0.25 mg (Number/Total)	P
Additional narcotics (other than codeine)	4/30	4/28	0.99
Antipruritics	4/30	12/28	0.018
Antiemetics	11/30	15/28	0.29

(Courtesy of Yang T, Breen TW, Archer D, et al: Comparison of 0.25 mg and 0.1 mg intrathecal morphine for analgesia after cesarean section. *Can J Anesth* 46:856-860, 1999.)

surgery. In addition, all had 500 mg naproxen twice daily begun on the evening of surgery and continued until hospital discharge.

Findings.—The 2 groups did not differ in Visual Analogue Scale (VAS) pain scores or in the proportion requesting an opioid other than codeine (Table 2). The 0.1 mg group had lower VAS pruritus scores in the first 24 hours (Fig 1). Fewer women in the 0.1-mg group than in the 0.25-mg group asked for nalbuphine to treat itching. Nausea scores were lower in the 0.1-mg group than in the 0.25-mg group.

Conclusions.—The analgesia provided by 0.1 mg IT morphine plus NSAIDs is comparable with that of 0.25 mg after cesarean section but with

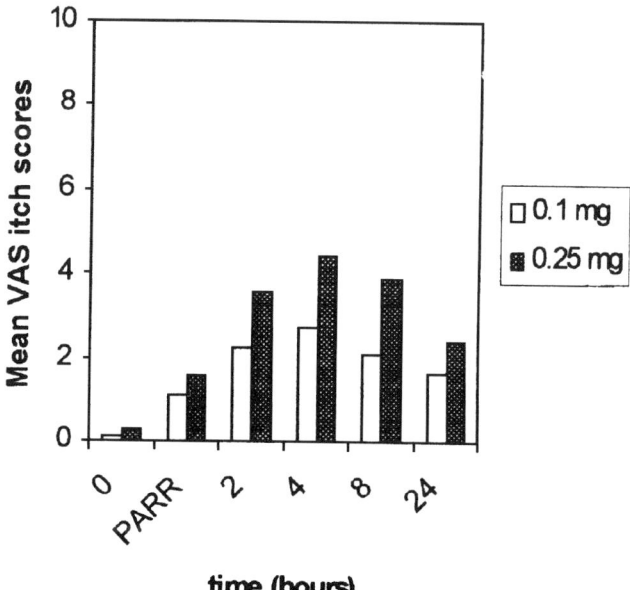

FIGURE 1.—Comparison of visual analog scale pruritus scores in the 0.1 mg group versus the 0.25 mg group postoperatively. (Courtesy of Yang T, Breen TW, Archer D, et al: Comparison of 0.25 mg and 0.1 mg intrathecal morphine for analgesia after cesarean section. *Can J Anesth* 46:856-860, 1999.)

fewer adverse effects. The authors recommend 0.1 mg IT morphine with NSAIDs in this setting.

▶ Others have concluded that 0.1 mg is the optimal dose of IT morphine for postcesarean analgesia. Likewise, other studies have demonstrated the efficacy of co-administration of an NSAID and intraspinal morphine. Such multimodal therapy likely results in a decreased incidence of side effects when compared with administration of a larger dose of intraspinal morphine alone.

D. H. Chestnut, MD

Patients With Complications

What Height of Block Is Needed for Manual Removal of Placenta Under Spinal Anaesthesia?

Broadbent CR, Russell R (John Radcliffe Hosp, Oxford, England)
Int J Obstet Anesth 8:161-164, 1999   2–37

Background.—Relatively little published information is available on the height of block required for maternal comfort during manual placenta removal with spinal block. This prospective, observational study was performed to determine the factors affecting maternal discomfort during this procedure.

Study Design.—Between November 1996 and March 1998, there were 8026 deliveries at the John Radcliffe hospital. Of these, 178 required manual placenta removal. Data were collected prospectively from 101 women who had manual placenta removal under spinal block. All women in the study group were of more than 24 weeks' gestation, and removal was less than 12 hours postpartum. None had received systemic pethidine or epidural analgesia during labor. None had regional block for assisted delivery. Maternal position, injection volume, block height, sensations of pain or pressure, the force applied by the surgeon, grade of the 42 anesthetists, time from injection to procedure, surgery duration, blood loss, volume of IV solution, and occurrence of hypotension were recorded.

Findings.—Factors significantly associated with maternal discomfort during manual removal of the placenta under spinal anesthesia were block height and the force applied by the surgeon. Only 2 women experienced discomfort with a block to cold of T6 or above. Factors that were not significantly related to maternal discomfort were obstetrician grade, anesthetist grade, position of mother, volume of injection, time from injection to procedure, and procedure duration. Intraoperative hypotension was not associated with maternal discomfort but was associated with greater maternal blood loss.

Conclusion.—Little information is available about the block height necessary for maternal comfort during manual removal of the placenta under spinal anesthesia. This prospective study suggests use of a block to cold to T6 or above to minimize maternal discomfort during this procedure.

▶ Readers of this abstract should be aware that the authors assessed the sensory level by determining the absence of cold sensation. Subarachnoid blocks that are assessed by the absence of cold sensation typically are judged to be 1 or 2 dermatomes higher than the same blocks assessed by pinprick.

In my practice, I have found that a T10 level—assessed by pinprick—reliably provides effective analgesia for manual removal of a placenta. In the present study, the authors noted that the obstetrician used "moderate force" in 63 of 101 patients. I wonder whether the results of this study would have differed if the authors had administered a small dose of nitroglycerin to facilitate uterine relaxation immediately before manual removal of the placenta.

D. H. Chestnut, MD

Assessment of Changes in Coagulation in Parturients With Preeclampsia Using Thromboelastography
Sharma SK, Philip J, Whitten CW, et al (Univ of Texas, Dallas)
Anesthesiology 90:385-390, 1999   2–38

Objective.—Preeclampsia increases the risk of hemostasis. Thromboelastography, commonly used to assess coagulation during cardiopulmonary bypass, was used to evaluate changes in coagulation compared with conventional tests of hemostasis in preeclamptic women.

Methods.—Thromboelastographic analysis and platelet counts were performed on 52 healthy pregnant women in active labor, 140 mild preeclamptic women, and 114 severe preeclamptic women.

Results.—Thromboelastography parameters were similar among healthy women, mild preeclamptic women, and severe preeclamptic women with a platelet count of at least 100,000/mm³. Mild preeclamptic women were significantly hypercoagulable, whereas severe preeclamptic women with a platelet count of less than 100,000/mm³ were significantly hypocoagulable. Ten severe preeclamptic women had a maximum amplitude (MA) of less than 54 mm, the lower MA limit for healthy women. None of the mild preeclamptic women had an MA greater than 54 mm. Whereas 5 severe preeclamptic women with a platelet count of less than 100,000/mm³ had an MA less than 54 mm, all 4 mild preeclamptic women with a platelet count of less than 100,000/mm³ had normal coagulation values.

Conclusion.—Compared with other preeclamptic women and healthy women, severe preeclamptic women with a platelet count of less than 100,000/mm³ were hypocoagulable.

▶ The role of thromboelastography in the preanesthetic assessment of preeclamptic women remains unclear. The platelet count probably remains the single best screening test for these patients. However, the severity of thrombocytopenia or hypocoagulability that contraindicates epidural analgesia remains unclear. Anesthesiologists must weigh the known benefits of epidural analgesia versus the small—but not zero—risk of epidural hematoma in preeclamptic women.

D. H. Chestnut, MD

Spinal Haematoma Following Epidural Anaesthesia in a Patient With Eclampsia
Yuen TST, Kua JSW, Tan IKS (Pamela Youde Nethersole Eastern Hosp, Chai Wan, China)
Anaesthesia 54:350-371, 1999   2–39

Background.—The true incidence of spinal hematoma after central neural blockade in obstetric patients has not been established and may be higher than believed. The authors described a woman with severe preeclampsia in whom spinal epidural hematoma developed after spinal anesthesia for cesarean section.

> *Case Report.*—Woman, 20, was hospitalized at 35 weeks' gestation with twin pregnancy because of hypertension and albuminuria. Severe pre-eclampsia was diagnosed, the platelet count being $71 \times 10^9.1^{-1}$. Cesarean section was performed. Epidural anesthesia was instituted after platelet transfusion. Postoperatively, the patient had a generalized tonic-clonic seizure, sparing the lower limbs, which enabled an early diagnosis of spinal epidural hematoma to be made. After laminectomy and clot removal, the patient recovered with no permanent neurologic sequelae.

Conclusions.—Clinicians must carefully weigh the risks and benefits of epidural and general anesthesia and explain these risks and benefits to the patient. A posttransfusion platelet count should be obtained to aid in decision-making about epidural block. Clinicians need to use as much care in removing the catheter as in placing it. After epidural block, monitoring of recovery from central neural blockade is essential. Saline solution should be used instead of air for loss of resistance as part of the epidural method.

▶ To my knowledge, this represents only the second published case of intraspinal hematoma after epidural anesthesia in a preeclamptic patient. Unfortunately, this case report provides more questions than answers. For example, the authors state that the platelet count was 71,000/mm³ on the third day of hospitalization, compared with a platelet count of 49,000/mm³ on the day of admission. What was the interval between the platelet count determination and the subsequent administration of epidural anesthesia? Why did the authors give 6 units of platelets to a patient with a platelet count of 71,000/mm³? Did the patient show clinical evidence of a bleeding abnormality? I question the wisdom of giving epidural anesthesia to a patient who had recently required the administration of 6 units of platelets.

D. H. Chestnut, MD

Spinal Versus Epidural Anesthesia for Cesarean Section in Severely Preeclamptic Patients: A Retrospective Survey
Hood DD, Curry R (Wake Forest Univ, Winston-Salem, NC)
Anesthesiology 90:1276-1282, 1999   2–40

Introduction.—The use of spinal anesthesia is controversial in patients with severe preeclampsia who need cesarean section delivery. Significant maternal hypotension is thought to be more likely with spinal anesthesia than with epidural anesthesia in this patient population. The blood pressure effects of spinal and epidural anesthesia were examined retrospectively in a large clinical series of women with severe preeclampsia who required cesarean section delivery.

Methods.—A computerized medical records database was examined for all nonlaboring patients with preeclampsia undergoing cesarean section between January 1, 1989 and December 31, 1996. Patients were grouped according to type of anesthesia, either epidural or spinal. Medical records for patients in both groups were compared for lowest recorded blood pressure for the 20-minute period before induction of regional anesthesia, the period from induction of regional anesthesia to delivery, and the period from delivery to the end of surgery.

Results.—Thirty-five women received epidural anesthesia, and 103 received spinal anesthesia. Changes in the lowest mean blood pressure (Fig

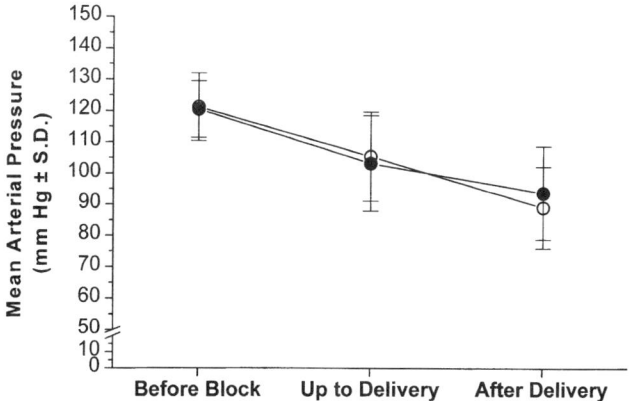

FIGURE 1.—Severely preeclamptic patients receiving 103 spinal (*open circles*) or 35 epidural (*closed circles*) anesthetic procedures for cesarean section. Data are mean ± SD. Lowest mean blood pressures recorded do not differ between groups. *Before Block,* 20 minutes before regional anesthesia induction; *Up to Delivery,* period from regional anesthesia induction to delivery; *After Delivery,* period from delivery to the end of surgery. (Courtesy of Hood DD, Curry R: Spinal versus epidural anesthesia for cesarean section in severely preeclamptic patients: A retrospective survey. *Anesthesiology* 90:1276-1282, 1999. Copyright American Society of Anesthesiologists, Inc. Used with permission of Lippincott-Raven Publishers.)

1) and use of intraoperative ephedrine were similar for patients in both groups. Patients who received spinal anesthesia received significantly more intraoperative crystalloid, compared with patients who received epidural anesthesia (1780 vs 1359 mL, respectively). There were no between-group differences in neonatal Apgar scores and incidence of maternal intensive care unit admission or postoperative pulmonary edema.

Conclusion.—Decreases in blood pressure were similar for both spinal and epidural anesthesia in patients with severe preeclampsia who underwent cesarean section. Maternal and fetal outcomes were similar for both groups. The possibility that the spinal and epidural groups were dissimilar in this retrospective review cannot be excluded.

▶ In recent years obstetric anesthesiologists have reevaluated the use of spinal anesthesia in women with severe preeclampsia. These patients often have decreased intravascular volume. Heretofore, many obstetric anesthesiologists have avoided spinal anesthesia in this population, because of concern that the abrupt onset of the sympathectomy might result in severe hypotension.

In this study, the authors observed similar outcome in women who received either spinal or epidural anesthesia for cesarean section. However, one of the limitations of most retrospective studies is the potential for selection bias. Is it possible that the women who received epidural anesthesia had more severe disease than the women who received spinal anesthesia? That is, is it possible that the anesthesiologists gave epidural anesthesia to the sickest patients, which might have reduced the likelihood of observing a better outcome in the epidural group? For example, in this study, women in the epidural group were more likely to have received antihypertensive therapy before induction of anesthesia than were women in the spinal group.

In my judgment, when time permits, epidural anesthesia remains preferable to spinal anesthesia for cesarean section in most women with severe preeclampsia. The slow onset of sympathetic blockade seems advantageous in this population. However, in cases of urgent cesarean section, spinal anesthesia may be a better choice. In such cases, administration of spinal anesthesia allows the anesthesiologist to avoid the risks of general anesthesia, with its attendant risk of airway complications.

D. H. Chestnut, MD

The Effect of Spinal Anesthesia on the Success Rate of External Cephalic Version: A Randomized Trial
Dugoff L, Stamm CA, Jones OW III, et al (Univ of Colorado, Denver)
Obstet Gynecol 93:345-349, 1999   2–41

Background.—The management of breech presentation can include external cephalic version, which has an average success rate of 58%. Successful external cephalic version can eliminate operative delivery and decrease maternal morbidity, although many patients find it uncomfortable. Some studies have reported that epidural anesthesia can increase the success rate of external cephalic version.

Methods.—This study included 102 women with singleton pregnancies with breech presentation at term. Patients were randomly assigned to receive spinal anesthesia or no anesthesia. External cephalic version was attempted up to 4 times and discontinued in cases of patient discomfort or fetal heart decelerations. Statistical analyses included χ^2 tests, Student's *t* tests, and multivariate analysis.

Results.—Of the 102 women, 50 received spinal anesthesia and 52 did not. Groups were similar in maternal age, maternal weight, parity, gestational age, amniotic fluid index, birth weight, placental location, type of breech presentation, and gestational age at delivery. External cephalic version was successful in 22 of 50 patients who received spinal anesthesia and 22 of 52 patients who did not. The success rate was similar in the 2 groups. In 4 patients who had spinal anesthesia and 1 patient who did not have anesthesia, spontaneous version occurred before external cephalic version was attempted; analysis included these 5 patients.

Discussion.—Spinal anesthesia has no effect on the success rate of external cephalic version in women with breech presentation after 36 weeks of gestation. Spinal anesthesia is not recommended for routine version unless the patient cannot tolerate the procedure without anesthesia.

▶ During my obstetrics and gynecology residency, few obstetricians performed external cephalic version. In those days, external cephalic version was considered a risky procedure. Subsequently, the use of real-time US and fetal heart rate monitoring enhanced the safety of the procedure. However, some obstetricians have argued that analgesia/anesthesia should be avoided during external cephalic version so that maternal discomfort will prevent the obstetrician from applying excessive force. In recent years, several studies have evaluated the use of either epidural or spinal analgesia/anesthesia during external cephalic version. These studies have provided conflicting results as to whether regional analgesia/anesthesia increases the likelihood of successful version. On the other hand, advantages of regional analgesia/anesthesia include decreased maternal discomfort and the ability to provide immediate anesthesia for cesarean section for those patients in whom external cephalic version is unsuccessful.

D. H. Chestnut, MD

Combined Spinal-Epidural in the Obstetric Patient With Harrington Rods Assisted by Ultrasonography

Yeo ST, French R (King Edward Mem Hosp, Subiaco, Australia; Christchurch Hosp, New Zealand)

Br J Anaesth 83:670-672, 1999
2–42

Background.—Regional anesthesia is difficult in laboring women with corrected scoliosis. The incidence of complications and of failure to obtain satisfactory analgesia is increased. The induction of epidural analgesia for labor in a women with severe scoliosis corrected partially with Harrington rods was reported.

Case Report.—Woman, 37, was referred to the anesthetic assessment clinic at 36 weeks' gestation. This was her first pregnancy. US at 32 weeks showed macrosomia, and induction at 37 weeks was planned. Her medical history was significant for severe congenital scoliosis, corrected partially with Harrington rods when she was 11 years of age. One week after her assessment, she was admitted for induction. During the next 48 hours, she received prostaglandins followed by Syntocinon infusion to augment contractions. Initial analgesia with intramuscular Entonox and pethidine was not adequate, and the patient, who had become very distressed, requested epidural analgesia. A single-shot spinal was attempted for initial pain control before epidural placement. Spinal palpation revealed no landmarks other than iliac crests. Two attempts at spinal analgesia, one with a 27-gauge Whitacre spinal needle and one with a Yale 18-gauge introducer, were unsuccessful. US was obtained, and the 2 Harrington rods were located in the thoracic region. These rods were followed down until the right rod disappeared just above the lumbar region. The left rod at the level of the iliac crests was used as a lateral marker for the vertebral midline. On the first attempt, cerebrospinal fluid was successfully aspirated with a 27-gauge Whitacre, and bupivacaine 2 mg with fentanyl 25 µg was administered. As the spinal block regressed, an epidural was sited at the same place, using a loss of resistance to saline with an 18-gauge Touhy needle and 20-gauge catheter, resulting in a patchy block insufficient for controlling pain. The epidural was removed, an intrathecal catheter was introduced, and intermittent bolus doses of bupivacaine 2 mg with fentanyl 25 µg were administered, producing excellent analgesia. Clonidine was added to prolong the block. Because of failure to progress, cesarean delivery was necessary. A 0.5% heavy bupivacaine 4 mL was delivered over 20 minutes in four 1-mL doses with fentanyl 15 µg. This produced an adequate block to T3. A baby girl, 4770 g, was born without complication. After surgery, morphine 200 µg was delivered through the intrathecal catheter. In addition, diclofenac 100 mg suppositories were given twice a day, with Panadeine Forte tablets when needed. The intrathecal catheter was removed before the patient was returned to the ward. The recovery period was uncomplicated, with good analgesia and no occurrence of a post-dural puncture headache. The patient was discharged 5 days after delivery.

Conclusions.—This patient with partially corrected severe scoliosis required epidural analgesia for labor. No palpable landmarks could be found. US enabled identification of the vertebral midline, which allowed provision of regional anesthesia.

▶ Administration of epidural anesthesia, spinal anesthesia, or both is problematic in patients with Harrington rod instrumentation. To my knowledge, this represents the first published report of the use of US to facilitate administration of combined spinal-epidural analgesia in a parturient with spinal column instrumentation. Other anesthesiologists have used US to facilitate administration of epidural anesthesia in obese parturients with normal spinal column anatomy.[1]

D. H. Chestnut, MD

Reference

1. Wallace DH, Currie JM, Gilstrap LC, et al: Indirect sonographic guidance for epidural anesthesia in obese pregnant patients. *Reg Anesth* 17:233-236, 1992.

Management of Labor in Eisenmenger Syndrome With Inhaled Nitric Oxide
Lust KM, Boots RJ, Dooris M, et al (Royal Brisbane Hosp, Herston, Australia; Royal Women's Hosp, Herston, Australia)
Am J Obstet Gynecol 181:419-423, 1999   2–43

Background.—Eisenmenger's syndrome has been defined as pulmonary hypertension from high pulmonary vascular resistance with a reversed or bidirectional shunt at the aortopulmonary, ventricular, or atrial level. The development of pulmonary hypertension complicating an atrial septal defect is relatively uncommon, usually not occurring until the fourth decade of life. However, Eisenmenger's syndrome can result from an atrial septal defect in young women during pregnancy. The management of Eisenmenger's syndrome with inhaled nitric oxide (NO) in a young woman in labor was reported.

> *Case Report.*—Woman, 29, with dyspnea was hospitalized from 26 weeks' gestation onward. Echocardiography had shown gross right ventricular dilation and a large atrial septal defect. She also had a right-to-left shunt and moderate tricuspid regurgitation with severe pulmonary hypertension. Fetal development and growth

was adequate. Hospital care consisted of bed rest, oxygen to maintain oxygen saturation at greater than 90%, and therapeutic systemic heparinization. As the pregnancy progressed, the patient's dyspnea increased and was associated with sudden onset of central chest pain. At 34 weeks' gestation, vaginal delivery was induced electively. The morning of induction, heparin infusion was stopped. Prophylaxis included intramuscular betamethasone for fetal lung maturity and amoxicillin and gentamicin for bacterial endocarditis. Prostaglandin E_2 was administered intravaginally to induce labor. Epidural anesthesia with fentanyl and 0.1% bupivacaine was started after labor onset. After the onset of contractions, the patient was moved to the ICU. Cardiotocography, echocardiography, oximetry, and pulmonary artery catheterization were used to monitor labor. NO, 900 ppm, was administered through a nasal cannula. Mixed expired gas was analyzed with a chemiluminescence monitor, and methemoglobin levels were determined hourly. The NO flow rate was titrated to a maximal decrease in pulmonary artery pressure and improved gas exchange. Oxygenation was well maintained during labor. However, pulmonary pressure increased to 117/36 mm Hg. At delivery, systemic pressure was 112/70 mm Hg. Nebulized prostacyclin to 20 ng/kg per minute did not reduce pulmonary arterial pressure. IV prostacyclin to 5 ng/kg per minute resulted in systemic hypotension and type II deceleration on the cardiotocogram, with no change in pulmonary arterial pressure. Ten units of synthetic oxytocin (Syntocinon) was administered with the delivery of the anterior shoulder, followed by infusion of 40 units for 8 hours. A healthy baby girl was delivered without complication.

After delivery, a fraction of inspired oxygen of 0.8 and NO at 10 ppm were continued. Pulmonary arterial pressure declined gradually, and cardiac output improved within 24 hours of delivery. On the second postpartum day, the patient had persistent heavy vaginal bleeding and supraventricular tachycardia, and there was no clinical change in oxygenation or evidence of heart failure. Pulmonary arterial pressure rose to 109/67 mm Hg and cardiac output to 6.2 L/min during supraventricular tachycardia. Synthetic oxytocin infusion settled the bleeding, and digoxin and amiodarone infusion settled the supraventricular tachycardia. Pulmonary arterial pressure and cardiac output stabilized. Synthetic oxytocin was delivered for 48 hours. No focal source of bleeding was found on vaginal examination. Heparin administration was stopped on days 7 to 9 because of persistent vaginal bleeding. Ten days after delivery, the patient needed a transfusion, after which therapeutic anticoagulation was resumed. On postpartum day 5, amiodarone infusion was stopped because of first-degree heart block. On postpartum day 7, a Johnson transtracheal oxygen catheter was inserted to continue NO at 10 ppm. Fourteen days after delivery, progressive hypoxemia developed, and there was increasing pulmonary arterial pressure. Echocardiography showed right ventricular function worsening, severe tricuspid regurgitation, and an estimated right ventricular systolic pressure of 110 to 120 mm Hg. IV prostacyclin, sublingual nifedipine, NO to 80 ppm, and aminophylline failed to decrease pulmonary arterial pressure. IV norepinephrine was begun because of progressive hypotension. Although the patient was accepted for heart–lung transplantation, her condition deteriorated. Twenty-one days postpartum, she died.

Conclusions.—In this patient with Eisenmenger's syndrome caused by an atrial septal defect, NO administration by inhalation during labor improved oxygenation and initial pulmonary arterial pressure. Although she delivered a healthy infant at 34 weeks' gestation, the patient subsequently died from worsening pulmonary hypertension and heart failure.

▶ Inhaled NO improved oxygenation and decreased pulmonary artery pressure in this patient. Unfortunately, this case report concludes with the all-too-familiar statement that the patient ultimately succumbed as a result of worsening pulmonary hypertension and heart failure.

D. H. Chestnut, MD

The Use of Propofol, Nitrous Oxide, or Isoflurane Does Not Affect the Reproductive Success Rate Following Gamete Intrafallopian Transfer (GIFT): A Multicenter Pilot Trial/Survey
Beilin Y, Bodian CA, Mukherjee T, et al (Mount Sinai School of Medicine, New York; Univ of Alabama at Birmingham; UMDNJ–Robert Wood Johnson Med Ctr, New Brunswick, NJ; et al)
Anesthesiology 90:36-41, 1999   2–44

Introduction.—There is controversy regarding the effects of anesthesia agents on pregnancy outcomes when gamete intrafallopian transfer (GIFT) is performed under general anesthesia. The effects of propofol, nitrous oxide, midazolam, and isoflurane on pregnancy outcome after GIFT were examined in a multicenter, retrospective pilot trial; the need for a larger, prospective randomized trial was also evaluated.

Methods.—An invitation was mailed to all 50 fertility programs in the United States that are members of the Society for Assisted Reproductive Technology and conduct over 30 GIFT procedures yearly. Participant programs were asked to contribute information from medical records of women who underwent GIFT from January 1993 to January 1994. They were asked to document whether propofol, nitrous oxide, midazolam, or isoflurane was administered during the GIFT procedure; whether the patient became pregnant; and whether she had delivered at least 1 live neonate.

Results.—Data on 455 women was contributed from 7 medical centers. The clinical pregnancy rate (number of pregnancies per total number of

GIFT procedures) was 35%. The delivery rate (number of women who delivered at least 1 live baby per total number of GIFT procedures) was 32%. There was no significant difference between the clinical pregnancy or delivery rates and those women who received propofol, nitrous oxide, midazolam, or isoflurane during GIFT and those who did not receive inhaled anesthetic.

Conclusion.—There was no indication of an agent-related difference in pregnancy or delivery rates when propofol, nitrous oxide, or isoflurane were used as part of the anesthetic technique for GIFT. A more extensive prospective trial is not warranted.

▶ The results of this study are welcome, given the advantages of propofol for outpatient surgery. However, the study specifically evaluated outcome for GIFT. Propofol may have a different effect when given for procedures that involve the transfer of embryos (for example, zygote intrafallopian transfer). In an earlier study, Vincent et al[1] observed that the incidence of ongoing pregnancies was lower among women given propofol-nitrous oxide anesthesia for zygote intrafallopian transfer when compared with a similar group of women who received thiopental–nitrous oxide–isoflurane anesthesia (29% vs 54%). Additional studies are needed to clarify the role of propofol for zygote intrafallopian transfer.

D. H. Chestnut, MD

Reference

1. Vincent RD, Syrop CH, Van Voorhis BJ, et al: An evaluation of the effect of anesthetic technique on reproductive success after laparoscopic pronuclear stage transfer. *Anesthesiology* 82:352-358, 1995.

Wolff-Parkinson-White Syndrome Simulating Inferior Myocardial Infarction in a Cocaine Abuser for Urgent Dilation and Evacuation of the Uterus
Lustik SJ, Wojtczak J, Chhibber AK (Univ of Rochester, NY)
Anesth Analg 89:609-612, 1999   2–45

Objective.—A patient with apparent recent myocardial infarction was diagnosed with Wolff-Parkinson-White (WPW) syndrome. Methods to differentiate WPW from myocardial infarction in a cocaine abuser and the anesthetic management of WPW are discussed.

Case Report.—Woman, 34, 17 weeks pregnant, was hospitalized for a dilation and evacuation. She reported having palpitations, lightheadedness, and chest pain 2 weeks previously that was successfully treated in the emergency department. She admitted to occasional cocaine use and described several episodes of substernal pain. She also smoked almost a pack of cigarettes per day and drank 3 beer 2 or 3 times weekly. Although her preoperative ECG showed possible myocardial infarction, the cardiologist diagnosed WPW syndrome, and she underwent successful dilation and evacuation. Postoperatively, testing revealed the presence of a posteroseptal accessory pathway, which was successfully treated with catheter ablation. Her inferior Q waves resolved.

Discussion.—The presence of delta waves in leads V_2 and V_3 were diagnostic of WPW. Negative delta waves in the inferior leads, present in 16% of WPW patients, look like infarction Q waves.

▶ I included this study because any history of cocaine abuse should raise all the cardiac red flags to the top of the pole. A worse problem may be the coronary spasm associated with this "dirty" old drug. I use the word "dirty" as pharmaceutical companies do, meaning an old drug with many, and generally unpredictable, side and unwanted effects.

J. H. Tinker, MD

3 Pediatric Anesthesia Topics

Ropivacaine vs Bupivacaine in Major Surgery in Infants
Ivani G, Lampugnani E, De Negri P, et al ("Regina Margherita" Children's Hosp, Turin, Italy; Casa Sollievo della Sofferenza, San Giovanni Rotondo, Italy; Karolinska Hosp, Stockholm; et al)
Can J Anesth 46:467-469, 1999   3–1

Introduction.—Ropivacaine is a new aminoamide local anesthetic that produces sensory blockade similar in duration to that of equipotent doses of bupivacaine in animals and adults but with less motor blockade. The onset time and duration of neuroblockade were evaluated and compared after ropivacaine and bupivacaine in infants undergoing major surgery in a prospective, double-blind investigation. The efficacy and safety of using ropivacaine rather than bupivacaine during operative anesthesia and post-operative analgesia were also examined.

Methods.—The age range of 28 infants undergoing elective major abdominal surgery was 1 to 12 months. They were randomized after induction of general anesthesia to receive either 0.1 mL/kg bupivacaine 0.25% (group B) or ropivacaine 0.2% (group R) by lumbar epidural block. Anesthesia onset time, total surgical time, and duration of analgesia were recorded.

Results.—There were no significant between-group differences in demographic data, hemodynamic variables, or duration of surgery. Sensory blockade onset was 13.1 and 11.7 minutes, respectively, for group B and group R. Duration of analgesia was 456 and 491 minutes, respectively, for group B and group R. Codeine and acetaminophen rescue were required at least once during the 24-hour evaluation period for 8 patients in group B and 6 in group R. No major side effects were reported for either group.

Conclusion.—Ropivacaine provided sensory and motor blockade similar to that of equal volumes of bupivacaine in onset, duration of action, and efficacy in infants undergoing major abdominal surgery using combined epidural/light general anesthesia.

▶ It is salutary to see clinical research evaluating new drugs in small infants. Clinical pharmacology in the pediatric population is a growth area for anesthesiologists.

M. Wood, MD

Development of a Nurse-Led Sedation Service for Paediatric Magnetic Resonance Imaging

Sury MRJ, Hatch DJ, Deeley T, et al (Great Ormond Street Hosp for Children NHS Trust, London; Inst of Child Health, London)
Lancet 353:1667-1671, 1999   3–2

Introduction.—MRI requires that patients be immobile for at least 20 minutes in a noisy and enclosed space. Most children will lie still for MRI examination only if they are made to sleep by sedation or anesthesia. Anesthesia resources are limited and the demand for sedation is rising with increasing use of MRI. The safety and efficacy of a nurse-led sedation service was examined during a 30-month period.

Methods.—A senior nurse with intensive care experience became the first nonmedical sedationist to lead a sedation unit within the radiology department of 1 medical institution. Both the radiologist and the sedationist reviewed physician request forms to determine patient fitness for sedation. The sedationist used agreed upon criteria to determine patients' fitness for sedation. Food was not allowed for 3 hours before sedation. Clear liquids were not restricted. Patients were monitored by the sedationist throughout the MRI process via continuous clinical observation, pulse oximetry, capnography, electrocardiography, and noninvasive blood pressure monitoring.

After completion of the procedure, the sedationist tested the ability of the children to open their mouths and breathe with the nostrils pinched shut. A continuous audit of nurse-led sedation was used to record the following: numbers of patients, failure rate, lowest pulse oximeter saturation, adverse respiratory events, requirement for IV diazepam top-ups, delayed recovery, use of oxygen, side effects, and inability to open the mouth in response to pinching of the nostrils after scanning was completed.

Results.—During a 30-month evaluation period, 1155 sedations were performed. Of these, 61 (5%) were not successful. There were no adverse events related to the airway or breathing. All children were able to open their mouths to maintain their airway in response to pinching the nostrils after scanning was completed.

Conclusion.—It is possible for nurse-led sedation to be used safely in children undergoing MRI.

▶ This study emphasizes the importance of sedation in pediatric patients outside the operating room environment. All departments are having to grapple with how to organize this on an economic basis. These authors suggest that nurses may administer this sedation service if in a designated area. They also emphasize the fact that sedation for more painful procedures is quite different and that the results for this study in an MRI setting should not be extrapolated to other situations.

M. Wood, MD

Atlantoaxial Rotatory Subluxation After a Pediatric Tonsillectomy

Dasen KR (Kaiser Permanente Med Ctr, Sacramento, Calif)
Anesth Analg 89:917-919, 1999   3–3

Objective.—Atlantoaxial subluxation leading to neurologic injuries after airway manipulation is usually the result of bone or ligament abnormalities. A case of postoperative atlantoaxial rotatory subluxation in 1 7-year-old boy after tonsillectomy and adenoidectomy was reported.

> *Case Report.*—Boy, 7 years, obese, with a history of snoring and recurrent tonsillitis, had a Mallampati class 2 airway. His range of motion was normal. The procedure was uneventful, and he was released without musculoskeletal or neurologic symptoms. On day 4, he came into the emergency department with "cock robin" head positioning, a painful neck, left torticollis, hoarseness, cough, uvular edema, and low-grade fever that had begun 24 hours after discharge. He was diagnosed with atlantoaxial rotatory subluxation. A CT scan revealed the spinous process of C1 left of the midline and the spinous process of C2 on the midline. Treatment with a hard cervical collar for 3 months, amoxicillin for infection, and acetaminophen for pain resulted in resolution of the condition within 13 days. The patient made a full recovery.

Conclusion.—The cause of his symptoms was probably pharyngeal inflammation caused by infection that led to a spasm of the deep cervical musculature (Grisel's syndrome). Minimizing head rotation may help to prevent this syndrome.

▶ I doubt that I actually ever heard of "atlantoaxial rotatory subluxation" before I read this study, but just the name scares the daylights out of me. I have for years preached to the residents to be gentle with the head and neck of a paralyzed or anesthetized patient. My view of the neck is that it is made up of dozens, maybe hundreds, of complex parts all put together in ways that have been complete mysteries to me since Anatomy in medical school. I teach the residents that to pull on it, or superextend it, or to do just about anything else with it, can be scary, especially in older folks.

J. H. Tinker, MD

4 Cardiothoracic and Vascular Anesthesia Patient Care Topics

The Impact of an Occluded Internal Carotid Artery on the Mortality and Morbidity of Patients Undergoing Coronary Artery Bypass Grafting
Tunio AM, Hingorani A, Ascher E (Maimonides Med Ctr, Brooklyn, NY)
Am J Surg 178:201-205, 1999   4–1

Background.—Stroke is a major problem in patients undergoing coronary artery bypass grafting (CABG). Although other mechanisms may be involved, concomitant carotid artery disease is likely a major contributor to perioperative stroke. The effects of internal carotid artery (ICA) stenosis or occlusion on perioperative stroke rate and mortality among patients with CABG were analyzed.

Methods.—The retrospective study included 3344 patients undergoing CABG at the authors' center during a 3.5-year period. Fifty-nine percent of the patients were men. In each case, a preoperative carotid artery duplex scan—performed at an ICAVL-accredited laboratory by a registered vascular technologist—was available for review. About 93% of patients (group A) had ICA stenosis of less than 60%, while 5% had ICA stenosis of 60% to 99% (group B), and 2% had ICA occlusion (group C). In group C, 87% of patients had less than 60% stenosis of the contralateral ICA, and the rest had stenosis of 60% to 99%. Forty percent of patients in group B and 3% of those in group C underwent carotid endarterectomy (CEA) along with CABG. Perioperative stroke rates and mortality were compared among groups.

Results.—The 3 groups were similar in terms of age, surgical indications, diabetes, hypertension, and smoking. The mean pump time was 125 to 138 minutes, and the aortic cross-clamp time 75 to 78 minutes. Thirty-day stroke rate was 1.6% in group A compared with 3.8% in group B and 6.5% in group C. The difference between groups B and C was nonsignificant. Within group C, the perioperative stroke rate was 25% for patients with contralateral stenosis compared with 3.8% for those without contralateral stenosis. Among patients undergoing concomitant CEA for severe stenosis in the contralateral ICA, the stroke rate was 100% in group C versus 4.2% in group B. Thirty-day mortality was 3.6% in group A versus 6.6% in group B and 8.6% in group C.

Conclusions.—Among patients undergoing CABG, the presence of ICA occlusion is associated with increased perioperative morbidity and mortality. This is the first large study of the effects of ICA occlusion on the outcomes of CABG. The findings support the safety of simultaneous CEA and CABG.

▶ Just as interesting, if not much more, are the patients who had severe carotid lesions and did not have perioperative strokes! Is there a subgroup of these folks who somehow become hypercoagulable? On about the second day after surgery? I think studies of the stress responses that occur following major surgery hold keys to understanding these devastating complications. Was there the slightest doubt that these patients, with occluded carotids, would fare worse after any kind of major surgery than those with relatively clean carotids?

J. H. Tinker, MD

Fast-Track Cardiac Anesthesia in Patients With Sickle Cell Abnormalities

Djaiani GN, Cheng DCH, Carroll JA, et al (Univ of Toronto)
Anesth Analg 89:598-603, 1999   4–2

Objective.—Patients with sickle cell hemoglobinopathies are at increased risk of perioperative complications. Perioperative management of 10 patients with sickle cell trait (SCT) who underwent fast-track cardiac anesthesia was retrospectively reviewed.

Methods.—Perioperative management data, duration of surgery, length of stay in the ICU, duration of hospitalization, and outcomes were compared for 10 patients (2 female) with SCT and 30 patients (5 female) without SCT undergoing first-time coronary artery bypass grafting. Fast-track cardiac anesthesia was induced using a combination of cold crystalloid and blood cardioplegia.

Results.—No patient had a sickling crisis, significant hypoxemia, hypercarbia, or acidosis. Urine output during cardiopulmonary bypass was 365 mL for the SCT group and 395 mL for the control group. Respective postoperative blood loss was 687 and 585 mL. Hb concentration was significantly reduced in both groups after surgery. Three SCT patients and 10 control patients required a blood transfusion. Mean postoperative blood loss and transfusion rate were similar for both groups. One SCT patient with a history of renal impairment, diabetes, mild stroke, and hypertension died on postoperative day 58. Postoperative extubation time and length of ICU and hospital stays were similar for both groups.

Conclusion.—Fast-track cardiac anesthesia is safe for patients with SCT.

▶ The term "fast-track" is a currently popular slogan. I rant and rave (another slogan) all the time against management by slogan. I think most "fast-track" programs that I've seen really didn't end up saving very much in the overall picture. Sicklers are a good example. What if just 1 goes into crisis after being "fast-tracked" out the door? Would you want that for a family member?

J. H. Tinker, MD

The Relationship of Myocardial Stroke Work to Coronary Flow Velocity Immediately After Aortic Valve Replacement
Jin XY, Gibson DG, Pepper JR (Royal Brompton Hosp, London)
Ann Thorac Surg 67:705-710, 1999   4–3

Objective.—The degree of myocardial injury after aortic valve replacement is difficult to quantify. There is some evidence that warm continuous blood cardioplegia is less protective than intermittent cold blood cardioplegia. Changes in left ventricular myocardial stroke work, left anterior descending coronary artery flow velocities, and the ratio of the 2 during and up to 20 hours after aortic valve replacement were investigated to discern any differences between the 2 cardioplegic methods.

Methods.—Elective isolated aortic valve replacement was performed in 26 patients (15 men) with an average age of 63 years. Fifteen patients received cold cardioplegia, and 11 had normothermic cardioplegia. Echocardiography was performed, and left ventricular pressure was recorded. Pressure and stress were determined during ejection and peak pressure increases and decreases, myocardial stroke work was calculated, and left ventricular hemodynamics and coronary flow velocities were determined perioperatively and at 1, 6, 12, and 20 hours.

Results.—Left ventricular stroke work decreased significantly and immediately after surgery from 26.1 to 15.0 m/min with cold paraplegia and from 32.8 to 14.4 m/min with warm blood cardioplegia. Values did not return to preoperative levels during the study. Regional myocardial stroke work decreased significantly after surgery from 228 to 160 mJ/mL per minute with cold cardioplegia and from 227 to 135 mJ/mL per minute with warm blood cardioplegia. Early diastolic left anterior descending coronary artery (LAD) flow velocities increased by a factor of 1.6, and late diastolic LAD flow velocities increased by a factor of 2 compared with baseline values. The ratio of myocardial stroke work to the LAD flow velocity time integral decreased significantly in both the cold and warm blood cardioplegia groups (4.3 vs 16.3 mJ/mL per meter per minute and 7.4 vs 17.9 mJ/mL per meter per minute, respectively) but was significantly lower with warm blood cardioplegia (7.8 vs 10.9 mJ/mL per meter per minute).

Conclusion.—The depression of myocardial function after cardiopulmonary bypass is followed by an abnormal increase in coronary flow velocities in the left ventricle for at least 20 hours after surgery. The ratio of myocardial stroke work to the LAD flow velocity time integral was significantly lower with warm blood cardioplegia than with cold blood cardioplegia.

▶ I selected this study more to make some fun of the well-known propensity of cardiac physiologists to multiply things with each other. "Work," to a cardiac physiologist, is pressure times flow. "Stroke work" is pressure times stroke volume. My residents insist on using "resistance," which is pressure divided by flow as if it was an inherent property of a physiologic system, or an indicator of something profound or even useful clinically. If you multiply all this by my social security number, you get the well-known Tinker's index, which is just as useful. Stroke work has little to do with oxygen demand or consumption (the same thing in the absence of ischemia), and it has little to do with cardiac well-being. To use it to assess 1 kind of magical cardioplegia over another is folly. Besides, it is well known that all you need for a good cardioplegia "brew" is to add a pinch of powdered toad bladder extract and a pinch of dried powdered bat wings.

J. H. Tinker, MD

Comparison of Vital Capacity Induction With Sevoflurane to Intravenous Induction With Propofol for Adult Ambulatory Anesthesia
Philip BK, Lombard LL, Roaf ER, et al (Harvard Med School, Boston)
Anesth Analg 89:623-627, 1999   4–4

Objective.—Inhaled induction of anesthesia is feasible with sevoflurane. The vital capacity inhaled induction (VCI) with sevoflurane was compared with IV induction with propofol in adults undergoing ambulatory anesthesia.

Methods.—Patients (n = 56) were randomly allocated to receive VCI with 8% sevoflurane in 75% nitrous oxide/oxygen (n = 32) or IV induction with 2 mg/kg bolus propofol (n = 24). Time to loss of consciousness, recovery times after surgery, and adverse events were recorded for both groups. Patients rated the quality of their anesthesia.

Results.—Induction times were significantly shorter for the VCI group than for the IV group with 59% of VCI patients losing consciousness in 1 breath. Induction adverse events were cough and hiccough for the VCI group and movement and blood pressure changes for the IV group. Patients in both groups would have the same type of anesthesia again. Duration of anesthesia, psychomotor function, wakefulness, and discomfort were similar for both groups. There were more patients in the VCI group than the IV group with nausea (78% vs 50%), although the difference was not significant. Discharge times were similar for both groups.

Conclusion.—Induction anesthesia with sevoflurane was significantly faster than with IV propofol. Adverse events, duration of anesthesia, recovery times, and discomfort were similar for both groups.

▶ Single-breath induction is indeed possible with sevoflurane, because of its low solubility and lack of pungency. I am not sure I agree with the authors who believe that this type of induction is as acceptable to the usual ambulatory patient as an induction with propofol, but maybe so. It is likely cheaper. It is likely just as safe. It is likely to prove quite easy to do.

J. H. Tinker, MD

An Assessment of the Safety of Short-term Amiodarone Therapy in Cardiac Surgical Patients With Fentanyl-Isoflurane Anesthesia
White CM, Dunn A, Tsikouris J, et al (Hartford Hosp, Conn; Univ of Connecticut, Storrs)
Anesth Analg 89:585-589, 1999   4–5

Objective.—Chronic amiodarone use, in combination with fentanyl anesthesias, may cause atrioventricular blockade, symptomatic bradycardia, sinus arrest, and severe hypotension. The effect of short-term amiodarone use has not been investigated. The effect on hemodynamics of fentanyl-containing anesthesia, administered to elderly patients receiving short-term amiodarone therapy before coronary artery bypass graft (CABG) or valvular surgery, was investigated in a prospective, randomized, double-blind, placebo-controlled trial.

Methods.—Elderly CABG patients were randomly allocated to receive 3.4 g over 5 days or 2.2 g over 24 hours of amiodarone (n = 45, 77.8% male) or placebo (n = 39, 79.5% male) before CABG. Fluid balance, use of dopamine, use of vasopressive catecholamines, and use of a phosphodiesterase inhibitor or intra-aortic balloon pump were recorded. Systolic, diastolic, and central venous blood pressures were measured before anesthesia induction, before cardiopulmonary bypass (CPB), and after CPB. Heart rates were recorded before induction of anesthesia and after CPB.

Results.—Fluid status increased by more than 2 L in 2 (4.4%) amiodarone patients and in 4 (10.3%) placebo patients. No patient required dopamine or an intra-aortic balloon pump. Epinephrine or a derivative was administered to 8 (17.8%) amiodarone and 5 (12.8%) placebo patients and milrinone to 1 (2.2%) and 2 (5.1%) patients, respectively. There were no significant differences between groups. Prefentanyl systolic blood pressure and post-CPB systolic blood pressure were significantly lower in amiodarone patients than in placebo patients. Amiodarone patients received less fluid and had a lower net increase in fluid status during surgery than the placebo group, although the differences were not significant.

Conclusion.—Short-term amiodarone therapy does not lead to hemodynamic instability in CABG patients receiving fentanyl anesthesia regimens.

▶ Amiodarone is that amazing drug that turns some patients purple! It has approximately the half life of DDT, namely until the twelfth of never. I teach that these patients should raise the red flag for us in anesthesia, not so much because of interactions between the drug and anesthesia, but because the internists would not be likely to give a healthy patient a drug that might turn him or her purple! I do think that as more and more experience accumulates, we will be less afraid of this drug than now. I included this study to have the chance to remind us all that our friendly cardiologists are liking this drug more and more these days, so I guess we're stuck with it. One thing is certain. Forget asking them to stop the drug before anesthesia and surgery. It won't help. I don't think it is possible for the body to eliminate the stuff!

J. H. Tinker, MD

Initial Experience With Beating Heart Surgery: Comparison With Fast-Track Methods
Ott RA, Gutfinger DE, Steedman R, et al (Anaheim Mem Med Ctr, Calif)
Am Surg 65:1018-1022, 1999   4–6

Objective.—Fast-track recovery methods after coronary artery bypass grafting (CABG) reduced postoperative hospital stays without increasing morbidity. New off-pump techniques and single-vessel CABG are reducing recovery times even more. A series of consecutive patients undergoing conventional CABG with a fast-track recovery method was retrospectively compared with the initial series of patients undergoing beating heart surgery with either the single-vessel minimally invasive approach or the off-pump multivessel bypass technique with a median sternotomy.

Methods.—Between January 1996 and September 1996, 104 patients underwent conventional CABG with cardiopulmonary bypass followed by a fast-track recovery method (group A), 29 underwent a single-vessel off-pump bypass (group B), and 25 patients underwent off-pump CABG with a median sternotomy (group C).

Results.—There were 3 (1.8%) deaths. Group B patients were significantly younger than group A and C patients, and group C patients had more risk factors than group A and B patients. Group A and C patients required 3 or more bypass grafts, but group B patients needed only 1. Average operative times were 2 hours for group B and 2.5 hours for groups A and C. Operative mortality, duration of hospital stay, and postoperative complication rates were similar for all groups. Postoperative hospital stays were 4.8 days for group A, 3.9 days for group B, and 5.2 days for group C.

Conclusion.—Short-pump CABG is recommended where extensive revascularization is required. The off-pump technique offers an advantage for patients at risk of postoperative organ system failure. Minimally invasive direct coronary artery bypass is the procedure of choice for patients who require a single bypass that is not amenable to interventional percutaneous techniques.

▶ Those who are forced by unfortunate circumstance to have to work closely with me know that I am continually carping and making fun of our national penchant for slogans, of which "fast track" is the latest in the heart room. This article shows how false some of this kind of amateur economics can get. Let's say we do the ultimate and get our patients out the door (not just out of the operating room or ICU) in a very short time. This will save money only if there is another patient who is patiently waiting to come *in* the door. If we simply get done early and then stand around, then whatever increased risk we may have subjected our patients to is simply invalid from an economic standpoint. In my several decades in our "business," I have learned to beware of glib, well-meaning folks bearing slogans.

J. H. Tinker, MD

Cardiac Output Can Be Reliably Measured Noninvasively After Coronary Artery Bypass Grafting Operation
Kööbi T, Kaukinen S, Turjanmaa VMH (Univ of Tampere, Finland)
Crit Care Med 27:2206-2211, 1999   4–7

Background.—Cardiac output can be measured in patients undergoing cardiac surgery by the thermodilution method, but it is an expensive procedure that carries a risk of complications. Whole-body impedance cardiography—in which electrodes are attached to the wrists and ankles, and the electrical current is assumed to pass through the main vascular trees—was evaluated as an alternative technique of measuring cardiac output after coronary artery bypass grafting (CABG).

Methods.—The prospective study included 82 patients undergoing CABG with insertion of a pulmonary artery thermodilution catheter. Postoperative cardiac-output measurements were made by means of both the thermodilution method and the whole-body impedance cardiography method in all patients. The simultaneous measurements were made at 2 times in 2 groups: within 3 hours after surgery in 41 patients (early ICU period) and both before surgery and in the second 12 hours after surgery in the other 41 patients (late ICU period).

Results.—The measurements showed good agreement in the preoperative period, bias 0.04 ± 1.64 L/min, and in the late ICU period, bias 0.00 ± 1.84 L/min. In more than 80% of patients, the thermodilution and whole-body impedance cardiography measurements were within 20% of each other. Agreement decreased to the satisfactory level in the early ICU period, bias 0.38 ± 2.74 L/min. Postoperative thermal instability may have contributed to measurement error with the thermodilution method. At all 3 times, repeatability was better with whole-body impedance cardiography. The 2 methods showed agreement similar to that achieved with invasive methods in comparable settings.

Conclusions.—Before and after CABG, cardiac output can be reliably measured by the use of whole-body impedance cardiography. The results of whole-body impedance cardiography are as reliable as those of invasive techniques. It is a highly repeatable measurement that is valuable for continuous postoperative monitoring.

▶ This article reminds me of an old cartoon that appeared in *Science* magazine years ago. It had 2 panels. It depicted the "William Tell" scenario, with a person with an apple on his head. In the first panel, the archer had shot 2 arrows close together into the apple. The caption under this panel read "Accuracy." You guessed it. In the second panel, the archer had placed the 2 arrows, just as close together, in the center of the forehead of the very unhappy "volunteer." The caption read "Precision."

These authors compared their resurrection of an ancient holy grail method of cardiac output measurement, namely, impedance plethysmography, to a notoriously inaccurate and technique-dependent method, thermodilution. In the cardiac operating room, during separation from bypass, the surgeon demands an "output." My resident "shoots" several. He gets a 6, then a 9, then a 4, then a 6 again. He tells the surgeon the output is "6." He has no more idea what the output is than he has knowledge about the China/Taiwan controversy—unless he is Chinese; then he knows a lot more about the latter! I will not hold my breath about impedance, especially since it requires frequent "calibrations" against—you guessed it—thermodilution.

J. H. Tinker, MD

5 Other Perioperative Patient Care Issues

Postoperative (Pressure) Alopecia: Report of a Case After Elective Cosmetic Surgery
Dominguez E, Eslinger MR, McCord SV (Naval Med Ctr, Portsmouth, Va)
Anesth Analg 89:1062-1063, 1999   5–1

Objective.—A case of rare postoperative alopecia was reported after general anesthesia in a cosmetic plastic surgery patient.

> *Case Report.*—Woman, 50, having bilateral breast reduction, received 90 mg propofol, 200 µg of fentanyl, and 50 mg of rocuronium IV with anesthesia maintained with isoflurane and nitrous oxide. The patient remained supine throughout the unremarkable procedure. She had soreness and tenderness over her eyes at 12 hours, and was discharged 23 hours after admission. She lost hair during a 2-week period. Within weeks, new hair began to grow, and at 6 months, her hair had regrown.

Discussion.—Pressure-related alopecia has been reported in 8 women after prolonged gynecologic procedures. There are reports of this complication also among patients of both sexes and all ages apparently caused by localized pressure-induced ischemia.

Conclusion.—Periodic repositioning of the patient's head during long surgeries can possibly prevent this complication.

▶ The key here is that this patient's head was "placed over folded sheets." If they really used "folded sheets," the latter are too firm and unforgiving in my opinion. There is a difference between what we call "bath blankets" as a pillow, and "sheets."

J. H. Tinker, MD

6 Anesthesia-Related Pharmacology and Toxicology

New Muscle Relaxants

Pharmacokinetics and Pharmacodynamics of Rapacuronium in Patients With Cirrhosis

Duvaldestin P, Slavov V, Rebufat Y (Henri Mondor Hosp, Creteil, France)
Anesthesiology 91:1305-1310, 1999
6–1

Introduction.—Delayed elimination kinetics of steroidal neuromuscular blocking agents have been seen in patients with cirrhosis. Rapacuronium is an aminosteroid nondepolarized neuromuscular blocking agent with a quicker onset and duration of action, compared with other currently available nondepolarized agents. Like other steroidal muscle relaxants, it may be partially eliminated by the liver. The pharmacokinetics and pharmacodynamics of rapacuronium were examined in patients with cirrhosis to determine the influence of liver disease on its neuromuscular blocking effect.

Methods.—Eight patients with liver cirrhosis without esophageal varices and 8 patients with normal liver function undergoing elective surgery or endoscopy with general anesthesia were evaluated. They received fentanyl, 2 µg/kg, and thiopental, 5 to 7 mg/kg, and were maintained with isoflurane (0.6%-0.8%, end-tidal), nitrous oxide (60% in oxygen), and repeated doses of fentanyl (1 µg/kg). Rapacuronium, 1.5 mg/kg, was administered IV before tracheal intubation was performed. Thumb adduction force evoked by supramaximal ulnar nerve stimulation was noted in 16 patients. Venous blood was collected at frequent intervals for 8 hours. Rapacuronium and its breakdown product, Org 9488, were measured in plasma using high-pressure liquid chromatography.

Results.—The mean plasma concentration of rapacuronium was significantly lower in patients with cirrhosis, compared with control subjects. The Org 9488 compound was detected in all plasma samples, with the highest concentration occurring at 2 minutes, then progressively diminishing. The central volume of distribution was significantly higher in patients with cirrhosis, compared with control subjects (median, 131 vs 75 mL/kg) (*P* < .01). The total apparent volume of distribution was also increased in patients with cirrhosis, compared with control subjects (median, 331 vs 221 mL/kg) (*P* < .05).

The median elimination half-life was 88 minutes in control subjects and 90 minutes in patients with cirrhosis (*P* < .05). Median plasma clearance was 6.9 mL/min per kilogram in patients with cirrhosis and 5.3 mL/min per kilogram in control subjects (*P* < .05). The rapacuronium neuromuscular blocking effect was similar for both groups. Median onset times were 65 and 60 seconds, respectively, in control subjects and patients with cirrhosis. Median times to return to 90% of thumb adduction force control value were 49 and 47 minutes in control subjects and patients with cirrhosis, respectively.

Conclusion.—The neuromuscular blocking effect of a single bolus dose of rapacuronium in patients with cirrhosis is similar to that seen in patients with normal hepatic function. No reduction in plasma clearance of rapacuronium was seen in patients with cirrhosis.

▶ I have chosen this article to highlight a new muscle relaxant, rapacuronium. Rapacuronium, as the name suggests, is a new nondepolarizing neuromuscular blocking agent that has both a rapid onset and short duration of action. Hence, it will probably be used for short procedures. Will it be a viable alternative to succinylcholine? Perhaps. We do not know. Will it be an alternative to miracuronium? Probably. Renal elimination is of minor importance, and this study completes the picture by demonstrating the effect of cirrhosis on the pharmacokinetics and dynamics of rapacuronium.

M. Wood, MD

A Pharmacodynamic Explanation for the Rapid Onset/Offset of Rapacuronium Bromide
Wright PMC, Brown R, Lau M, et al (Univ of Newcastle-upon-Tyne, England; Univ of California, San Francisco)
Anesthesiology 90:16-23, 1999   6–2

Background.—Preliminary studies have indicated that onset of rapacuronium bromide and recovery at the adductor pollicis is more rapid than with other nondepolarizing muscle relaxants. Whether pharmacokinetic or pharmacodynamic characteristics explain this rapid onset and recovery was determined.

Study Design.—Participants were 10 healthy volunteers, aged 20 to 42 years, who were anesthetized. Twitch tensions of the adductor pollicis and laryngeal muscles were assessed. Rapacuronium, 1.5 mg/kg, was administered and twitch tension assessment was repeated. Arterial and venous blood samples were collected. Concentrations of rapacuronium and its primary metabolite, ORG9488, were determined by high-pressure liquid chromatography–mass spectrometry. Arterial and venous concentrations

Adductor Pollicis   Laryngeal Adductors

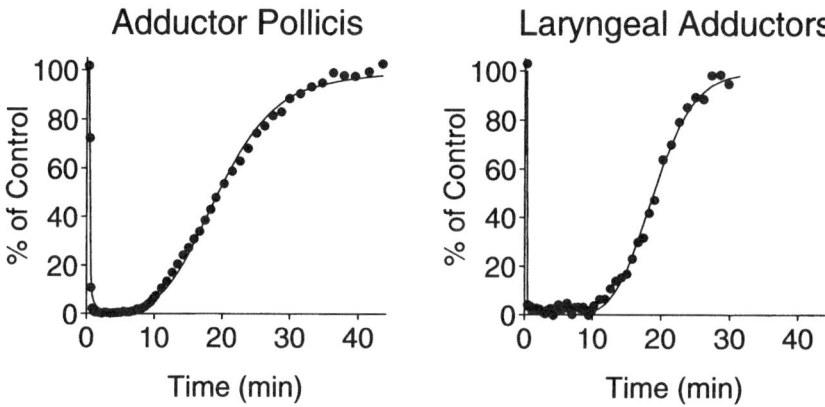

FIGURE 3.—A representative *post hoc* fit of the pharmacodynamic model (based on an ORG9488:rapacuronium potency ratio of 2) to the effect data for the adductor pollicis and the laryngeal adductors. *Circles* represent measured values; the *line* represents the fitted function. (Courtesy of Wright PMC, Brown R, Lau M, et al: A pharmacodynamic explanation for the rapid onset/offset of rapacuronium bromide. *Anesthesiology* 90:16-23, 1999. Copyright American Society of Anesthesiologists, Inc. Used with permission of Lippincott-Raven Publishers.)

of rapacuronium were plotted against time. The magnitude and time until maximal twitch depression and recovery were determined.

Results.—Equilibrium between rapacuronium plasma concentration and both effect sites occurred rapidly. Equilibrium was reached more rapidly at the laryngeal adductor muscles than at the adductor pollicis. The steady-state plasma concentration that depressed twitch tension by 50% and the Hill factor were similar for these 2 muscles (Fig 3).

Conclusion.—The onset and offset of rapacuronium are rapid at both the adductor pollicis and laryngeal adductor muscles. Rapacuronium has a rapid onset compared with other nondepolarizing muscle relaxants because of a more rapid equilibration between plasma concentrations and effect sites. Laryngeal muscles did not appear to be resistant to rapacuronoium. Rapacuronium appears to be very useful for the facilitation of tracheal intubation.

Influence of Renal Failure on the Pharmacokinetics and Neuromuscular Effects of a Single Dose of Rapacuronium Bromide
Szenohradszky J, Caldwell JE, Wright PMC, et al (Univ of California, San Francisco; Univ of Newcastle-upon-Tyne, England)
Anesthesiology 90:24-35, 1999   6–3

Background.—Rapacuronium is a newer nondepolarizing muscle relaxant, with a rapid onset and offset. Because renal function influences muscle relaxant clearance, new muscle relaxants must be tested in patients with renal failure. Rapacuronium was administered to patients with renal failure and to healthy control subjects to examine its pharmacokinetics in these 2 populations.

Healthy Volunteers

Patients with Renal Failure

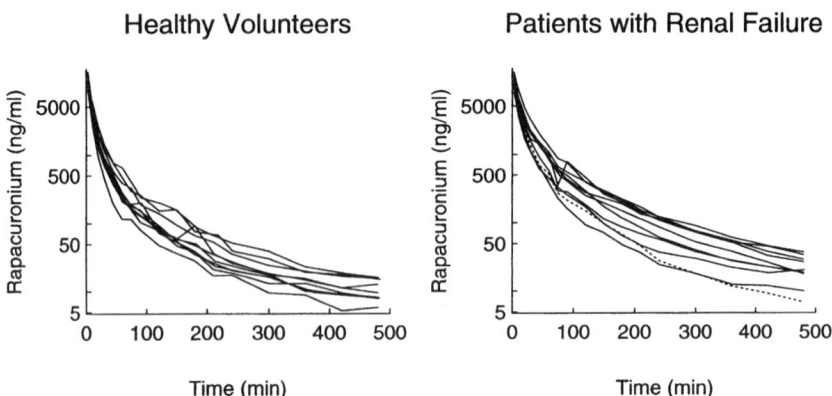

FIGURE 1.—Values for the plasma concentrations of rapacuronium after administration of 1.5 mg/kg rapacuronium are shown for 10 healthy volunteers (**left**) and 10 patients with renal failure (**right**). Values for the patient who received phenytoin before anesthesia are shown with a *dashed line*. (Courtesy of Szenohradszky J, Caldwell JE, Wright PMC, et al: Influence of renal failure on the pharmacokinetics and neuromuscular effects of a single dose of rapacuronium bromide. *Anesthesiology* 90:24-35, 1999. Copyright American Society of Anesthesiologists, Inc. Used with permission of Lippincott-Raven Publishers.)

Study Design.—Ten healthy volunteers and 10 patients with chronic renal failure were studied. Volunteers underwent anesthesia without surgery, whereas patients with renal failure had nontransplant surgical procedures, to eliminate the possibility that a transplanted kidney might confound the analysis. All study subjects were anesthetized with propofol, and the stable mechanical twitch response of the adductor pollicis muscle was recorded. Rapacuronium was administered and the twitch response was again recorded until T1 recovered completely. Venous blood was sampled in all participants, and urine was sampled in the healthy volunteers. Population approach, mixed-effects modeling (NONMEM) was used to determine the pharmacokinetics of rapacuronium and its primary metabolite, ORG9488. The magnitude of the maximal twitch depression, time from administration to maximal twitch depression, and time until recovery of T1 were determined for all study participants and compared between patients and healthy volunteers.

Results.—Twitch depression 1 minute after rapacuronium administration was less in patients with renal failure than in healthy volunteers. The times to maximal twitch depression and to twitch recovery were similar for patients and healthy volunteers. Clearance of rapacuronium was 32% less in the patients (Fig 1). The steady-state distribution volume was 14% less in women versus men and 16% less in patients versus healthy volunteers. For the rapacuronium metabolite, ORG9488, clearance was decreased by 85% in patients.

Conclusion.—Onset and offset of the nonpolarizing muscle relaxant rapacuronium are similar in healthy volunteers and in patients with renal failure. Although plasma concentrations of rapacuronium are initially similar between these 2 groups, plasma concentrations of rapacuronium decrease more slowly and plasma concentrations of its metabolite,

ORG9488, decrease minimally in patients with renal failure. Although the time course of a single rapacuronium dose is not strongly affected by renal failure, recovery from repeated doses may be affected by reduced clearance in these patients.

▶ Rapacuronium (Abstracts 6–2 and 6–3) may well be the new muscle relaxant of the year 2000, and all anesthesiologists will wish to use it to see whether it measures up to the gold standard, succinylcholine. If it is successful, other new muscle relaxants will disappear from clinical practice, and have enjoyed a very short life.

M. Wood, MD

Molar Potency Is Predictive of the Speed of Onset of Neuromuscular Block for Agents of Intermediate, Short, and Ultrashort Duration

Kopman AF, Klewicka MM, Kopman DJ, et al (New York Med College; St Vincent's Hosp, New York; Columbia Univ, New York)
Anesthesiology 90:425-431, 1999   6–4

Background.—In 1988, Bowman et al reported that fast onset and brief duration may be achieved only with muscle relaxants of low potency. This relationship has been confirmed for long-acting neuromuscular blockers but has not been confirmed for nondepolarizing muscle relaxants of shorter duration. The time to peak efficiency was assessed for rocuronium, vecuronium, cisatracurium, mivacurium, and succinlycholine to examine the correlation between molar potency and onset time.

Study Design.—Participants were 99 healthy adult patients who were undergoing elective surgical procedures. Anesthesia was induced with alfentanil plus propofol. Tracheal intubation was accomplished without muscle relaxants. Anesthesia was maintained with nitrous oxide and desflurane plus narcotics, as necessary. The evoked electromyographic response to single stimuli was continuously recorded. Drug doses were selected to produce about 95% twitch depression. The time to 50% to 90% of peak effect was plotted as a function of dose administered to the patient for each muscle relaxant.

Findings.—There was no difference in onset profiles of mivacurium and vecuronium. There was no difference in the time to 50% of peak effect between succinylcholine and rocuronium. For all other parameters, onset times were succinlycholine < rocuronium < vecuronium-mivacurium < cisatracurium. When the log of the ED_{95} in micromoles per kilogram for all 5 drugs was plotted against the log of onset time to 50% peak effect, the R^2 values for the best fit line was greater than 0.98.

Conclusions.—For rocuronium, vecuronium, cisatracurium, mivacurium, and succinylcholine, the speed of onset to 50% to 90% of maximal effect was a function of molar potency. The inverse correlation between molar potency and speed of onset previously described for long-duration muscle relaxants also appears to apply to nondepolarizing agents of shorter duration.

▶ This is a very nice study demonstrating clinically that Bill Bowman was correct in stating that fast onset and brief duration are related to low potency for muscle relaxants.

M. Wood, MD

Remifentanil and Other Opioids

Remifentanil's Effect Is Not Prolonged in a Patient With Pseudocholinesterase Deficiency
Manullang J, Egan TD (Univ of Utah, Salt Lake City)
Anesth Analg 89:529-530, 1999   6–5

Background.—Remifentanil, a new synthetic opioid, provides rapid onset of analgesia with an ultrashort duration of action that is apparently not affected by pseudocholinesterase deficiency in vitro. However, this has not been demonstrated in vivo. The current study reports a patient with a previously undiagnosed pseudocholinesterase deficiency who needed prolonged mechanical ventilation after succinylcholine administration but who had no prolongation of remifentanil's effects.

Case Report.—Woman, 23, had undergone an oculoplastic procedure under general anesthesia after trauma to the eye 1 year earlier. She was otherwise healthy. The patient's anesthetic included a succinylcholine bolus injection and a remifentanil infusion. An enzyme deficiency was suspected after a single succinylcholine dose produced prolonged neuromuscular blockade, which necessitated mechanical ventilation after surgery. Subsequently, the patient's mother recalled a similar anesthetic experience when the patient was a child. Laboratory testing verified an atypical pseudocholinesterase phenotype diagnostic of a genotype homozygous for pseudocholinesterase deficiency (Table 1). Within a few minutes of discontinuation of remifentanil in the recovery room, the patient

TABLE 1.—Postoperative Laboratory Testing Results

Laboratory Test	Patient Results	Normal Values
Pseudocholinesterase level (U/L)	1,088	52,000–12,800
Dibucaine number	16	>75
Estimated phenotype	SS	UU

Abbreviations: SS, Homozygous for pseudocholinesterase deficiency, *UU,* normal.
(Courtesy of Manullang J, Egan TD: Remifentanil's effect is not prolonged in a patient with pseudocholinesterase deficiency. *Anesth Analg* 89[2]:529-530, 1999.)

recovered completely from its sedative and respiratory depressant effects.

Conclusions.—The current report suggests that patients with pseudocholinesterase deficiency have a normal response to remifentanil. This is consistent with in vitro data demonstrating that remifentanil metabolism is not related to pseudocholinesterase activity.

▶ This very nice case report demonstrates that the effects of succinylcholine (and mivacurium) will be prolonged in a patient with deficient pseudocholinesterase but that the effects of remifentanil will not. Thus, the metabolism of remifentanil is unrelated to pseudocholinesterase activity; rather, nonspecific red cell esterases are involved in its rapid metabolism and short duration of effect.

M. Wood, MD

Determination of the Potency of Remifentanil Compared With Alfentanil Using Ventilatory Depression as the Measure of Opioid Effect
Glass PSA, Iselin-Chaves IA, Goodman D, et al (Duke Univ, Durham, NC; Glaxo Inc, Durham, NC)
Anesthesiology 90:1556-1563, 1999   6–6

Background.—Remifentanil, a new opioid, has properties similar to those of other μ-specific agonists. The potency of this agent was compared with that of alfentanil.

Methods.—Thirty healthy young men were enrolled in a double-blind study. Remifentanil or alfentanil was given intravenously for 180 minutes, with the use of a computer-assisted continuous infusion device. Ventilation depression was assessed by the minute ventilatory response to 7.5% carbon dioxide given by a "bag in the box" system. The target concentration of the study drug was adjusted to maintain 40% to 70% depression of baseline minute ventilation.

Findings.—Data on 28 volunteers were sufficient for modeling median effective concentration (EC_{50}) values. The EC_{50} for depression of minute ventilation with remifentanil was 1.17 ng/mL. For alfentanil, the EC_{50} was 49.4 ng/mL.

Conclusions.—When whole-blood concentrations are compared, remifentanil is about 40 times more potent than alfentanil. Because alfentanil is typically measured as a plasma concentration, remifentanil is about 70 times more potent than alfentanil when remifentanil whole-blood concentration is compared with alfentanil plasma concentration.

▶ It is very important to know exactly how potent remifentanil is as a respiratory depressant. The answer is that it is very potent, given that alfentanil is also quite potent compared with other opioids. Remifentanil is approximately 40 times more potent than alfentanil on the basis of blood concentration. However, it is also important to recognize that the range was 26 to 65 or, more exactly, that the 95% CI was 26 to 65, indicating large interindividual variability. There is very little margin between respiratory depression and analgesic effect; thus, to some extent, measuring respiratory depression does give some indication of opioid potency as well.

M. Wood, MD

Metabolism of Remifentanil During Liver Transplantation
Navapurkar VU, Archer S, Gupta SK, et al (Addenbrooke's Hosp, Cambridge, England; Glaxo Wellcome, Triangle Park, NC)
Br J Anaesth 81:881-886, 1998   6–7

Objective.—Remifentanil, with its ester linkage, has an ultrashort duration of action and its elimination is independent of hepatic and renal function. Orthotopic liver transplantation (OLT) provides an opportunity to determine whether a drug is metabolized in other organs. The pharmacokinetic profiles of remifentanil were compared after a single bolus infusion dose during the dissection and anhepatic phases of liver transplantation to investigate extrahepatic metabolism and to determine whether the drug is metabolized or sequestered in the lungs in an open-label, single-dose study.

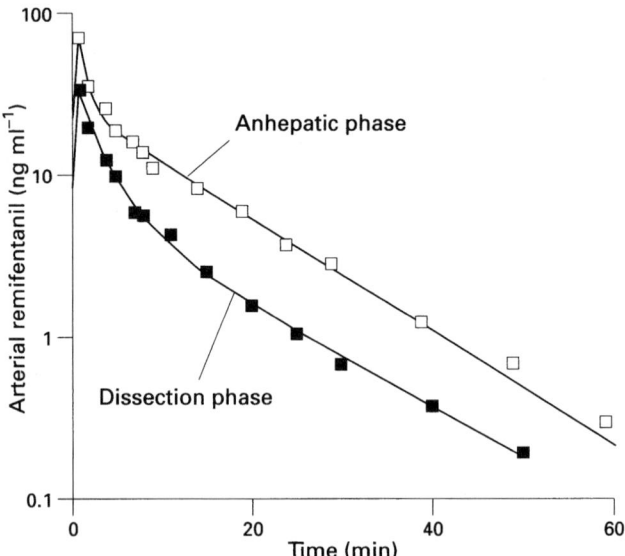

FIGURE 1.—Arterial blood concentration-time profile of remifentanil for patient 1 during the hepatic and anhepatic phases. The symbols are actual data, and the *solid line* is the predicted line. (Courtesy of Navapurkar VU, Archer S, Gupta SK, et al: Metabolism of remifentanil during liver transplantation. *Br J Anaesth* 81:881-886, 1998, by permission of Oxford University Press.)

Methods.—OLT was performed in 6 patients given a single bolus infusion of remifentanil 10 μg/kg per minute at the beginning of the dissection and anhepatic phases of OLT. Arterial concentrations of remifentanil and its metabolite GR90291 were determined over time.

Results.—Blood remifentanil clearance followed the 2-compartment model (Fig 1). Remifentanil clearance was significantly greater in the dissection phase than in the anhepatic phase (79.54 vs 39.57 ml/min per kilogram). Average maximum arterial concentrations of GR90291 were significantly lower in the dissection phase than in the anhepatic phase. The remifentanil area under the curve for the anhepatic phase was twice the size of the average area under the curve for the dissection phase. Patients required significantly more fluids during the dissection phase.

Conclusion.—Remifentanil is metabolized outside the liver. Its distribution and elimination half-life in healthy volunteers are similar to those of patients undergoing OLT.

▶ Pharmacokinetic studies during transplantation are extremely difficult to perform because of blood loss, fluid replacement, hemodynamic changes, and so on, and yet the anhepatic phase of liver transplantation provides a rare opportunity to study in vivo hepatic metabolism in human patients. This is, therefore, not a perfect study, but extrahepatic metabolism of remifentanil appears to occur, in keeping with its ester hydrolysis by blood and tissue esterases.

M. Wood, MD

The Effect of Fentanyl on Sevoflurane Requirements for Somatic and Sympathetic Responses to Surgical Incision
Katoh T, Kobayashi S, Suzuki A, et al (Hamamatsu Univ, Japan)
Anesthesiology 90:398-405, 1999   6–8

Introduction.—In a previous report, authors of this study found that fentanyl reduced requirements for sevoflurane for loss of consciousness and surgical incision. Fentanyl led to a reduction in the minimum alveolar concentration (MAC) of isoflurane and desflurane required to block adrenergic response (BAR) to surgical incision in 50% of patients (MAC-BAR). In this study of patients scheduled for elective surgery, investigators sought to determine the MAC and MAC-BAR reduction of sevoflurane by fentanyl with and without nitrous oxide (N_2O).

Methods.—The 226 patients included in the study were 20 to 50 years of age. All were classified as American Society of Anesthesiologists physical status 1 and were to undergo surgery on the abdomen, extremities, or body surface. Initial randomization was to a sevoflurane group (n = 96) or a sevoflurane/N_2O group (n = 86). Each group was further allocated to 1 of 5 fentanyl concentration subgroups. Those in the sevoflurane group were anesthetized with sevoflurane and fentanyl; patients in the sevoflurane/N_2O group received sevoflurane, fentanyl, and N_2O (66 vol%). Blood samples were obtained 5 minutes before and within 30 seconds after incision to measure the concentration of fentanyl in plasma. Somatic and sympathetic responses to incision were noted for MAC and MAC-BAR assessment at predetermined concentrations of sevoflurane.

Results.—Findings in 91 patients were analyzed. Postincision concentrations of fentanyl, which were used in the statistical analyses, ranged from 0 to 9.66 ng/mL. There was a marked reduction in MAC with increasing concentrations. Thus, the reduction of MAC was approximately 37% and 61% at fentanyl concentrations of 1 and 3 ng/mL, respectively. A concentration of 6 ng/mL produced only a 13% further reduction in MAC. The 3 ng/mL concentration of fentanyl resulted in an 83% reduction in MAC-BAR. Both the MAC and the MAC-BAR of sevoflurane, in the presence of 66 vol% N_2, were reduced with greater concentrations of fentanyl.

Conclusion.—Similar decreases in MAC and MAC-BAR occurred with increasing concentrations of fentanyl in plasma. An initial steep reduction was followed by a ceiling effect. There were similar decreases in the presence of N_2O, but no ceiling effect was observed. Even without sevoflurane, the combination of N_2O and fentanyl suppressed somatic and sympathetic response after skin incision.

▶ Fentanyl reduces the dose of isoflurane and desflurane needed to block the adrenergic response to surgical incision in 50% of patients—termed MAC-BAR. This well-performed study shows that the above holds true for sevoflurane. Are increases in arterial blood pressure and heart rate in response to surgical incision an indication of "light anesthesia" or of inadequate anesthesia? Not necessarily, and there may not be a good correlation between MAC-BAR and MAC (ie, there may be no MAC-BAR response and yet a somatic response may occur). However, the take-home message from this article is that low fentanyl concentrations, (ie, 3 µg/mL) reduced MAC-BAR and that giving even more fentanyl did little to further reduce MAC and MAC-BAR. Hence, fentanyl does reduce sevoflurane requirements for the somatic and sympathetic response to surgical incision, but if it does not work, increasing the amount of fentanyl may be ineffective.

M. Wood, MD

Morphine-Sparing Effect of Acetaminophen in Pediatric Day-Case Surgery
Korpela R, Korvenoja P, Meretoja OA (Univ of Helsinki, Finland)
Anesthesiology 91:442-447, 1999   6–9

Introduction.—Children who undergo day-case surgery are sometimes undertreated for surgical pain. Acetaminophen is often used as an adjuvant for postoperative analgesia to reduce the need for opioids. A randomized study was conducted to examine the efficacy of different doses of rectal acetaminophen in children scheduled for day-case surgery.

Methods.—Forty-two boys and 78 girls, aged 1 to 7 years, were included in the study. All were classified as American Society of Anesthesiologists physical status 1. Herniorrhaphy was the most frequently performed procedure (71 cases). In a double-blinded design, children were allocated after the induction of anesthesia to receive suppositories containing 0, 20, 40, or 60 mg/kg acetaminophen. Opioids or local anesthetics were not used. Investigators who were unaware of the dose of acetaminophen followed up each child for 2 hours in the postanesthesia care unit (PACU). Pain was evaluated by observers who used behavioral assessment and physiologic measurements. At the discretion of the nursing staff, rescue pain medication consisting of IV morphine (0.1 mg/kg) was administered in the PACU. Parents were telephoned 24 hours after the child's discharge to determine the incidence of pain, nausea, and vomiting. Rescue analgesia at home consisted of rectal ibuprofen (10 mg/kg).

Results.—The administration of acetaminophen provided a clear dose-dependent morphine-sparing effect. Only 23% of the patients who received 60 mg/kg acetaminophen required morphine; only those treated with placebo or 20 mg/kg acetaminophen experienced severe pain. Eighty percent of the children in the placebo group experienced pain at home, and 33% had postoperative nausea and vomiting. In contrast, 17% to 20% of the children in the high-dose acetaminophen groups had pain at home, and 0% to 3% had nausea and vomiting.

Conclusion.—A single dose of 40 or 60 mg/kg of acetaminophen, when administered at the induction of anesthesia, had a clear morphine-sparing effect in children undergoing day-case surgery. Rescue morphine, required more often by children in the placebo and 20-mg/kg acetaminophen groups, was associated with postoperative nausea and vomiting.

▶ This is a very nicely conducted clinical study. Simple measures used carefully throughout and carried through may be of immense benefit in treatment of postoperative pain. The study also highlights that morphine is associated with postoperative nausea and vomiting and that reducing the dose of morphine may reduce the incidence of these effects.

M. Wood, MD

Gender Differences and Anesthetic Pharmacology

Sex Differences in Morphine-Induced Ventilatory Depression Reside Within the Peripheral Chemoreflex Loop

Sarton E, Teppema L, Dahan A (Leiden Univ, The Netherlands)
Anesthesiology 90:1329-1338, 1999   6–10

Introduction.—In a previous report, the authors of this study found that, compared with morphine in men, morphine in women caused significantly more depression of both the steady-state response to carbon dioxide and the semi-steady-state or peak ventilatory response to acute hypoxia. The present study used a mathematical model of the ventilatory

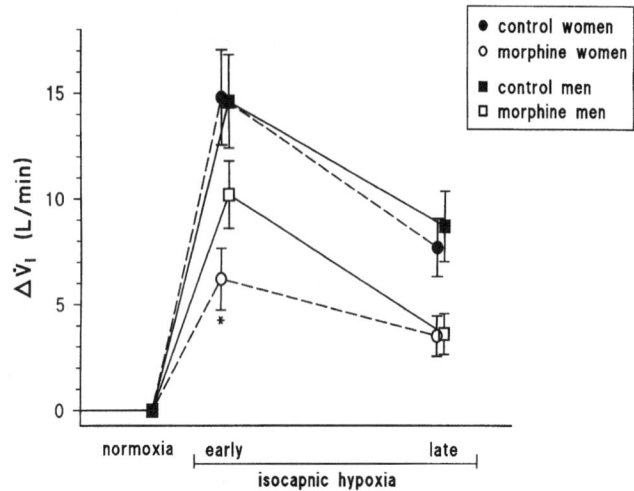

FIGURE 5.—The influence of morphine on the ventilatory response to sustained isocapnic hypoxia in men and women. Change in inspired minute ventilation (V_I) is the increase in V_I above normoxic V_I. After morphine, ventilatory responses to acute hypoxia but not to sustained hypoxia differed between men and women. Women versus men: *P < .01. (Courtesy of Sarton E, Teppema L, Dahan A: Sex differences in morphine-induced ventilatory depression reside within the peripheral chemoreflex loop. *Anesthesiology* 90:1329-1338, 1999. Copyright American Society of Anesthesiologists, Inc. Used with permission of Lippincott-Raven Publishers.)

controller to gain information regarding the sites of the sex-related ventilatory effects of morphine within the ventilatory control system.

Methods.—Experiments were performed in healthy young volunteers (9 men and 7 women). Control (carbon dioxide and hypoxic) studies preceded the morphine studies. Before and during the infusion of morphine, dynamic ventilatory responses to square-wave changes in end-tidal carbon dioxide tension (7.5-15 mm Hg) and step decreases in end-tidal oxygen tension (step from 110 to 50 mm Hg; duration of hypoxia, 15 minutes) were obtained. Morphine was administered as an IV bolus dose of 100 μg/kg, followed by 30 μg/kg per hour. Hypercapnic responses were separated into fast peripheral and slow central components, yielding central (G_c) and peripheral (G_p) carbon dioxide sensitivities.

Results.—Three women were observed in the follicular phase and 4 in the luteal phase of their menstrual cycles, but the influence of menstrual cycle was not studied. In carbon dioxide studies in men, morphine reduced G_c from a mean of 1.61 to a mean of 0.12 L/min per mm Hg^{-1}; G_p was not affected. Carbon dioxide studies in women showed that morphine reduced G_c from a mean of 1.51 to a mean of 1.17 L/min and G_p from a mean of 0.54 to a mean of 0.39 L/min per mm Hg. Men and women exhibited equivalent morphine-induced changes in G_c, but changes in G_p were greater in women. Whereas morphine depressed the hyperventilatory response at the initiation of hypoxia more in women than in men, the ventilatory response to sustained hypoxia did not differ between the sexes

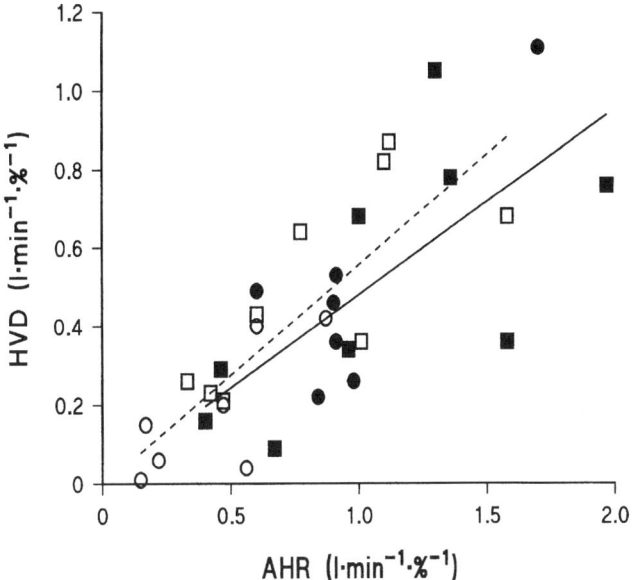

FIGURE 6.—The hypoxic ventilatory decrease against the acute hypoxic response in men (*squares*) and women (*circles*). *Closed symbols*, Control studies; *open symbols*, morphine studies. Linear regression was performed on the control data (*solid line*) and on the morphine data (*broken line*). For the regression analysis, the data of men and women were pooled. *Abbreviations: HVD*, hypoxic ventilatory decline; *AHR*, acute hypoxic response. (Courtesy of Sarton E, Teppema L, Dahan A: Sex differences in morphine-induced ventilatory depression reside within the peripheral chemoreflex loop. *Anesthesiology* 90:1329-1338, 1999. Copyright American Society of Anesthesiologists, Inc. Used with permission of Lippincott-Raven Publishers.)

(Fig 5). Individuals with large acute hypoxic responses had a larger magnitude of hypoxic ventilatory decline and vice versa (Fig 6).

Conclusion.—Sex differences exist in the morphine-induced depression of responses mediated via the peripheral chemoreflex pathway, with women showing more depression. Responses mediated via the central chemoreflex pathway did not differ according to sex. In neither men nor women did morphine alter the translation of the initial hyperventilatory response to short-term hypoxia into the secondary decrease in inspired minute ventilation caused by sustained hypoxia.

Women Emerge From General Anesthesia With Propofol/Alfentanil/Nitrous Oxide Faster Than Men
Gan TJ, Glass PS, Sigl J, et al (Duke Univ, Durham, NC; Aspect Med Systems, Natick, Mass; Emory Univ, Atlanta, Ga; et al)
Anesthesiology 90:1283-1287, 1999   6–11

Background.—Recovery from general anesthesia is dependent on both drug sensitivity and drug disposition. Gender has not been reported to be a factor in the speed of recovery from general anesthesia. As part of a

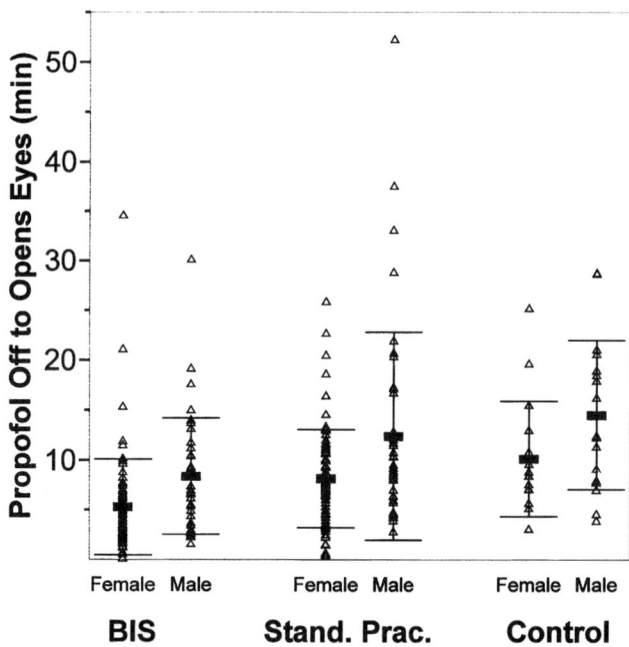

FIGURE 1.—The time in minutes (raw data and mean ± SD) to eye opening after discontinuation of propofol administration in bispectral index (*BIS*), standard practice, and control groups. Gender and randomization group are both independent predictors of time to eye opening (both *P* < .01). There was no statistically significant difference in the prerecovery BIS between gender within each group. (Courtesy Gan TJ, Glass PS, Sigl J, et al: Women emerge from general anesthesia with propofol/alfentanil/nitrous oxide faster than men. *Anesthesiology* 90:1283-1287, 1999. Copyright American Society of Anesthesiologists, Inc. Used with permission of Lippincott-Raven Publishers.)

multicenter study designed for a different purpose, a large, unexpected difference was noted in the recovery time from general anesthesia of men and women.

Study Design.—Participants were 96 men and 178 women scheduled for procedures at 4 institutions involving general anesthesia that would last at least 1 hour. All participants were premedicated with midazolam and received induction with propofol and alfentanil. After loss of consciousness, patients were infused with propofol, alfentanil, and nitrous oxide. The study was designed to test the hypothesis that use of the bispectral index (BIS) would improve titration of hypnotic drugs. Patient consciousness level was monitored with the BIS. Time from discontinuation of anesthesia to eye opening and response to verbal command was evaluated for all patients. When it became apparent that there was a gender difference in average recovery time, an *a posteriori* analysis of this gender effect was performed.

Results.—The use of BIS improved the titration of hypnotic drugs and improved recovery time. Gender was an independnet predictive factor for recovery time. Women woke significantly faster than men (Fig 1). Only 5%

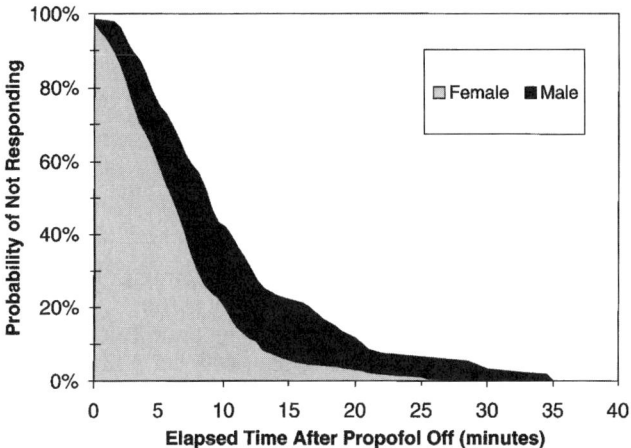

FIGURE 2.—Comparison of cumulative probability of patients remaining unconscious after discontinuation of propofol anesthesia in men and women patients (women = *light hatched area*, men = *solid dark area*). Cumulative probability was determined using Kaplan-Meier survival analysis. Log-rank differences between 2 groups were highly significant. (Courtesy Gan TJ, Glass PS, Sigl J, et al: Women emerge from general anesthesia with propofol/alfentanil/nitrous oxide faster than men. *Anesthesiology* 90:1283-1287, 1999. Copyright American Society of Anesthesiologists, Inc. Used with permission of Lippincott-Raven Publishers.)

of female patients had especially long recovery times compared with more than 20% of male patients (Fig 2).

Conclusion.—This is the first study to report that women recover faster from general anesthesia than do men. A combination of pharmacodynamic and pharmacokinetic factors appear to be involved. Studies of the effects of anesthesia and recovery from anesthesia should be designed to incorporate gender differences. More studies are required to investigate the mechanism of this gender difference and determine its generalizability.

Sevoflurane-Induced Reduction of Hypoxic Drive Is Sex-Independent

Sarton E, van der Wal M, Nieuwenhuijs D, et al (Leiden Univ, The Netherlands; Imperial College School of Medicine, London)
Anesthesiology 90:1288-1293, 1999 6–12

Background.—These authors have previously shown that the μ-opioid receptor agonist, morphine, has a different effect on respiratory depression in men versus women. It is not known whether this gender difference is specific to morphine or also applies to other anesthetic agents. The effect of the volatile anesthetic sevoflurane on the ventilatory response to iso-capnic hypoxic pulses in male versus female volunteers was compared.

Methods.—The study group consisted of 10 healthy male and 10 healthy female adult volunteers. Resting end-tidal carbon dioxide tension (PET_{CO_2}) levels were measured, then PET_{CO_2} was increased by about 4 mm Hg. A series of hypoxic pulses was repeated without sevoflurane (control) and one with inhaled 0.25% end-tidal sevoflurane. These 2 studies were performed in a randomized order and there was a 20-minute rest period between them. The average values of the last 10 breaths before hypoxia was induced and at the end of the 3 minutes of hypoxia were compared with calculated hypoxic ventilatory sensitivity.

Results.—Hypoxic arterial hemoglobin oxygen saturation demonstrated a significant effect of gender. Sevoflurane significantly reduced both the bispectral index (BIS) and the hypoxic ventilatory sensitivity in men and women to an equal extent.

Conclusions.—Inhalation of a subanesthetic amount of sevoflurane produced identical BIS values, reduced hypoxic ventilatory sensitivity, and produced lower hypoxic saturation in both men and women. These findings are in contrast to the sex differences observed with morphine anesthesia.

▶ It is increasingly being recognized that there are gender differences in the pharmacologic effects of the opioids, especially in the postoperative period (Abstracts 6–10, 6–11, and 6–12). We now know that there are differences between men and women in the effect of morphine on ventilatory depression, and that women emerge from general anesthesia faster. Why should this be so? For all positive pharmacodynamic effects, it is important to exclude a pharmacokinetic effect, and that is why pharmacologists like to quote a change in end point normalized to plasma concentration. However, I believe that as journals of gender-specific medicine become popular, and studies funded by the National Institutes of Health must include men and women, we are going to see more and more differences in pharmacology between men and women. However, what is even more fascinating is that we do not know why!

M. Wood, MD

Propofol

Mechanisms of Bronchoprotection by Anesthetic Induction Agents: Propofol Versus Ketamine

Brown RH, Wagner EM (Johns Hopkins School of Public Health, Baltimore, Md)
Anesthesiology 90:822-828, 1999   6–13

Objective.—Propofol and ketamine can decrease the risk of bronchospasm during tracheal intubation in patients with severe asthma. To determine whether the drugs act on airway smooth muscle or have neural effects, the anesthetic agents were administered directly to the airways of sheep via the bronchial artery.

Methods.—A tracheostomy and a left thoracotomy were performed on 8 anesthetized, ventilated sheep. The esophageal and thoracic tracheal branches of the bronchoesophageal artery were ligated, and the bronchial branch was cannulated and perfused. Propofol, ketamine, and thiopental were infused in random order at rates of 0.06, 0.20, and 0.60 mL/min. Airway resistance R_{aw} was measured after 10 minutes by forced oscillation before and during constriction, and airway reactivity was calculated from R_{aw} before and after infusion of methacholine into the bronchial artery. After recovery, the infusion experiment was repeated at the next rate. Vagal nerves were stimulated simultaneously, causing bronchoconstriction and a decrease in heart rate. The concentration of anesthetic drug in bronchial circulation was determined, and the dose that caused a 50% decrease in baseline response was calculated.

Results.—Baseline systemic blood pressure and baseline airway resistance did not vary significantly during the experiment. Infusions of ketamine and propofol protected against bronchoconstriction induced by vagal nerve stimulation, reducing bronchoconstriction by 8% and 26%, respectively. Propofol and ketamine attenuated the effect of methacholine-induced bronchospasm. Propofol significantly decreased methacholine-induced bronchoconstriction at the highest concentration (43%).

Conclusion.—Propofol and ketamine exert bronchoprotective effects through neural mechanisms. Ketamine is more effective at preventing bronchoconstriction.

▶ Choice of an IV anesthetic induction agent in a patient with asthma is key. According to this study, propofol and ketamine protect against induced bronchoconstriction as compared with thiopental—the gold standard for an intravenous induction drug. We also now know that the most important mechanism for bronchoprotection is through neurally mediated mechanisms and not by direct effects. Do these agents have relaxant effects in their own right? And can they reverse bronchoconstriction? Inhalational agents probably can cause bronchodilation, but whether propofol and ketamine have this ability remains controversial.

M. Wood, MD

Antinauseants

Effects of Anticholinergics on Postoperative Vomiting, Recovery, and Hospital Stay in Children Undergoing Tonsillectomy With or Without Adenoidectomy

Chhibber AK, Lustik SJ, Thakur R, et al (Univ of Rochester, NY)
Anesthesiology 90:697-700, 1999   6–14

Objective.—The incidence of postoperative nausea is increased 2-fold in adults receiving glycopyrrolate rather than atropine sulfate. The effect of atropine and glycopyrrolate on postoperative emesis in children undergoing tonsillectomy, with or without adenoidectomy, was evaluated in a double-blind trial.

Methods.—After general inhalation anesthesia was induced with 70% nitrous oxide, 30% oxygen, and increasing concentrations of halothane, 93 children (42 girls) were randomly allocated to receive 15 µg/kg atropine or 10 µg/kg glycopyrrolate. After surgery, neuromuscular block was reversed with 60 µg/kg neostigmine and 10 µg/kg glycopyrrolate or 15 µg/kg

TABLE 2.—Measures of Recovery and Incidence of Vomiting

	Atropine Group (n = 43)	Glycopyrrolate Group (n = 47)
PACU stay (min)	25 ± 13	28 ± 13
ASC stay (min)	316 ± 108	335 ± 88
Admitted to hospital	1 (2%)	4 (9%)
Vomiting		
Hospital and/or home (in 24 h postop)	24 (56%)	38 (81%)*
Home only	2 (5%)	4 (9%)
Hospital	22 (51%)	34 (72%)

Note: Values are mean ± standard deviation.
*$P < .05$.
Abbreviations: PACU, Postanesthesia care unit; ASC, ambulatory surgical center.
(Courtesy of Chhibber AK, Lustik SJ, Thakur R, et al: Effects of anticholinergics on postoperative vomiting, recovery, and hospital stay in children undergoing tonsillectomy with or without adenoidectomy. Anesthesiology 90:697-700, 1999. Copyright American Society of Anesthesiologists, Inc. Used with permission of Lippincott-Raven Publishers.)

atropine. Heart rate was determined before and after drug administration. Incidence of emesis was recorded.

Results.—Ninety children completed the study. The atropine group had a significantly lower incidence of vomiting than the glycopyrrolate group (Table 2). Patients who vomited stayed significantly longer in the pastanesthesia care unit (31 vs 21 minutes) or in the ambulatory surgical center (384 vs 294 minutes) than patients who did not vomit. All patients who received postoperative narcotics vomited. Heart rate was unaffected by atropine or glycopyrrolate.

Conclusion.—Use of atropine rather than glycopyrrolate is associated with a lower incidence of postoperative vomiting.

▶ This is a fascinating study, not because atropine may be a better drug to use for reversal than glycopyrrolate but because of what it tells us about the importance of the central cholinergic nerve system in the etiology of postoperative nausea and vomiting. Glycopyrrolate does not have the ability to cross the blood-brain barrier because it is a quarternary compound.

M. Wood, MD

Supplemental Oxygen Reduces the Incidence of Postoperative Nausea and Vomiting

Greif R, Laciny S, Rapf B, et al (Univ of California–San Francisco; Donauspital-SMZO, Vienna; Apotheus Labs, Lubbock, Tex)
Anesthesiology 91:1246-1252, 1999   6–15

Introduction.—Even with the introduction of new antiemetic medications and short-acting opioids and anesthetics, the postoperative incidence of nausea and vomiting (PONV) persists in between 20% and 70% of patients. No reports have specifically examined the effect of inspired oxygen concentration on the incidence of postoperative gastrointestinal

TABLE 3.—Nausea and Vomiting Incidence and Severity
During the First 24 Postoperative Hours

		30% Oxygen	80% Oxygen	P*
0-6 h after surgery	PONV (number/%)	18/15.1	9/8	0.141
	Nausea (number/%)	18/15.1	9/8	0.077
	None/mild/severe	101/10/8	103/8/1	
	Vomiting (number/%)	2/1.7	0	0.169
	None/mild/moderate/severe	117/0/0/2	112/0/0/0	
6-24 h after surgery	PONV (number/%)	24/22.2	11/9.8	0.045†
	Nausea (number/%)	21/17.6	10/8.9	0.066
	None/mild/severe	98/12/9	102/3/7	
	Vomiting (number/%)	7/5.9	2/1.8	0.108
	None/mild/moderate/severe	112/1/4/2	110/1/0/1	
Entire 24-h period	PONV (number/%)	36/30.3	19/17	0.027†
	Nausea (number/%)	33/27.7	18/16	0.034†
	None/mild/severe	86/20/13	94/11/7	
	Vomiting (number/%)	7/5.9	2/1.8	0.108
	None/mild/moderate/severe	112/1/4/2	110/1/0/1	

*P value for *PONV* calculated by χ-square test; severity of nausea or vomiting calculated by Mann-Whitney test.
†Statistically significant differences between the 2 study groups.
(Courtesy of Greif R, Laciny S, Rapf B, et al: Supplemental oxygen reduces the incidence of postoperative nausea and vomiting. *Anesthesiology* 91:1246-1252, 1999. Copyright American Society of Anesthesiologists, Inc. Used with permission of Lippincott-Raven Publishers.)

complications. The effect of supplemental oxygen on the incidence of PONV was assessed in 231 patients undergoing elective colon or rectal resection.

Methods.—Patients underwent anesthesia induction with fentanyl and isoflurane. They were randomly assigned to receive during surgery and for the first 2 postoperative hours either 30% oxygen and balance nitrogen or 80% oxygen and balance nitrogen (119 and 112 patients, respectively). Nurses blinded to group assignment and oxygen consumption assessed the incidence of nausea and vomiting in the first 24 postoperative hours.

Results.—Factors known to affect nausea and vomiting were similar for the 2 groups. Both groups had perioperative and first postoperative morning oxygen saturation levels that were well within normal limits. Supplemental oxygen decreased the incidence of nausea or vomiting from 30% in patients who received 30% oxygen to 17% in patients who received 80% oxygen (Table 3).

Conclusion.—Supplemental oxygen diminished the incidence of PONV almost twofold after colorectal surgery. It is not known why this occured; perhaps subtle intestinal ischemia has a role. Because oxygen is inexpensive and essentially risk-free, supplemental oxygen may be an effective way to decrease PONV.

▶ This group of investigators has published 2 important articles describing some very interesting effects of supplemental oxygen that, I have to admit, surprised me. (See Abstract 1–7.) Why supplemental perioperative oxygen should reduce the incidence of PONV is unknown. The authors did study a control group that received 30% oxygen balance nitrogen using a mask, so it could not be attributed to a placebo effect.

M. Wood, MD

Antiemetic Prophylaxis Does Not Improve Outcomes After Outpatient Surgery When Compared to Symptomatic Treatment
Scuderi PE, James RL, Harris L, et al (Wake Forest Univ, Winston-Salem, NC)
Anesthesiology 90:360-371, 1999   6–16

Background.—Postoperative nausea and vomiting (PONV) are unpleasant but rarely harmful to the patient. Patient outcome for prophylactic antiemetic treatment was compared with that for symptomatic treatment of PONV in a group of surgical patients to determine whether prophylaxis results in better outcomes.

Methods.—A total of 575 surgical patients, aged 18 to 65 years, undergoing outpatient surgery requiring general anesthesia were enrolled in a double-blind, randomized, placebo-controlled study. The patients were stratified into 8 subgroups based on risk factors for PONV. Before surgery, patients were randomly assigned to receive either the antiemetic, ondansetron, or saline (placebo) with anesthesia. Patients were also randomly assigned to receive either placebo or treatment if PONV occurred after admission to the postanesthesia care unit (PACU). Additional treatment for PONV was at the discretion of the anesthesiologist. Nausea was evaluated every 30 minutes in the PACU. PONV and its treatment were also recorded. Questionnaires were used to rate patient satisfaction with PONV management.

Results.—There were no significant differences in time to discharge, rate of unanticipated admissions, or time to return to normal activity between the prophylaxis and treatment groups. Reported patient satisfaction was equivalent for these 2 groups. Female patients with a history of motion sickness or PONV who were undergoing highly emetogenic procedures reported higher levels of satisfaction with prophylaxis, but their overall level of satisfaction with the outpatient surgical experience was equivalent to that of other patients.

Conclusions.—Although PONV is unpleasant for patients, routine prophylaxis does not appear to confer any objective clinical benefit compared with treatment of PONV symptoms after outpatient surgery.

▶ When should we administer drugs prophylactically to reduce PONV, and when should we administer antiemetic drugs to treat the symptoms of PONV? PONV is unpleasant, and patients clearly do not like the misery that it entails, even if they come to no long-term harm. End points in clinical trials vary; therefore, we must ask why we treat PONV—to reduce patient discomfort or to move the patient more efficiently through the system? Depending on the answer to this question, the outcomes may differ. Some investigators question whether the number of episodes of vomiting is a valid end point, and argue that it is a surrogate for a true outcome (eg, unplanned hospital admission). Thus, many authors argue that prophylaxis is of little benefit. Finally, all drugs carry risks, and one also has to assess the side effects of antiemetic prophylaxis administration to someone with no symptoms.

M. Wood, MD

Oral Granisetron Prevents Postoperative Vomiting in Children
Fujii Y, Toyooka H, Tanaka H (Univ of Tsukuba, Tsukuba City, Japan; Toride Kyodo Gen Hosp, Toride City, Japan)
Br J Anaesth 81:390-392, 1998   6–17

Background.—Without prophylaxis, the incidence of vomiting after tonsillectomy in children is high. The efficacy of granisetron, a selective 5-hydroxytryptamine type 3 receptor antagonist, in preventing postoperative vomiting in this population was investigated.

Methods.—One hundred sixty children, aged 4 to 10 years, were enrolled in the randomized, double-blind, placebo-controlled study. All were ASA I. The children were given placebo or granisetron, 20, 40, or 80 µg/kg, by mouth 1 hour before surgery. A complete response was defined as no emesis and no need for another rescue antiemetic in the first 24 hours after anesthesia.

Findings.—Forty percent of the placebo recipients had a complete response, compared with 48%, 85%, and 90% of the patients given 20, 40, or 80 µg/kg, respectively. No clinically important adverse events occurred.

Conclusions.—Preoperative oral granisetron can effectively prevent vomiting in children after tonsillectomy. Doses of more than 40 µg/kg are required.

Prophylactic Oral Antiemetics for Preventing Postoperative Nausea and Vomiting: Granisetron Versus Domperidone
Fujii Y, Saitoh Y, Tanaka H, et al (Univ of Tsukuba, Tsukuba City, Japan; Toride Kyodo Gen Hosp, Toride City, Japan)
Anesth Analg 87:1404-1407, 1998   6–18

Background.—Preoperative oral granisetron has been shown to prevent postoperative nausea and vomiting (PONV) after gynecologic surgery. However, no one has compared the efficacy of this agent with that of another commonly used oral antiemetic in preventing PONV. The efficacies of granisetron and domperidone were compared in a prospective, randomized, double-blinded study.

Methods.—One hundred women undergoing major gynecologic surgery were enrolled. Half received granisetron, 2 mg, and half received domperidone, 20 mg. Complete response was defined as no PONV and no need for rescue antiemetic medication for up to 3 hours after anesthesia.

Findings.—Complete response occurred in 88% of the granisetron recipients and in 52% of the domperidone recipients. Between 3 and 24 hours after anesthesia, these values were 86% and 48%, respectively. None of the groups had any clinically important adverse events.

Conclusions.—Oral granisetron is more effective than domperidone in preventing PONV after major gynecologic surgery. With granisetron, 88% of the women were free of nausea and vomiting in the first 3 hours after surgery.

▶ I selected these two articles (Abstracts 6–17 and 6–18) to exemplify the fact that we are seeing more and more 5-hydropytryptamine type 3 (5-HT₃) antagonists on the market to treat or prevent PONV, and granisetron is yet another one of which anesthesiologists should be aware. It belongs to the ondansetron group, and the article by Fujii et al compared the drug with domperidone, which is not a 5-HT₃ antagonist but a dopamine antagonist related to the butyrophenones. In the second study from the same group, a placebo comparison group was studied, so it is not unexpected that prophylactic granisetron would be effective.

M. Wood, MD

Patient-Controlled Antiemesis: A Randomized, Double-Blind Comparison of Two Doses of Propofol Versus Placebo

Gan TJ, El-Molem H, Ray J, et al (Duke Univ, Durham, NC)
Anesthesiology 90:1564-1570, 1999   6–19

Background.—The role of propofol in the management of postoperative nausea and vomiting (PONV) is unclear. The efficacy of small doses of propofol administered by patient-controlled device in treating PONV was investigated.

Methods and Findings.—Sixty-nine patients with significant nausea or emesis within 1 hour of arrival in the recovery room after ambulatory surgery were assigned randomly to repeated doses of propofol, 20 mg (P-20); propofol, 40 mg (P-40); or placebo on demand. Mean nausea scores for the P-20 and P-40 groups were 25% and 29% less, respectively, than those for the placebo group score (Fig 1). Differences were evident 15 minutes after initiation of treatment. Fifty-six percent of placebo recipients vomited, compared with 12% in the P-20 group and 23% in the P-40 group. Seventy percent of the placebo group needed rescue antiemetics, compared with 17% and 23% in the P-20 and P-40 groups, respectively. The 3 groups had comparable sedation scores. Propofol recipients had briefer stays in the postanesthetic care unit and greater satisfaction with their control of PONV than placebo recipients. Two episodes of oversedation occurred in the P-40 group.

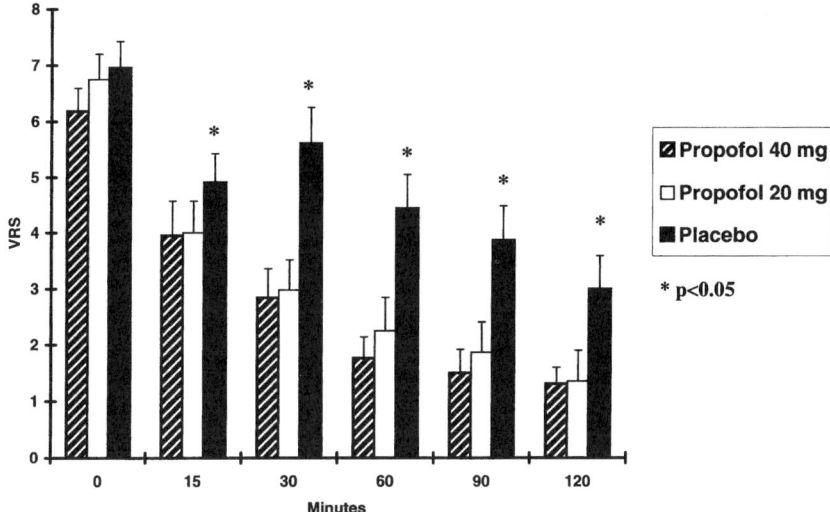

FIGURE 1.—Nausea scores versus time (mean ± SD). (Courtesy of Gan TJ, El-Molem H, Ray J, et al: Patient-controlled antiemesis: A randomized, double-blind comparison of two doses of propofol versus placebo. *Anesthesiology* 90:1564-1570, 1999. Copyright American Society of Anesthesiologists, Inc. Used with permission of Lippincott-Raven Publishing.)

Conclusions.—Propofol is effective in the management of PONV. A demand dose of 20 mg propofol appears to be more appropriate than the 40 mg dose, which may cause oversedation.

▶ It does appear that propofol is effective in managing PONV—a very important and interesting finding.

M. Wood, MD

Toxicity of Desflurane and Sevoflurane

Severe Carbon Monoxide Poisoning During Desflurane Anesthesia
Berry PD, Sessler DI, Larson MD (Univ of California, San Francisco)
Anesthesiology 90:613-616, 1999   6–20

Introduction.—Recent studies have shown that severe carbon monoxide (CO) toxicity can occur as a result of degradation of volatile anesthetics by desiccated carbon dioxide absorbents. In the anesthetized patient, the clinical features of intraoperative CO exposure may not be evident. The diagnosis in the case reported here was suggested by a combination of moderately decreased oxygen saturation by pulse oximetry (Sp_{O2}) and an erroneous gas analyzer reading.

Case Report.—Woman, 24, with American Society of Anesthesiologists physical status I, was anesthetized for a clinical research
study. As part of the same study, she had undergone an identical
general anesthestization 2 weeks earlier with no complications.

Both epidural and general anesthesia were administered during the study. An IV cannula was inserted, and 3 mL lidocaine 1.5% was infiltrated into the T10-T11 interspace. General anesthesia was induced with 180 mg IV propofol, followed by 10 mg IV vecuronium. The woman was then mask ventilated with desflurane in oxygen at a tidal volume near 15 mL/kg at approximately 12 breaths per minute for approximately 3 minutes. Intubation of the trachea was achieved without difficulty. Ten minutes after induction of anesthesia, the end-tidal gas analyzer indicated the presence of enflurane, followed after a few minutes by a "mixed agent." No enflurane vaporizer was attached to the anesthetic machine.

CO toxicity was then suspected, and the Baralyme was immediately replaced with fresh Baralyme. Fifteen minutes later an arterial blood sample showed oxygenated hemoglobin 63%, carboxyhemogloblin 36%, and methemoglobin 1%. The study protocol was then aborted, and the woman was ventilated with 100% oxygen. Twenty minutes after the Baralyme replacement, the anesthetic analyzer indicated an end-tidal desflurane concentration of 5% to 5.5%, consistent with the vaporizer setting. The Sp_{O2} had returned to the 99% preoperative reading. No abnormal sequelae were apparent after the woman emerged from anesthesia, and there had been no changes in motor control when she was interviewed 6 months after the incident.

Discussion.—The anesthetic machine in this case had not been used for several days and had probably been left switched on and connected to the oxygen pipeline. There is no routinely available method to reliably identify the presence of CO within the breathing circuit. Severe intraoperative CO exposure was suggested here by an unexpectedly low Sp_{O2} and an erroneous gas analyzer reading.

▶ This is a very important case report, highlighting a serious adverse effect of desflurane administration. All anesthesiologists should be aware of this important potential complication.

M. Wood, MD

Amsorb: A New Carbon Dioxide Absorbent for Use in Anesthetic Breathing Systems
Murray JM, Renfrew CW, Bedi A, et al (The Queen's Univ of Belfast, Northern Ireland)
Anesthesiology 91:1342-1348, 1999   6–21

Background.—A carbon dioxide absorbent for use in anesthesia, consisting of calcium hydroxide with calcium chloride, a compatible humectant, has been developed. This mixture, called Amsorb, does not contain sodium or potassium hydroxide but does have 2 setting agents—calcium sulfate and polyvinylpyrrolidine—to improve hardness and porosity. Testing of Amsorb was described.

Methods.—The new absorbent was subjected to standardized tests for hardness, porosity, and carbon dioxide absorption. It was also exposed in vitro to sevoflurane, desflurane, isoflurane, and enflurane to assess whether these anesthetics were degraded to either compound A or carbon monoxide. The performance data and the inertness of the absorbent were compared with 2 currently available brands of soda lime.

Findings.—Amsorb conformed to US Pharmacopeia specifications in its carbon dioxide absorption, granule hardness, and porosity. On exposure to sevoflurane 2% in oxygen at a flow rate of 1 L/min, compound A concentrations did not increase to above those of the parent drug. Mean concentrations of compound A were noted when both traditional brands of soda lime were used. After dehydration of the traditional soda limes, immediate exposure to desflurane 6%, enflurane 2%, and isoflurane 2% produced mean carbon monoxide concentrations of 600, 580, and 620 ppm, respectively. However, carbon monoxide concentrations were negligible when Amsorb was exposed to the same anesthetics.

Conclusions.—Amsorb is an effective carbon dioxide absorbent. It does not react chemically with sevoflurane, enflurane, isoflurane, or desflurane.

▶ It is becoming clear that carbon dioxide can be removed from our breathing circuits without the strong bases sodium or potassium hydroxide! This is great news because it means that there will be considerably less breakdown of sevoflurane. Dr Eger's fears of some terrible effect of compound A (not yet seen after many millions of cases), will fade further into the museum of "straw men."

J. H. Tinker, MD

Effects of Xenon on Hemodynamic Responses to Skin Incision in Humans
Nakata Y, Goto T, Morita S (Teikyo Univ, Chiba, Japan)
Anesthesiology 90:406-410, 1999   6–22

Introduction.—Concerns about the use of nitrous oxide (N_2O) have led to an increased interest in xenon anesthesia. Although previous studies suggest that the cardiovascular effects of xenon are minimal, the effects of surgical stimulation on the cardiovascular system during xenon anesthesia are not fully known. A randomized study evaluated the hemodynamic suppressive effects of xenon in combination with sevoflurane at skin incision in patients undergoing surgery.

Methods.—Forty adult patients took part in the study. All were classified as American Society of Anesthesiologists physical status 1 or 2 and were scheduled for elective lower abdominal surgery. Anesthesia was induced with single vital capacity inhalation of 5% sevoflurane; IV vecuronium was used to facilitate tracheal intubation. Patients were assigned to

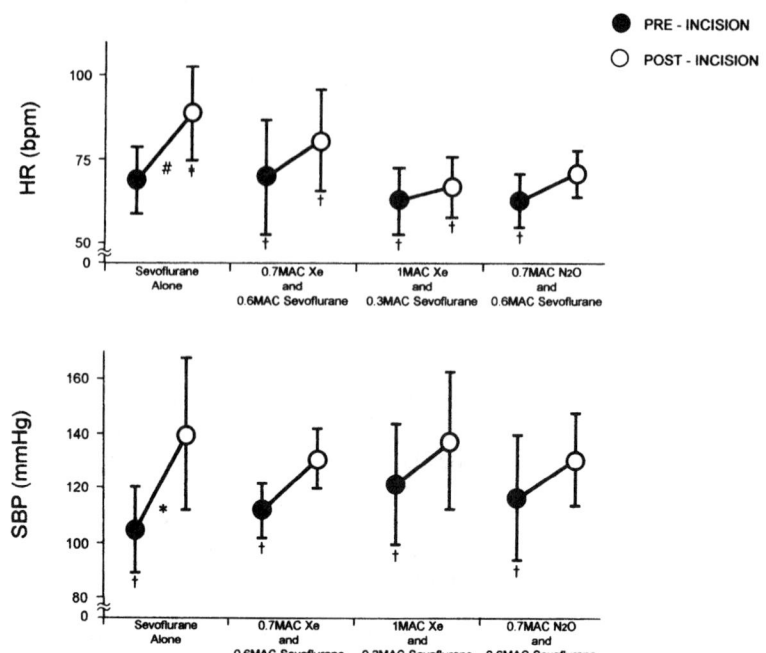

FIGURE 1.—Changes in heart rate (*upper*) and systolic blood pressure (*lower*) from before to after incision. Data are expressed as the mean ± SD. *Increase in SBP significantly higher than the 0.7 MAC xenon, 1 MAC xenon, and N₂O groups. †Significantly lower than the baseline within the group. ‡Significantly higher than the baseline within the group. #Increase in HR significantly higher than in the 1 MAC xenon and N₂O groups. *Abbreviations: MAC,* minimum alveolar concentration; *HR,* heart rate; *SBP,* systolic blood pressure. (Courtesy of Nakata Y, Goto T, Morita S: Effects of xenon on hemodynamic responses to skin incisions in humans. *Anesthesiology* 90:406-410, 1999. Copyright American Society of Anesthesiologists, Inc. Used with permission of Lippincott-Raven Publishers.)

1 of 4 groups: 1.3 minimum alveolar concentration (MAC) sevoflurane; 0.7 MAC xenon with 0.6 MAC sevoflurane; 1 MAC xenon with 0.3 MAC sevoflurane; or 0.7 MAC N₂O with 0.6 MAC sevoflurane. Patients were monitored by means of an electrocardiograph, a pulse oximeter, and a noninvasive blood pressure cuff.

Results.—Patients in the 4 groups were similar in gender, age, weight, and hemodynamic variables before the administration of inhaled anesthetics. Alterations in hemodynamic variables in response to incision were less with sevoflurane in combination with xenon and N₂O than with sevoflurane alone. Heart rate decreased significantly after anesthesia in the 0.7 and 1 MAC xenon groups and remained at that level even after skin incision. Whereas heart rate remained stable after anesthesia in the sevoflurane group, it increased significantly after incision. There was a significant decrease in heart rate after anesthesia and a return to baseline levels after incision in the N₂O groups. Increases in heart rate at incision were significantly greater in the sevoflurane groups than in the 1-MAC xenon and N₂O groups. Systolic blood pressure decreased after anesthesia and returned to the baseline level after skin incision in all 4 groups (Fig 1).

Conclusion.—Xenon and N$_2$O, when used with sevoflurane, can reduce hemodynamic responses to skin incision compared with sevoflurane alone. This effect may be attributed to a similarity of analgesic properties in xenon and N$_2$O, although the exact mechanism has not been determined.

▶ Is xenon an anesthetic? Is xenon an analgesic? Will xenon be of use clinically? Difficulty of use and cost militate against xenon's use in the near future, and it is important to recognize that IMAC xenon is 71%, so that hypoxia limits increased MAC administration. Xenon research may also yield information into the mechanisms of action of general anesthetics, especially N$_2$O, which would allow manufacturers to target drugs to the site of action and attenuate side effects of general anesthetics.

M. Wood, MD

Direct Cerebral Vasodilatory Effects of Sevoflurane and Isoflurane
Matta BF, Heath KJ, Tipping K, et al (Addenbrooke's Hosp, Cambridge, England)
Anesthesiology 91:677-680, 1999   6–23

Objective.—Although both desflurane and isoflurane produce more cerebral vasodilation than halothane, findings for sevoflurane are inconsistent. The intrinsic vasodilatory effect of 0.5 and 1.5 minimum alveolar concentration (MAC) sevoflurane and isoflurane were compared in humans.

Methods.—Twenty patients, aged 20 to 62 years, received propofol (2.5 mg/kg), fentanyl (2 µg/kg), and atracurium (0.5 mg/kg) and a propofol infusion before undergoing routine spinal surgery. Blood flow velocity in the middle cerebral artery was measured using transcranial Doppler US, and brain electrical activity was measured at the isoelectric point using electroencephalography at baseline and after 2 consecutive 15-minute periods of unchanged end-tidal concentrations between which sevoflurane or isoflurane concentrations were increased or decreased as appropriate.

Results.—Sevoflurane increased the blood flow velocity in the middle cerebral artery at 0.5 and 1.5 MAC significantly less than isoflurane.

Conclusion.—The dose-dependent cerebral vasodilatory effect of sevoflurane is significantly less than isoflurane.

▶ Sevoflurane is less a cerebral vasodilator than isoflurane. A useful piece of information? Is it good or bad with respect to whether you should choose sevoflurane? Does the vasodilation of isoflurane confer any protective effects? They are always talking about retractor pressure in neurology. Sevoflurane sounds better with respect to increased intracranial pressure, but what is best is not obvious.

J. H. Tinker, MD

The Elimination of Sodium and Potassium Hydroxides From Desiccated Soda Lime Diminishes Degradation of Desflurane to Carbon Monoxide and Sevoflurane to Compound A but Does Not Compromise Carbon Dioxide Absorption

Neumann MA, Laster MJ, Weiskopf RB, et al (Univ of California, San Francisco; Johann Wolfgang Goethe Univ, Frankfurt, Germany)
Anesth Analg 89:768-773, 1999   6–24

Objective.—Carbon dioxide (CO_2) absorbents degrade enflurane, isoflurane, and desflurane to carbon monoxide (CO) when water content is significantly decreased. Sevoflurane is degraded to nephrotoxic compound A. Whether the bases—calcium, sodium, potassium, and barium hydroxide—present in the absorbents differ in their capacity to degrade anesthetic gases to toxic substances was investigated.

Methods.—Eight samples of soda lime absorbents containing hydrated calcium hydroxide $Ca(OH)_2$ with varying amounts of different bases were supplied in 2 forms: one with a normal water content and one without water. Equal volumes of anesthesia gases were passed through each desiccated lime sample. Degradation products were collected and analyzed.

Results.—Moist absorbents did not produce significant amounts of CO. CO production in dry absorbents depended on the bases present, with absorbents high in potassium hydroxide (KOH) and sodium hydroxide (NaOH) producing the highest levels of CO. The lowest levels of CO were generated with lime containing only $Ca(OH)_2$, and CO production decreased with time. The amount of compound A generated when sevoflurane is passed through an absorbent increases slightly, but significantly, when KOH and NaOH are present. Removal of KOH and NaOH reduces CO production by a factor of 10 and reduces production of compound A by as much as 41%. The amount of breakthrough CO_2 increased slightly, but nonsignificantly, with $Ca(OH)_2$-only absorbents.

Conclusion.—Generation of CO and compound A is significantly decreased by absorbents that contain only $Ca(OH)_2$.

▶ I was taught that the bases, namely sodium, potassium chloride, or both, are essential in the absorption of CO_2, because they are needed as intermediaries to form the appropriate bicarbonates first. Next, they were considered to reform as bases, because they catalyzed the reaction to form the carbonates from the calcium or barium hydroxides. It was so neat. It is very effective at its task, namely CO_2 absorption. I tried to invent a type of absorber using various tertiary and quaternary amines similar to those used on submarines. I discovered that the thins would have to be about 3 feet in diameter to work as well as ours do today! I never thought of removal of the strongest bases! These folks may be on to something!

J. H. Tinker, MD

Effect of Dexmedetomidine on the Minimum Alveolar Concentration (MAC) of Sevoflurane in Adults Age 55 to 70 Years

Fragen RJ, Fitzgerald PC (Northwestern Univ, Chicago)
J Clin Anesth 11:466-470, 1999   6–25

Objective.—Animal studies have shown that the use of dexmedetomidine premedication decreases the amount of anesthetic required. The effect of 2 dexmedetomidine infusions on minimum alveolar concentration (MAC) of sevoflurane was determined in a prospective, randomized, placebo-controlled study in older adults.

Methods.—Either dexmedetomidine (0.3 or 0.6 ng/mL) or placebo was infused into 45 patients ASA physical status 1 and 2, undergoing elective surgery with at least a 3-inch incision. After 15 minutes, patients received sevoflurane and oxygen by face mask. Patients were intubated, and sevoflurane anesthesia was decreased to the target concentration and maintained for 15 minutes while infusion of dexmedetomidine or placebo was continued. Plasma concentrations of dexmedetomidine were determined at baseline and at time of incision.

Results.—Plasma concentrations of dexmedetomidine were 0 at baseline, 0 in the placebo group, and 0.39 and 0.70 ng/mL in the low-dose and high-dose dexmedetomidine groups. Sevoflurane MACs of the placebo and the low- and high-dose dexmedetomidine groups were 1.77%, 1.79%, and 1.46% by the Dixon and Mood method and 1.83%, 1.78%, and 1.51% by the logistic regression method.

Conclusion.—High-dose dexmedetomidine decreased the MAC of sevoflurane by 17% compared with placebo and low-dose dexmedetomidine.

▶ Dexmedetomidine ("dex") is a drug looking for a use. I cannot understand why I would want to lower the volatile agent requirement by substituting what is certain to be a more expensive drug. Such logic might go well on "I Love Lucy." The old and cherished idea that you could reduce the doses of drugs by giving several drugs is not likely to be true, because you add whatever risks there are with the new drug! I hope "dex" turns out to be worth something to us, but for now I cannot see what that would be.

J. H. Tinker, MD

7 Anesthesia Techniques and Monitors

Anesthesia for Intranasal Surgery: A Comparison Between Tracheal Intubation and the Flexible Reinforced Laryngeal Mask Airway
Webster AC, Morley-Forster PK, Janzen V, et al (Univ of Western Ontario, London)
Anesth Analg 88:421-425, 1999   7–1

Objective.—Prototype flexible reinforced laryngeal mask airways (LMAs), because they do not directly stimulate the larynx, reduce the respiratory and cardiovascular reflex responses to placement and removal. A study was undertaken to determine whether the use of the flexible reinforced LMA for anesthesia in intranasal surgery can reduce the incidence of airway complications without compromising airway protection as compared with tracheal intubation, and the incidence of complications of tracheal extubation was compared in awake and anesthetized patients.

Methods.—Outpatients undergoing endoscopic intranasal surgery or septoplasty were randomly allocated to size 4 flexible reinforced LMA with spontaneous breathing and removal while awake (group 1, n = 35), tracheal intubation with a right atrial enlargement preformed cuffed endotracheal tube with intermittent positive pressure ventilation and extubation while awake (group 2, n = 34); and tracheal intubation with spontaneous breathing and extubation while deeply anesthetized (group 3, n = 32). Incidence of coughing, sore throat, hoarseness, blood loss, and oxyhemoglobin desaturation at removal were recorded.

Results.—The incidence of laryngospasm was 0 in group 1, 6% in group 2, and 19% in group 3. The incidence of oxyhemoglobin desaturation was 0 in group 1, 26% in group 2, and 16% in group 3. The differences between group 1 and groups 2 and 3 were significant. The differences between groups 2 and 3 were not significant. The time between discontinuation of anesthesia and departure from the operating room was significantly less in group 1 than in group 2 and group 3 (10.74 vs 14.85 vs 12.16 min). Whereas all groups reported a high incidence of sore throat on the first postoperative day, the incidence of hoarseness was significantly lower in group 1 than in groups 2 and 3.

Conclusion.—The flexible reinforced LMA is safe and more effective than endotracheal anesthesia for use during intranasal surgery.

Recurrent Laryngeal Nerve Injury Caused by a Laryngeal Mask Airway
Lowinger D, Benjamin B, Gadd L (St Luke's Hosp, Sydney, Australia)
Anaesth Intensive Care 27:202-205, 1999   7–2

Objective.—There are reports of laryngeal nerve damage after use of the laryngeal mask airway (LMA). A rare case of permanent unilateral vocal cord paralysis that required thyroplasty for voice restoration is reported.

> *Case Report.*—Man, 44, employed as an announcer, underwent ligation of varicose veins. After anesthesia was induced, a size 4 LMA was inserted. The cuff inflated with about 20 mL of air, but cuff pressure was not monitored. After uneventful surgery, the LMA was removed. In the next 24 hours, the patient experienced dysphonia that progressed to aphonia with no pain by day 2. Although his left cord was immobile, no other neurologic abnormality was revealed. Left cord paralysis was diagnosed at 6 months without arytenoid cartilage dislocation or other glottic disorder. A trial injection of Gelfoam at 9 months restored good voice for a few weeks. At 12 months, thyroplasty was performed with a 4-mm hydroxyapatite prosthesis. The patient's voice improved, even though cord paralysis persisted.

Conclusion.—Whereas the LMA is generally safe and effective, in rare cases it can lead to persistent dysphonia, probably as a result of extensive local ischemia with demyelination and neural loss.

▶ I selected these articles (Abstracts 7–1 and 7–2) to highlight the fact that we are continually seeing new uses and modifications of the LMA. However, these devices are not entirely without risk.

M. Wood, MD

First Clinical Implications of Perioperative Red Cell Volume Measurement With a Nonradioactive Marker (Sodium Fluorescein)
Orth VH, Rehm M, Thiel M, et al (Ludwig-Maximilians-Universität, München, Germany)
Anesth Analg 87:1234-1238, 1998   7–3

Background.—The sodium fluorescein method of measuring red blood cell volume (RCV) has recently been improved by Haller and colleagues, who used flow cytometry to count cells and achieved a good reproducibility. The current study assessed the effects of different sampling and storage methods to improve the Haller technique for clinical use.

Methods.—RCV in 30 patients undergoing gynecologic surgery was measured by the SoF method. Sixteen patients underwent isovolemic hemodilution (IHD) before surgery. RCV was measured before and after IHD and at the end of surgery. To establish the validity of the simplified sodium fluorescein method, RCV in the IHD bags (bag RCV) was compared with the difference in RCV before and after preoperative IHD.

Findings.—Measures of bag RCV acquired during preoperative IHD using SoF had a 4.2% precision. Intraoperatively estimated and measured blood loss differed significantly. Blood loss tended to be underestimated. In some patients, blood loss was substantially underestimated or overestimated. Hematocrit values before and after surgery provided an imprecise estimation of RCV.

Conclusions.—Measurement RCV by means of sodium fluorescein is a precise technique for monitoring RCV changes during preoperative IHD and surgery. Large differences between intraoperatively estimated and measured blood loss were commonly noted. Preoperative hemotocrit values yielded an imprecise estimate of patients' RCV.

▶ At the present time, we assess RCV and blood loss on the basis of clinical condition and laboratory parameters such as hematocrit and hemoglobin levels. The decision to transfuse during the perioperative period is in reality based on clinical acumen. During fluctuating physiologic conditions, laboratory estimates can be misleading. A new test that has been recently introduced is one for RCV measurement that uses a nonradioactive marker, sodium fluorescein, instead of radioactive tracers, such as chromium-51 and technetium-99m. Repeated measurements using radioactive tracers are not possible because of long half-lives, whereas the sodium fluorescein test can be performed every hour. I thought it interesting to read also about two other studies describing a new noninvasive method of indocyanine green (ICG) pulse dye-densitometry that allows measurement of circulating blood volume.[1,2] ICG is rapidly distributed within the circulating central compartment and then is eliminated by the liver in about 20 minutes. Thus, it is possible to obtain information on circulating blood volume every 20 minutes and, as Steven Barker[3] suggests in his editorial, the "pulse method" may become the next intraoperative monitor. These two new systems are in the early stages of testing, but they may be very useful for fluid management during anesthesia and surgery. We will have to wait and see.

M. Wood, MD

References

1. Haruna M, Kumon N, Yahagi N, et al: Blood volume measurement at the bed-side using ICG pulse spectrophotometry. *Anesthesiology* 89:1322-1328, 1998.
2. Lijima T, Iwao Y, Sankawa H: Circulating blood volume measured by pulse dye-densitometry: Comparison with ^{131}I-HSA analysis. *Anesthesiology* 89:1329-1335, 1998.

3. Barker SJ: Blood volume measurement: The next intraoperative monitor? *Anesthesiology.* 89:1310-1312, 1998.

The Effect of Propofol on Oxidative Stress in Platelets From Surgical Patients

De La Cruz JP, Zanca A, Carmona JA, et al (Univ of Málaga, Spain; Hosp Costa del Sol, Málaga, Spain)
Anesth Analg 89:1050-1055, 1999   7–4

Objective.—Propofol's antioxidant properties have been shown to reduce plasma lipid peroxide formation in animal studies. In humans, the highest levels of peroxides occur in cell membranes. The effect of propofol anesthesia on components of oxidative stress in platelets was studied in surgical patients.

Methods.—Platelets were obtained from 12 healthy volunteers (5 men) with an average age of 30 years, given an IV bolus dose of 10% fat emulsion in a volume equivalent to that used for administration of propofol, and from 60 surgical patients (17 men) with an average age of 36 years, who had anesthesia induced with an IV bolus dose of 4 mg/kg thiopental (n = 18), an IV bolus dose of 2 mg/kg propofol (n = 18), or an IV bolus dose of propofol plus a 1-hour infusion (n = 24). Platelet oxidative stress was determined by measuring levels of thiobarbituric acid reactive substances, glutathione, and glutathione peroxidase, reductase, and transferase.

Results.—Although thiopental did not significantly alter any measure of oxidative stress, propofol significantly inhibited production of thiobarbituric acid reactive substances by 25.7%, significantly reduced the percentage of glutathione in oxidized form by 29.5%, decreased glutathione peroxidase activity by 28.3%, and significantly increased total glutathione content by 24.6% and glutathione reductase activity by 44.5%. Propofol had little effect on glutathione reductase activity. Intralipid infusion in volunteers did not alter any of the variables. Results after bolus injection of propofol were similar to those for patients given an IV bolus dose of propofol.

Conclusion.—The antioxidant effects of propofol in humans may mitigate free radical and ischemic damage in patients during surgery.

▶ These authors studied something they call "oxidative stress" in platelets. I have long believed that studies of various aspects of the "stress" of anesthesia and surgery will eventually unlock the secrets to the major complications, such as perioperative myocardial infarction, stroke, and other thrombotic complications. Infections also will be shown related to various aspects of this "stress." Undoubtedly, anesthesia management has roles to play. In this study, propofol seems better than pentothal in the sense that propofol was associated with real inhibition of cellular oxidative damage.

This kind of study is the wave of the future in the sense that there will be many such elucidations of the stresses to which we subject our patients.

J. H. Tinker, MD

Randomized Trial of Hypotensive Epidural Anesthesia in Older Adults
Williams-Russo P, Sharrock NE, Mattis S, et al (Cornell Med College, New York; Hillside Hosp, New York; Lenox Hill Hosp, New York)
Anesthesiology 91:926-935, 1999   7–5

Objective.—Hypotensive anesthesia reduces intraoperative blood loss, but increases the patient's risk of ischemic injury. Cognitive outcome after total hip replacement (THR) surgery using a new technique for induced hypotension with epidural anesthesia with preserved or augmented cardiac output was investigated in a randomized, controlled clinical trial of 235 older adults with comorbid illnesses.

Methods.—Patients (50% female), aged 50 to 88 years, with cardiac disease, hypertension, or diabetes mellitus, were randomly allocated to a hypotensive mean arterial blood pressure of 45 to 55 mm Hg (n = 117) or to a range of 55 to 70 mm Hg (n = 118) during THR. Cognitive testing was performed perioperatively and at 1 week and 4 months after surgery. Changes in cognitive function and in comorbid conditions were compared between groups.

Results.—A total of 216 (92%) patients had long-term follow-up. There were no significant differences in cognitive or noncognitive outcomes between groups at any time points before or after surgery.

Conclusion.—The level of intraoperative blood pressure management during epidural anesthesia for THR made no difference in short- or long-term cognitive or noncognitive outcomes in older adults.

▶ I always cringe a bit at studies like this that invariably conclude whatever they were studying is okay to do. "Controlled" is more "deliberate" in my hands and has been controversial since the massive studies by David Little in the mid 1950s. The problem is always the same. If the possible complication is rare, but devastating, such as quadriplegia, how many must you do before you get one? In a way, it is like flying. The chances of dying in a plane crash are quite small, but non-zero. The chances of dying are the individual per-flight risk times the total number of flights. No way around that. If you get a patient with paraplegia, will you be perfectly willing to go back into the operating room and do the same procedure again? Reminds me of the fellow who got caught carrying a bomb onto an airliner. Asked why he did it, he said, "I know that the chances of a bomb being carried onto an airliner are very small. But the chances of there being two bombs on the same plane? Now that is really small!" It boils down to how much risk of a devastating complication you are willing to accept.

J. H. Tinker, MD

An Environmental Survey of Compliance With Occupational Exposure Standards (OES) for Anaesthetic Gases

Henderson KA, Matthews IP (Univ of Wales, Cardiff)
Anaesthesia 54:941-947, 1999   7–6

Objective.—A survey of compliance with Occupational Exposure Standards for anesthesia gases was performed.

Methods.—Static monitoring and personal sampling of nitrous oxide (N_2O) and isoflurane were performed in the operating, anesthesia, and recovery rooms of all 8 hospitals with surgical suites in South Wales.

Results.—Findings showed compliance with standards. Levels of N_2O were lowest in the operating rooms. Higher levels of N_2O were found in radiology and delivery suites, where there was no scavenging of gases and inadequate ventilation.

Conclusion.—Levels of N_2O exceeded standards in radiology and delivery suites with inadequate ventilation and no gas scavenging.

▶ In the x-ray department, they all wear film badges, because in the final analysis, it matters not how much radiation was released, but only who got what! Several individual exposure devices have been touted for doing this for our personnel in operation rooms, with little success and a lot of scare tactics. Really, this is indeed what is needed, however. If I measure any operating room at the wrong time, I can find unacceptable levels. If I measure the operating room at 3 AM in the upper west corner, I will find virtually nothing. Do you really purge the nitrous before you take the mask off to intubate? Good practice helps a lot here and is often discounted. Another problem is where did they get the so-called "standards?" Look it up, and you will *not* be impressed!

J. H. Tinker, MD

Which Clinical Anesthesia Outcomes Are Important to Avoid? The Perspective of Patients

Macario A, Weinger M, Carney S, et al (Stanford Univ, Calif; Univ of California, San Diego)
Anesth Analg 89:652-658, 1999   7–7

Objective.—How patients rate low morbidity outcomes after anesthesia has not been assessed. Patients were surveyed about their rank order of preference for avoiding specific anesthesia outcomes and were asked how they perceive common adverse events.

Methods.—Patients were asked to rank 10 common anesthesia outcomes from most to least desirable and place a value on how undesirable the less desirable outcomes were.

Results.—Of 195 surveys distributed, 130 were returned, and 101 (40 males, aged 19-83 years) were completed. There were 62 patients who reported experiencing at least 1 of the studied outcomes. Vomiting was the least desirable outcome with 56% of respondents reporting that relief of nausea was more important than relief of shivering. Ranking and subjective value ratings were significantly correlated (r^2). Other outcomes in decreasing importance were gagging on endotracheal tube, pain, nausea, recall without pain, residual weakness, shivering, sore throat, and somnolence.

Conclusion.—When clinical anesthesia outcomes were compared with patient preferences, vomiting was rated as the least desirable anesthesia outcome. These data may help anesthesiologists improve on individual patients' outcomes by considering their preferences and expectations.

▶ This study makes an interesting and invalid assumption, namely that some complications are more desirable to eliminate than others; ie, we need to somehow prioritize our work toward the elimination of certain complications, and we can afford to let others slide, because they don't seem to bother the patients that much. I believe in patient satisfaction surveys as much as the next person, but this is a bit much, don't you think?

J. H. Tinker, MD

Lloyd-Davies Position With Trendelenburg: A Disaster Waiting to Happen?
Horgan AF, Geddes S, Finlay IG (Glasgow Royal Infirmary, Scotland)
Dis Colon Rectum 42:916-920, 1999   7–8

Objective.—Lower limb compartment syndrome (LLCS) is a serious complication of prolonged elevation of the legs during surgery. Blood flow to the legs was monitored in patients undergoing major colorectal pelvic procedures to determine whether the position of the patient's legs influenced perfusion and subsequent risk of development of LLCS.

Methods.—Lower limb perfusion was measured at 15-minute intervals, using intra-arterial blood pressure monitoring, laser doppler flowmetry, and pulse oximetry in 12 consecutive patients undergoing prolonged colorectal procedures. In 3 patients, parameters were also recorded in the recovery room.

Results.—The median operating time was 210 minutes, and the median head-down position time was 35 minutes. No patient experienced LLCS. After positioning the legs in the lithotomy position, tilting the head down at 15° resulted in a significant decrease in leg perfusion. Repositioning the legs after the procedure gradually restored leg perfusion. Intracompartmental blood flow increased by a factor of 10 above preoperative values in 3 patients after surgery. Skin perfusion and intra-arterial pedal pressure did not increase in these patients.

Conclusion.—Although the lithotomy position did not lead to leg ischemia, lowering the head resulted in significant ischemia followed by hyperfusion after the procedure in 3 patients when the legs were lowered. These patients could be at increased risk for LLCS.

▶ I know of 2 of these compartment syndromes from prolonged modified lithotomies with the patients' legs unattended for many hours. If you had a patient in an ICU, and he or she was unconscious, you would insist that a physical therapist develop a program of frequent range-of-motion manipulations and changes of position. During long cases in the operating room, we can, but seldom do this, too. I know of a 36-hour hand surgery during which a physical therapist came into the operating room and performed these maneuvers on all available parts of the patient every few hours. Makes sense, doesn't it?

J. H. Tinker, MD

Cerebral Microembolism Diagnosed by Transcranial Doppler During Total Knee Arthroplasty: Correlation With Transesophageal Echocardiography
Sulek CA, Davies LK, Enneking FK, et al (Univ of Florida, Gainesville)
Anesthesiology 91:672-676, 1999   7–9

Objective.—Pulmonary embolism is common after tourniquet removal following total knee arthroplasty (TKA). The incidence of cerebral microembolism after tourniquet release was investigated using transcranial Doppler US.

Methods.—Transcranial Doppler US was performed in 22 patients (9 men) undergoing TKA after induction of anesthesia and during and after tourniquet inflation. Emboli were counted. Echogenic material in the left atrium was evaluated. Patients were examined preoperatively and before discharge.

Results.—Seven patients had bilateral TKA. Emboli were detected in 9 (60%) patients with unilateral TKA and in 4 (57%) patients with bilateral TKA. Although the likelihood of emboli in the 2 groups were not significantly different, the average number of emboli in the bilateral TKA group was significantly higher than in the unilateral TKA group (right TKA, 31; left TKA, 56; bilateral TKA, 87). Bilateral TKA patients with emboli had significantly longer tourniquet times than other patients (230 vs 198 minutes). Eight patients had echogenic material in left atrium (6 from the pulmonary vein and 2 through a patent foramen ovale), and all had emboli. There were no neurologic sequelae.

Conclusion.—A significant number of patients had cerebral emboli following tourniquet release after TKA, particularly if they had bilateral TKA. Emboli were most likely released through the left atrium and to a lesser extent by transatrial passage.

▶ I know of a case of massive and fatal cerebral fat embolism that became obvious after bilateral TKA. Issues in the case had to do with whether and when the anesthesiologist could or should recognize that this is happening and, perhaps, ask the surgeon to abort and not do the second side. I agree with the authors that these fat globules probably can slither through the pulmonary capillaries without the need for a patent foramen ovale. It should be remembered, however, that probe-patent foramen ovale occurs in about 28% of people at autopsy.

J. H. Tinker, MD

Compound A Does Not Accumulate During Closed Circuit Sevoflurane Anaesthesia with the Physioflex
Funk W, Gruber M, Jakob W, et al (Univ of Regensburg, Germany)
Br J Anaesth 83:571-575, 1999   7–10

Objective.—Although minimizing fresh gas flow in rebreathing anesthesia systems saves money, it increases the risk of accumulation of compound A, a degradation product of sevoflurane. The inspiratory and end-tidal gas compositions in the Physioflex closed system anesthesia apparatus were analyzed to elucidate possible exposure and uptake of compound A during closed circuit anesthesia.

Methods.—Sevoflurane was administered to 5 patients and isoflurane was administered to 2 patients. After tracheal intubation, ventilation was provided using 40% oxygen in air (tidal volume 10 mL/kg) with a valveless high flow (70 L/min) Physioflex closed circle system. The system contained an absorbent canister with 1 L of fresh soda lime with or without 2.9% potassium hydroxide. The end-tidal PCO_2 of 4.3 to 4.8 kPa. The surgeries lasted longer than 2 hours.

Results.—The temperature increased from 24.7°C to 31.2°C and was higher at the top of the canister. Relative humidity increased from 67% to 69% to 90% after 1 hour and decreased to 78% to 82% during the second hour. Although no compound A was detected when isoflurane was administered, compound A appeared 10 minutes after the use of sevoflurane began. The highest concentration of compound A detected was 7.6 ppm. Compound A did not accumulate, and flushing reduced inspiratory and end-tidal concentrations by 50%. Calculated patient intake of compound A was 4.4 ppm/h. Neither compound B nor methanol was detected.

Conclusion.—The amount of compound A detected during closed circuit administration of sevoflurane was below nephrotoxic levels reported in the literature.

▶ The Physioflex uses high flows of fresh gas. It is very logical that its use would not be accompanied by the liberation of compound A, because the latter's formation requires heat and a strong base. I selected this study to point out that there are at least a few folks who are still beating the (hopefully) dead horse of compound A, despite the fact that after, as the late Carl Sagan loved to say, "Millions and millions of sevoflurane anesthetics, little in the way of toxicity has yet emerged."

J. H. Tinker, MD

Peripheral Neuropathy in Healthy Men Volunteers Anesthetized With 1.25 MAC Sevoflurane for 8 Hours

Goldberg ME, Larijani GE, Eger EI II (Univ of Medicine and Dentistry of New Jersey, Camden; Univ of California, San Francisco)
Pharmacotherapy 19:1173-1176, 1999   7–11

Objective.—Although no incidents of injury to the nervous system have been reported after sevoflurane administration, 2 cases of peripheral neuropathy were reported in 2 male volunteers after prolonged administration of sevoflurane during a study assessing the capacity of sevoflurane and compound A to influence renal function.

> *Case 1.*—Man, 27, was anesthetized at 1.25 minimum alveolar concentration (3%) of sevoflurane at 2 L/min for 8 hours. He had an old rotator cuff injury and denied using steroids. The mean concentration of compound A was 44.5 ppm. The patient complained of incapacitating shoulder pain at 35 minutes and was given 30 mg ketorolac. On the next day, the incapacitating pain had shifted to the scapula and deltoid muscles, then to the hamstring muscle attachments and right thigh. Pain and numbness gradually went away over a period of several weeks.
>
> *Case 2.*—Man, 23, with an old shoulder injury, complained of finger numbness after waking from the same kind of anesthesia. His hand was swollen, and pain, numbness, and dysesthesia were localized to the median nerve. He had allodynia, unusual sensitivity to touch, and proprioceptive hallucinations. His arm swelled, and he lost sensation in the lower part of his arm. Right median nerve compression was diagnosed. His sensory and motor potentials continued to decrease over the next 5 months. At 8 months he underwent surgery to release adhesions of the median nerve At 12 months, he had a right thoroscopic sympathectomy to decrease pain.

Discussion.—Other volunteers had similar but less severe neurologic complaints.

Conclusion.—The cause of the neuropathies resulting from prolonged sevoflurane anesthesia is not known but may be associated with compound A or other substances generated during anesthesia.

▶ Talk about beating a dead horse. Dr Eger's quest to find something bad to link to compound A has gone to new lengths here. Will flatfeet and bunions be his next target? He has decided that compound A *must do something bad.* This is science?

J. H. Tinker, MD

8 Complications and Mishaps in Anesthesia

Latex Anaphylaxis Causing Heart Block: Role of Ranitidine
Patterson LJ, Milne B (Queen's Univ, Kingston, Ont)
Can J Anesth 46:776-778, 1999   8–1

Objective.—Because myocardium contains H_1 and H_2 receptors, treatment with H_2 receptors may lead to heart block. The case of a woman treated with ranitidine who had a 3:1 heart block secondary to latex anaphylaxis was discussed.

Case Report.—Woman, 38, having a radical hysterectomy for cervical cancer, was obese, had a history of sleep apnea, orthopnea, smoking, petit mal epilepsy, gastroesophageal reflux, and sciatica. She was premedicated with ranitidine, metoclopramide, and sodium citrate. The surgeons and nurse wore latex gloves. About 10 minutes into the surgery, the patient had a 3:1 heart block that was successfully treated with epinephrine. She was diagnosed with a possible latex allergy. The surgery was abandoned, the abdomen was closed, and the patient became unstable again. She was diagnosed with a latex allergy and treated successfully again. She required mechanical ventilation for pulmonary edema. An intradermal injection of latex confirmed her latex allergy. A tryptase level of 120 ng/mL confirmed an anaphylactic reaction.

Conclusion.—The patient's anaphylactoid reaction to latex resulted in a 3:1 heart block. Preoperative H_2 antihistamine administration probably contributed to the development of the heart block.

▶ I do not understand why anaphylaxis is linked here with heart block. Perhaps, it was simply the result of hypoxia. I selected this study to point out once again to anyone who still thinks that latex allergy is some sort of "nursing disease," that it is a very real threat to our patients.

J. H. Tinker, MD

An Unexpected Complication of the Intubating Laryngeal Mask

Branthwaite MA (Temple, London)
Anaesthesia 54:166-171, 1999

8–2

Objective.—A fatality resulting from use of the intubating laryngeal mask is discussed.

> *Case Report.*—Woman, 77, operated under general anesthesia for cataract extraction, had had uneventful contralateral cataract extraction 8 months previously using a size 4 laryngeal mask. She agreed to participate in a multicenter trial of the intubating laryngeal mask. She was 1 of several patients to use the mask the day of surgery. Intubation was achieved on the fifth try. Blood was aspirated from the pharynx and a nasogastric tube. After surgery, the patient complained of back pain. She had crepitus in the neck. A chest radiograph revealed air in soft tissues on both sides of the mediastinum. Esophageal rupture was diagnosed and confirmed. The patient did not respond to conservative treatment. During the next few days, atrial fibrillation, bilateral pleural effusions, and respiratory failure necessitating mechanical ventilation developed. A CT scan revealed barium and air in the right pleural cavity and barium in the right paravertebral area. A month later her esophageal perforation had sealed. A feeding jejunostomy was performed, and her gallbladder was decompressed. At 5 weeks, a CT scan showed dilatation of the proximal esophagus and demonstrated contrast material in the mediastinum, down to the aorta, and into the right hemithorax. Mechanical ventilation was discontinued, but her pseudomembranous colitis recurred, and she died 9 weeks after surgery. An autopsy found extremely severe colitis, an intra-abdominal abscess, and a healed esophageal perforation.

Conclusion.—A difficult intubation using the intubating laryngeal mask resulted in esophageal perforation in an elderly patient who subsequently died.

▶ I note that Dr Branthwaite has graduated (defected?) from the ranks of highly productive academic anesthetist to "barrister at law." If indeed the "M. A." is the same M. A. Branthwaite who has written so elegantly for years in anesthesiology. When I first heard a presentation on the laryngeal mask, I responded with my usual cynical skepticism. In fact, the thing works. The "intubating" version, may give us more trouble. Sounds like somebody tried to force things.

J. H. Tinker, MD

Is Cardiopulmonary Bypass Still the Cause of Cognitive Dysfunction After Cardiac Operations?

Taggart DP, Browne SM, Halligan PW, et al (John Radcliff Hosp, Oxford, England; Oxford Univ, England; Rivermead Rehabilitation Centre, Oxford, England)
J Thorac Cardiovasc Surg 118:414-421, 1999   8–3

Objective.—Cognitive impairment, not caused by embolism, accounts for two thirds of patients who experience cerebral injury after cardiac surgery, and persists in one third of patients for at least 1 year after surgery. The impairment has been attributed to cardiopulmonary bypass (CPB). Neuropsychologic performance was measured in patients before coronary artery bypass grafting (CABG), at discharge, and at 3 months after CABG with and without CPB to determine the impact of CPB on cognitive functioning.

Methods.—Ten neuropsychologic tests and functional assessments were performed at discharge and 3 months after CABG in 25 patients (88% male) who did not have CPB and in 50 patients (88% male) who had CPB. One surgeon performed all procedures, and all patients had the same anesthetic regimen. Between-group differences were analyzed.

Results.—The CPB group had significantly more grafts than the non-CPB group (2.7 vs 1.5). The average operating time for CPB patients was a significant 50 minutes shorter than for the non-CPB group. Although most test results demonstrated deterioration in both groups at discharge, there was no significant difference between groups. At 3 months, all test results were significantly improved in both groups with no significant difference in scores between groups.

Conclusion.—CPB does not appear to cause cognitive dysfunction after cardiac surgery.

▶ Now that coronary bypass can be done without bypass, it was a simple matter to plan and execute a study to see if the well-known cognitive dysfunction that is so vexing post bypass is just as bad if bypass was not used. Obviously, there are selection biases here; ie, the healthier patients might have had the non-bypass operations. That is not obvious here, however. Most experts here believe that multiple microemboli are the culprits with respect to cognitive dysfunction post cardiac surgery. Are there fewer of these without bypass? It is surely logical that there should be, but medicine is full of logical ideas that didn't necessarily pan out.

J. H. Tinker, MD

Xenon Does Not Trigger Malignant Hyperthermia in Susceptible Swine
Froeba G, Marx T, Pazhur J, et al (Universität München, Germany)
Anesthesiology 91:1047-1052, 1999   8–4

Background.—Xenon, a noble gas with anesthetic properties, is currently being studied for use in humans. A study was undertaken to determine whether xenon would trigger malignant hyperthermia in a model of susceptible swine.

Methods.—Nine swine sensitive to malignant hyperthermia were anesthetized with pentobarbital and then ventilated with 70% xenon in oxygen for 2 hours. Several parameters were measured every 10 minutes during xenon-oxygen ventilation and after a 30-minute xenon washout phase followed by subsequent administration of halothane and succinylcholine.

Findings.—Xenon exposure resulted in no changes in metabolic or hemodynamic parameters. There were no increases in plasma catecholamine levels that would indicate an episode of malignant hyperthermia. By contrast, episodes of fulminant and fatal malignant hyperthermia began within 20 minutes of halothane and succinylcholine administration in all swine.

Conclusions.—In this swine model, xenon produced no hemodynamic, gas-exchange, or metablic responses that indicated malignant hyperthermia during the 2 hours of administration. These findings cannot necessarily be generalized to human beings.

▶ Xenon as an anesthetic is in somebody's strategic plan for development. This was the second xenon article I found interesting enough to include in this year's YEAR BOOK. The fact that it does not trigger malignant hyperthermia is not surprising. The work was supported by a German company. I will bet that we will be seeing some fancy innovative xenon anesthesia administration apparatus for sale soon. I think this will be exciting. We need these kinds of new developments in our specialty.

J. H. Tinker, MD

9 Critical Care Medicine

Resource Use and Quality of Life Issues

Effects of an Organized Critical Care Service on Outcomes and Resource Utilization: A Cohort Study

Hanson CW III, Deutschman CS, Anderson HL III, et al (Univ of Pennsylvania, Philadelphia; Univ of California, Irvine)

Crit Care Med 27:270-274, 1999   9–1

Introduction.—Practice patterns are under scrutiny at both institutional and national levels to eliminate inefficiency, lower costs, and improve clinical results. Critical care medicine would seem to be particularly susceptible to the current forces of change. It is not, largely because critical care medicine is difficult to describe. The cost and effectiveness of 2 patterns of critical care practice in an academic medical center were examined to determine whether the presence of an on-site, organized, supervised critical service improves care and reduces resource utilization.

Methods.—Two patient cohorts admitted to a surgical intensive care unit (SICU) between July 1994 and June 1995 were compared (Table 3). One cohort received care from an on-site critical care team supervised by

TABLE 3.—Demographics

Category	CCS	NCCS	*p* Value
Age (yr)	61.33 ± 1.5	59.4 ± 1.3	NS
Gender (female/male)	44:56	40:60	—
ICU admission APACHE II score	13.9 ± 0.5	11.8 ± 0.4	<.01
ICU length of stay (days)	2.0 ± 0.3	2.8 ± 0.4	<.05
Complications/ICU stay	0.5 ± 0.1	1.7 ± 0.3	<.01
Equipment-days	6.5 ± 0.9	9.9 ± 0.4	NS
Arterial blood gases (n)	3.0 ± 0.4	6.1 ± 1.0	<.01
Blood products (units)	1.2 ± 0.3	2.0 ± 0.5	NS
Days of ventilation	0.7 ± 0.3	1.2 ± 0.3	<.01
Number of consultations	1.6 ± 0.1	2.8 ± 0.2	<.01
Hospital length of stay (days)	20.3 ± 2.0	23.6 ± 2.3	<.05
Medicare-adjusted charges*	34.5 ± 3	47.5 ± 5	<.01
Deaths during hospitalization	4	6	NS

*Values are in thousands of US dollars.

Abbreviations: CCS, Critical care service; *NCCS,* no critical care service; *NS,* not significant; *APACHE,* Acute Physiology and Chronic Health Evaluation.

(Courtesy of Hanson CW III, Deutschman CS, Anderson HL III, et al: Effect of an organized critical care service on outcomes and resource utilization: A cohort study. *Crit Care Med* 27[2]:270-274, 1999.)

an intensive care specialist. Controls received care from a team with patient care responsibilities in multiple sites supervised by a general surgeon. The primary outcome measures were duration of stay, resource utilization, and complication rates.

Results.—Patients treated by the critical care service had higher Acute Physiology and Chronic Health Evaluation II (APACHE II) scores, yet they spent less time in the SICU, used fewer resources, had fewer complications, and had lower total hospital charges. These differences were most evident in patients with the worst APACHE II scores.

Conclusion.—The critical care service model offered more efficient care to patients in the SICU. The difference in the 2 comparison groups became more pronounced with increased severity of illness.

Organizational Characteristics of Intensive Care Units Related to Outcomes of Abdominal Aortic Surgery
Pronovost PJ, Jenckes MW, Dorman T, et al (Johns Hopkins Univ, Baltimore, Md)
JAMA 281:1310-1317, 1999   9–2

Objective.—ICUs at different institutions vary widely in terms of morbidity and mortality rates. The effects of ICU structure and care processes on these outcomes are not known. The effects of ICU organization on the clinical and economic outcomes for patients undergoing abdominal aortic surgery were studied.

Methods.—The observational study included hospital discharge data from all hospitals in the state of Maryland in which abdominal aortic surgery was performed from 1994 through 1996. Data on a total of 2987 patients were analyzed. Data on organizational characteristics were obtained from the ICU medical directors. The main outcomes assessed were in-hospital mortality and length of hospital and ICU stay.

Results.—The in-hospital mortality rates ranged from 0% to 66%. ICUs that did not have daily rounds by an ICU physician showed a 3-fold increase in in-hospital deaths after adjustment for patient demographic characteristics, co-morbidity, severity of illness, hospital and surgeon volume, and hospital characteristics. Other outcomes, including cardiac arrest, acute renal failure, septicemia, and reintubation, were also more likely at centers without daily rounds by an ICU physician.

Conclusions.—The mortality rate after abdominal aortic surgery appears to be increased at ICUs that do not have daily rounds by an ICU physician. Several organizational aspects of ICU care may be modified to improve patient outcomes, although further studies would be needed to assess the results of these modifications.

▶ Historically, surgeons have held firm to their belief that postoperative critical care should be solely under the direction of the primary surgeon. Consultation with other services would be accepted, provided that ultimate control of patient care was dictated by the surgeon. Many articles and editorials written over the last decade have implored surgeons to continue to play an active role in intensive care units and not to relinquish care to consultant intensivists. However, as critical care has evolved as a specialty, recognizing the expanded knowledge and skills necessary to care for patients with complex illnesses, surgeons need to recognize the harsh reality that intensivists play a vital role in the care of their patients. Both of these articles (Abstracts 9–1 and 9–2) reflect a decreased length of stay, a decreased complication rate, and, in the latter study, a decreased mortality rate when a full-time intensivist participates in the care of a critically ill surgical patient. Although these two articles substantiate a belief that I have held for some time as a practicing intensivist, a number of questions are raised by both studies. In the first study, an increased length of stay was noted in patients who died in the intensive care unit and who were managed by the critical care service versus those who had not been managed by the critical care service. Although the authors do not comment on this finding, the devil's advocate in me would pose the question as to whether the critical care service merely prolonged the dying process in this subset of patients.

Finally, in the latter study it should be noted that 4 of the 5 physicians who participated in this study were either officers in or consultants to a newly formed company designed to provide clinical intensive care services to hospitals. It is uncertain whether the company developed as a result of the article or vice versa. Irrespective of this, the overall results are still compelling.

D. M. Rothenberg, MD, FCCM

Pharmacist Participation on Physician Rounds and Adverse Drug Events in the Intensive Care Unit
Leape LL, Cullen DJ, Clapp MD, et al (Harvard School of Public Health, Boston; Massachusetts Gen Hosp, Boston; Brigham and Women's Hosp, Boston)
JAMA 282:267-270, 1999   9–3

Objective.—Although studies show that pharmacist review of ICU prescription orders prevents mistakes and lowers drug costs by reducing drug use, there have been no studies of the benefit of having a pharmacist present in the ICU at the time drugs are prescribed. The efficacy of pharmacist participation in a medical ICU in preventing adverse drug events (ADEs) was tested in a controlled clinical trial.

Methods.—Between February 1, 1993 and July 31, 1993 (phase 1, preintervention) and October 1, 1994 and July 7, 1995 (phase 2, postintervention), the effect of pharmacist intervention was tested in a 17-bed ICU (the study unit) and compared with no pharmacist intervention in a 15-bed coronary care unit with a similar occupancy rate which served as the control unit. ADEs were compared for 75 randomly selected patients in each of 3 groups: all patients admitted to the study unit during phase 1 and phase 2, all patients admitted to the control unit during phase 2. In addition, there were 50 randomly selected patients from all those admitted to the control unit during phase 1.

An experienced consulting pharmacist made rounds with ICU medical personnel in the mornings. A pharmacist was available for consultation but did not make morning rounds with medical personnel in the coronary care unit. Outcome measures included measurement of ADEs, the types of interventions pharmacists made, and the acceptance by physicians and nurses of pharmacist participation.

Results.—The overall rate of preventable ordering ADEs/1000 patient-days decreased significantly in the study unit by 66% (from 10.4 to 3.5) from phase 1 to phase 2, an estimated savings of $2000 to $2500 per incident. During the same period, the decrease in the study unit compared with the control unit was a significant 72%. The rate of ADEs decreased significantly to 11.6 in the ICU from phase 1 to phase 2 but increased significantly by 34.3% (from 34.7 to 46.6) in the control unit. Of the 398 pharmacist interventions reported, 366 were related to ordering, and 362 (99%) were accepted by the physicians. Pharmacist-initiated clarification or correction of incomplete orders, wrong dose, wrong frequency, inappropriate choice, or duplicate therapy accounted for 46%. Drug interactions or drug allergic reactions were prevented in 22 cases.

With the cost of a preventable ADE estimated at $4685, the total annual reduction in this unit was about $270,000. The presence of the pharmacist flagged unsafe conditions, identified process improvement needs, and was well accepted by medical personnel.

Conclusion.—The participation of a pharmacist on medical rounds significantly lowers the risk of ADEs and results in substantial cost savings.

▶ The mortality associated with ADEs has become the focus of national attention, with the White House mandating that physicians and hospitals develop policies to prevent such mishaps. Within the setting of an ICU, the employment of a dedicated pharmacist with expertise in the use of vasoactive agents, antibiotics, sedatives, analgesics, and neuromuscular relaxants would appear to be not only beneficial from a patient care aspect, but from an economic aspect as well.

D. M. Rothenberg, MD, FCCM

The Influence of Access to a Private Attending Physician on the Withdrawal of Life-Sustaining Therapies in the Intensive Care Unit
Kollef MH, Ward S (Washington Univ, School of Medicine, St. Louis, Mo)
Crit Care Med 27:2125-2132, 1999   9–4

Objective.—Patient outcomes frequently depend on socioeconomic status. The relationship between withdrawal of life-sustaining therapies in the ICU and patient access to a private attending physician was investigated in a prospective cohort study.

Methods.—Between July and December 1996, data were collected prospectively on all 501 patients (48.7% men), aged 18 to 95 years, admitted to the ICU of a university-affiliated private teaching hospital. Private attending physicians, as the attending physicians of record, were responsible for approving all significant treatment changes or interventions in the ICU. Relative risks for withdrawal of life-sustaining therapies were calculated for patients with and without a private attending physician.

Results.—Private physicians attended 300 (59.9%) of patients. Patients with a private physician were significantly more likely to die, be white, have a malignant disease, be immunosuppressed, have end-stage organ failure, have advanced medical directives, have private health insurance, and have a more serious illness and were less likely to have drug or alcohol abuse problems compared with patients without a private physician. Patients with a private attending physician had significantly longer ICU and hospital stays, longer mechanical ventilation, more organ system derangements, and greater hospital mortality rates than patients without a private attending physician.

The 22% of patients who died in the hospital had significantly longer ICU and hospital stays (20.3 vs 25.2 days), longer mechanical ventilation, more organ system derangements, and greater hospital mortality rates than nonsurvivors without a private attending physician, despite similar Acute Physiology and Chronic Health Evaluation II scores. Patients without private attending physicians were significantly more likely than those with private attending physicians to have life-sustaining therapies withdrawn before death (80.0% vs 29.9%). Most (65.4%) of the 26 patients with private attending physicians who had life-support therapies withdrawn had life-support withdrawn by their attending physician. ICU and hospital costs for all patients with private attending physicians, and the nonsurvivor subset of these patients, were significantly higher than for patients without private attending physicians.

Conclusion.—Dying patients without a private attending physician were 3 times as likely to have life-sustaining therapies withdrawn before death than those patients with a private attending physician and to incur significantly lower costs.

Incorporating Palliative Care Into Critical Care Education: Principles, Challenges, and Opportunities
Danis M, Federman D, Fins JJ, et al (NIH, Bethesda, MD; Harvard Med School, Boston; Cornell Univ, Ithaca, NY; et al)
Crit Care Med 27:2005-2013, 1999   9–5

Objective.—The best approach to educating medical personnel about end-of-life care in the ICU was examined with the idea of developing a report for those who design curricula for and certify medical students and medical trainees.

Methods.—Critical care, palliative care, medical ethics, consumer advocacy, and communications personnel met at the Medical Education for Care Near the End of Life National Consensus Conference to study how death and dying are manifested in the ICU, the unique opportunities and barriers for teaching end-of-life care in the ICU, the model of care to be presented, the specific topics to be covered, the teaching approaches to be used, and the institutional changes necessary to effect the process.

Results.—Physicians in the ICU are faced with the task of providing life-sustaining care and of helping patients and families cope with the possibility of impending death. Although there is little uniformity to the way patients die, many deaths are preceded by sequential withholding of life-sustaining therapies. Although new technology provides the capability of sustaining life, it also provides a multidisciplinary decision-making environment that teaches teamwork. ICU physicians need to have critical care skills and yet be sensitive to the patient's need for palliative, compassionate treatment. A variety of teaching approaches need to be utilized throughout the medical curriculum. Institutional support from sympathetic hospital and medical school administrators is critical to the success of an end-of-life curriculum. Hospital care may need to be reoriented in the case of dying patients to provide a gradual transfer of care as the patient's need for compassionate, intensive, palliative care increases.

Conclusion.—Cooperation among subspecialty organizations, care and teaching facilities, and funding processes will be necessary to institute formal training in palliative care for dying patients.

▶ The ability to teach compassionate and palliative care in the ICU is solely limited by physicians who are unable to do so either because of constraints in the design of their ICU or lack of formal training in end-of-life issues (Abstracts 9–4 and 9–5). The article by Kollef and Ward (Abstract 9–4) would suggest that physicians who are trained in end-of-life issues improve the quality of care by more appropriately managing the dying patient. This article also demonstrates that an intensivist is most likely to be the individual physically responsible for withdrawing of life support, even when a private practitioner is the attending physician of record.

D. M. Rothenberg, MD, FCCM

Quality End-of-Life Care: Patient's Perspectives
Singer PA, Martin DK, Kelner M (Univ of Toronto)
JAMA 281:163-168, 1999   9–6

Objective.—It is important to develop a conceptual framework for quality end-of-life care. The elements of quality end-of-life care were identified and described by patients.

Methods.—Patients from 3 studies, those on dialysis (n = 48), infected with HIV (n = 40), and in long-term care facilities (n = 38), had in-depth, open-ended, face-to-face interviews about quality end-of-life care. Results were categorized and analyzed.

Results.—Patients identified 5 domains: adequate pain and symptom management, no prolongation of dying, achieving a sense of control, relieving burden, and strengthening of relationships with loved ones. Patient perspectives were in accord with 3 expert perspective models, although the patient perspective model was simpler, more straightforward, more specific, and more outcomes focused. The patient perspective model is also more authentic because it was developed by the patients themselves. Pain is still a problem for many patients; 4 out of 10 dying patients have severe pain most of the time. Clear guidelines defining appropriate pain care and differentiating it from euthanasia would be helpful to clinicians.

Conclusion.—Patient-defined quality end-of-life care domains provide a framework for research and clinical practice.

▶ Patients' perspectives detailed in this study confirm what the vast majority of physicians have concluded are the most important aspects of end-of-life care. Although not specifically addressed, the 5 domains of end-of-life care described apply as well to the care of the critically ill patient. As intensivists, we may be proficient in pain and symptom management; rarely, however, do we focus on supporting patient-family relationships, minimizing the loss of patient self-control, or assuring that our most intensive care does not merely prolong the dying process. Quality critical and end-of-life care must be directed toward meeting these, as well as the spiritual needs, of our patients and their families.

D. M. Rothenberg, MD, FCCM

Evaluation of Prognostic Criteria for Determining Hospice Eligibility in Patients With Advanced Lung, Heart, or Liver Disease
Fox E, for the SUPPORT Investigators (George Washington Univ, Washington, DC; et al)
JAMA 282:1638-1645, 1999   9–7

Background.—Dying patients usually must have a life expectancy of less than 6 months to be eligible for hospice care. Although cancer has a relatively predictable course, other diseases rarely demonstrate a progressive decline. A variety of criteria for determining the prognosis for predicting death within 6 months for seriously ill patients with advanced chronic disease was evaluated.

Methods.—Data from the Study to Understand Prognoses and Preferences for Outcomes and Risks of Treatments (SUPPORT) were analyzed for patients with an aggregate mortality rate of more than 50% who were admitted to 1 of 5 medical centers. Their diagnoses included chronic obstructive pulmonary disease (COPD; n = 1016), congestive heart failure (CHF; n = 1404), and end-stage liver disease (ESLD; n = 534). Variables analyzed included readmission within 2 months, home care after discharge, activities of daily living dependency of 3 or greater, weight loss of 2.3 kg or more within 2 months, albumin level of less than 25 g/L, partial pressure of oxygen of 55 mm Hg or less. Other variables analyzed were cor pulmonale while receiving oxygen in patients with COPD, an ejection fraction of 20% or less and arrhythmia in patients with CHF, and cachexia and a creatinine level of 153 μmol/L or greater in patients with ESLD. The analysis was used to define low, medium, and high thresholds for hospice eligibility.

Results.—A total of 347 patients, 116 (11%) with COPD, 92 (7%) with CHF, and 139 (26%) with ESLD died in the hospital. Of the remaining 2607, 54 were admitted to a hospice program, and 655 (25%) died within 6 months. Those patients who preferred palliative care (44%) had an increased likelihood of dying within 6 months. Among the hospice patients, 22% were alive at 6 months. The sensitivities of the broad, intermediate, and narrow inclusion criteria were low (41.7%, 16.2%, and 1.4%, respectively).

Conclusion.—The prognostic variables tested in this study were not able to predict which seriously ill patients were likely to die within 6 months. Six-month survival rates of patients with COPD, CHF, or ESLD, meeting various combinations of criteria, ranged from 53% to 70%.

▶ There can be no question that the societal debate over physician-assisted suicide and subsequent enactment of the Death with Dignity Act in Oregon have focused attention on the need for better palliative care. Unfortunately, there are no clear-cut algorithms or "clinical pathways" to assist patients, families, and physicians in initiating palliative care. This study from the SUPPORT group delineates our difficulty in predicting death in these otherwise severely ill patients. As such, the ability to enroll patients with end-stage heart, lung, or liver disease in hospice programs will continue to be a dilemma for both patient and physician.

D. M. Rothenberg, MD, FCCM

Mechanical Ventilation and Airway Management

Patient Responses During Rapid Terminal Weaning From Mechanical Ventilation: A Prospective Study
Campbell ML, Bizek KS, Thill M (Detroit Receiving Hosp; Henry Ford Health System, Detroit)
Crit Care Med 27:73-77, 1999   9–8

Objective.—Patient responses to rapid terminal weaning from mechanical ventilation were described and analyzed in a prospective, descriptive, correlational study.

Methods.—Surrogates of 31 adult non–brain-dead patients experiencing withdrawal of mechanical ventilation in a 300-bed, inner-city emergency/trauma hospital in a university-affiliated medical center, and the Comprehensive Supportive Care Team collaboratively made the decision for ventilator withdrawal. No patients were able to participate in this de-

TABLE 3.—Morphine Use

Administration Method	Mean	No. of Patients
Bolus (mg)	8.3 ± 1.07	16
Infusion (mg/hr)	5.5 ± 0.68	17
Cumulative dose (mg/24 hrs)	36 ± 9.69	17

(Courtesy of Campbell ML, Bizek KS, Thill M: Patient responses during rapid terminal weaning from mechanical ventilation: A prospective study. *Crit Care Med* 27[1]:73-77, 1999.)

cision. Physiologic data (arterial oxyhemoglobin saturation, end-tidal pressure of carbon dioxide, heart rate, respiratory rate and cerebral function), comfort data (Bizek Agitation Scale [BAS], and the COMFORT scale, monitored at baseline and every 5 minutes for as long as 2 hours or until death), and wakefulness data (measured by a portable cerebral function monitor) were collected before and during ventilator support and as long as 2 hours after ventilator support was withdrawn. Patient self-report data were collected, if applicable. Patients received no paralytic drugs but were premedicated with analgesic or anxiolytic agents or sedatives. Weaning was gradual and was determined by patient response, beginning with a synchronized intermittent mechanical ventilation mode with pressure-support ventilation followed by a gradual reduction in minute ventilation accomplished by decreasing the rate, decreasing the forced inspiratory oxygen fraction of inspired oxygen, and finally ending the wean with placement on a t-bar setup with humidified room air.

Results.—The average weaning time was 14 minutes. Most patients (84%) had oral or naso-endotracheal tubes (OET/NET), and 16% had tracheostomies. Postwean extubation was performed in 35% of patients. Survival was significantly longer in extubated patients than in patients who retained an OET/NET (85.30 vs 12.95 h). About 38% of family members remained at the bedside during the weaning process. Sixty-five percent of patients required analgesia/sedation; 35% did not (Table 3). BAS and COMFORT scales were significantly correlated ($r = 0.5966$). Bispectral index of cerebral function data, available for 11 patients, were significantly correlated with BAS ($r = 0.5279$) and COMFORT scales ($r = 0.5807$). After the wean, the average survival was 24.20 hours, ranging from 2 minutes to 183 hours, with a median of 2.3 hours. Two patients survived and were discharged to a hospice.

Conclusion.—An accurate picture of patient comfort is necessary during weaning because most patients are unable to self-report. BAS, COMFORT, and bispectral index of cerebral function scales are significantly correlated and effective assess patient distress.

▶ This article describes a detailed approach to terminal weaning of patients in whom withdrawal of life support has been deemed appropriate. A clear distinction is made between rapid terminal extubation and rapid terminal weaning, with the latter considered to be more likely to provide adequate comfort care at the end of life. Unfortunately, the authors attempt to correlate subjective scales for evaluating patients' distress with the bispectral index monitor. Given that none of the patients awakened to describe their ordeals and whether they received adequate comfort care, the authors' conclusion regarding their subjective scales and this so-called "objective monitor" is unsubstantiated. Studies regarding the use of bispectral analysis as a monitor to gauge sedation or comfort care in a critically ill patient have yet to be determined.

Finally, the authors comment on the possibility that terminal weaning may allow for rapid accumulation of carbon dioxide, which, in turn, may promote patient comfort by a "narcotic effect." This effect, to my knowledge, has never been proven and continues to be misquoted in the literature.[1]

D. M. Rothenberg, MD, FCCM

Reference

1. Carroll GC, Rothenberg DM: Carbon dioxide narcosis: Pathological or "pathillogical"? *Chest* 102:986-988, 1992.

Assessing Sedation During Intensive Care Unit Mechanical Ventilation With the Bispectral Index and the Sedation-Agitation Scale
Simmons LE, Riker RR, Prato BS, et al (Maine Med Ctr, Portland)
Crit Care Med 27:1499-1504, 1999   9–9

Background.—There is little information on the appropriate levels of sedation for patients receiving mechanical ventilation. Subjective methods such as the Sedation-Agitation Scale (SAS) and objective methods such as the bispectral index (BIS) have been used to assess the depth of sedation. The level of sedation of a heterogeneous group of ICU patients requiring

TABLE 1.—Sedation-Agitation Scale

7	Dangerous agitation	Pulling at ETT, trying to remove catheters, climbing over bedrail, striking at staff, thrashing side to side
6	Very agitated	Does not calm despite frequent verbal reminding of limits, requires physical restraints, biting ETT
5	Agitated	Anxious or mildly agitated, attempting to sit up, calms down to verbal instructions
4	Calm and cooperative	Calm, awakens easily, follows commands
3	Sedated	Difficult to arouse, awakens to verbal stimuli or gentle shaking but drifts off again, follows simple commands
2	Very sedated	Arouses to physical stimuli but does not communicate or follow commands, may move spontaneously
1	Unarousable	Minimal or no response to noxious stimuli, does not communicate or follow commands

Abbreviation: ETT, endotracheal tube.
(Courtesy of Simmons LE, Riker RR, Prato BS, et al: Assessing sedation during intensive care unit mechanical ventilation with the Bispectral Index and the Sedation-Agitation Index. *Crit Care Med* 27[8]:1499-1504, 1999.)

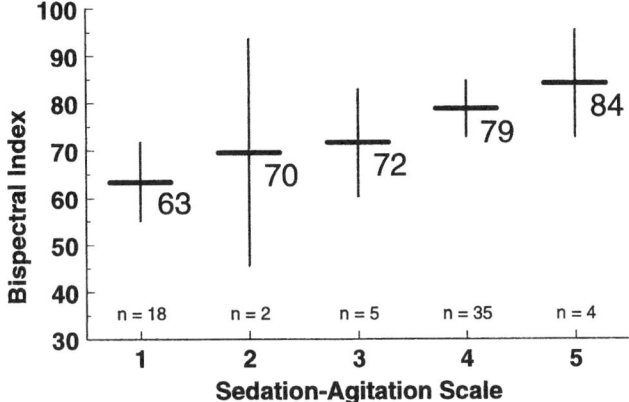

FIGURE 2.—Mean BIS values (*horizontal bars*) ± the 95% CI (*vertical bars*) for each Sedation-Agitation Scale value for each patient at baseline. (Courtesy of Simmons LE, Riker RR, Prato BS, et al: Assessing sedation during intensive care unit mechanical ventilation with the Bispectral Index and the Sedation-Agitation Index. *Crit Care Med* 27[8]:1499-1504, 1999.)

mechanical ventilation was prospectively quantitated in a pilot study using subjective and objective methods.

Methods.—A trained investigator, who quantified sedation by using the revised SAS, was present during a minimum of 2 hours of electroenceph-alographic monitoring of 64 episodes of ventilatory support involving 63 patients. An investigator blinded to SAS scores used continuous electro-encephalographic readings to assign the BIS at baseline, during stimulated activities, and during administration of bolus medications.

Results.—Subjective (SAS) sedation scores ranged from 1 (very deep sedation) to 5 (mild agitation) (Table 1). BIS scores ranged from 43 to 100. Subjective scoring of sedation by the SAS correlated better with the average BIS score ($r^2 = 0.21$) than with the baseline BIS score ($r^2 = 0.14$) (Fig 2). The correlation was better for trauma patients than for other patients and for patients receiving opiates than for patients not receiving opiates.

Conclusion.—The level of sedation for ICU patients was objectively and subjectively quantified by using the BIS as a measure of hypnotic drug effects, as well as the revised SAS.

▶ The need for reliable and consistent objective measures of sedation in critically ill patients is necessary to avoid the adverse effects of prolonged sedation or accidental recall, particularly in those patients receiving neuro-muscular blockade. Recent public fear of awareness during anesthesia has focused the attention on the development of a monitor to prevent this occurrence. BIS monitoring has been purported to be of use in gauging the level of sedation and anesthesia in the operating room and would, thus, appear to be a logical choice as an awareness monitor for critically ill patients as well. Given the subjective nature of rudimentary sedation scales and scoring systems, such as the Ramsay Sedation Scale, a more objective measurement of awareness in critically ill patients would appear to be welcomed. Although this study falls far short of a universal endorsement of BIS monitoring, it does raise the possibility of its use in limited circumstances.

D. M. Rothenberg, MD, FCCM

Effect of Mechanical Ventilation on Inflammatory Mediators in Patients With Acute Respiratory Distress Syndrome: A Randomized Controlled Trial
Ranieri VM, Suter PM, Tortorella C, et al (Università di Bari, Italy; Université de Genèva; Univ of Toronto)
JAMA 282:54-61, 1999   9–10

Introduction.—Mechanical ventilation can augment or cause an inflammatory response and acute lung injury. The influence of mechanical ventilation on the lung and systemic cytokine levels was assessed in patients with acute respiratory distress syndrome in a randomized, controlled trial.

Methods.—The mean age of 44 patients with acute respiratory distress syndrome was 50 years. Patients were enrolled from 2 ICUs between November 1995 and February 1998. Seven patients with adverse events were excluded. At baseline, volume-pressure curves were measured, and patients underwent bronchoalveolar lavage and venipuncture for laboratory testing. Nineteen and 18 patients, respectively, were randomly assigned to either a control or a lung-protective strategy group. For control subjects, the tidal volume was targeted to obtain normal values of arterial carbon dioxide tension of between 35 and 40 mm Hg; positive endexpiratory pressure (PEEP) was set to produce the greatest improvement in arterial oxygen saturation without worsening hemodynamics. The tidal volume and PEEP in the protective strategy group were based on the volume-pressure curve. These measurements were repeated at 24 to 30 hours and 36 to 40 hours after randomization.

Results.—At baseline, physiologic characteristics and cytokine concentrations were similar. There were significant between-group differences in tidal volume, end-inspiratory plateau pressures, and PEEP (11.1 vs 7.6 mL/kg, 31.0 vs 24.6 cm H_2O, and 6.5 vs 14.8 cm H_2O for the control and lung-protective strategy groups, respectively). The control group had increased bronchoalveolar lavage concentrations of interleukin (IL)-1β, IL-6, and IL-1 receptor agonist. Bronchoalveolar lavage and plasma concentrations of tumor necrosis factor (TNF)-α, IL-6, and TNF-α receptors were detected in both groups over 36 hours. Patients in the lung-protective strategy group had diminished bronchoalveolar lavage concentrations of polymorphonuclear cells, TNF-α, IL-1β, soluble TNF-α receptor 55, and IL-8. Diminished concentrations of IL-6, soluble TNF-α receptor 75, and IL-1 receptor antagonist were discovered in bronchoalveolar lavage and serum concentrations. The concentration of the inflammatory mediators 36 hours after randomization was markedly lower in the lung-protective strategy group compared with the control group.

Conclusion.—Mechanical ventilation can produce a cytokine response that may be diminished by minimizing overdistention and recruitment/derecruitment of the lung.

▶ This study adds considerably to the understanding of ventilator-induced lung injury in patients with acute respiratory distress syndrome. In addition to showing that ventilator-induced lung injury does, indeed, occur in humans, the study also provides evidence for a mechanism of action. By showing a decrease in this concentration of cytokines in bronchoalveolar lavage in the lung-protected strategy group, the authors may have established the lung as a site of inflammatory mediator production. This, in turn, could lead to the systemic inflammatory response syndrome and multiorgan system failure, the usual causes of death in these patients. Future questions regarding the optimal levels of tidal volume and PEEP need to be addressed.

D. M. Rothenberg, MD, FCCM

Effect of Enteral Feeding With Eicosapentaenoic Acid, γ-Linolenic Acid, and Antioxidants in Patients With Acute Respiratory Distress Syndrome
Gadek JE, and the Enteral Nutrition in ARDS Study Group (Ohio State Univ, Columbus; et al)
Crit Care Med 27:1409-1420, 1999   9–11

Background.—Low-carbohydrate, high-fat nutritional support for ventilated patients reduces demands on the respiratory system. Dietary fatty acids decrease the severity of inflammatory injury by modulating the availability of arachidonic acid. Animal studies show that diets rich in eicosapentaenoic acid (EPA), γ-linolenic acid (GLA), and antioxidants can moderate inflammation. The effect of enteral feeding with a diet supplemented with EPA, GLA, and antioxidants in reducing pulmonary inflammation and improving gas exchange and clinical outcomes in acute respiratory distress syndrome (ARDS) was compared with that of a standard control diet in a prospective, double-blind, randomized, controlled, multicentered trial.

Methods.—Between July 1993 and March 1997, 146 patients, aged 18 to 80 years, at risk for ARDS, were randomly assigned to a high-fat, low-carbohydrate, enteral control diet (n = 47) or an isonitrogenous, isocaloric enteral (EPA + GLA) diet (n = 51) beginning within 24 hours of entering the study (Table 2). Both diets provided a minimum caloric delivery of 75% of basal energy expenditure × 1.3 for at least 4 to 7 days. Arterial blood gasses were measured and recorded at baseline and during the study period. Gas exchange was calculated, and neutrophil recruitment was assessed.

Results.—Compared with patients receiving the control diet, patients receiving the test diet required significantly fewer days of ventilatory support, in the ICU, and on supplemental oxygen, and significantly fewer

TABLE 2.—Analyzed Composition of Enteral Diets

Nutrient	Control	EPA+GLA
Protein		
% of total calories	16.7	16.7
g/L	62.6	62.5
Source	87% sodium caseinate	87% sodium caseinate
Carbohydrate	13% calcium caseinate	13% calcium caseinate
% of total calories	28.1	28.1
g/L	105.7	105.5
Source	46% maltodextrin	45% maltodextrin
Lipids	54% sucrose	55% sucrose
% of total calories	55.2	55.2
g/L	92.1	93.7
Source	96.8% corn oil	31.8% canola oil
	3.2% soy lecithin	25% MCT
		20% borage oil
		20% fish oil
		3.2% soy lecithin
Vitamins		
Vitamin E (IU/L)	47.6	317
Vitamin C (mg/L)	317	844
β-Carotene (mg/L)	—	5.0
Taurine (mg/L)	—	316
L-Carnitine (mg/L)	—	181
Caloric density (kcal/mL)	1.5	1.5
Osmolality (mOsm/kg/H_2O)	465	493

Note: Each liter of both formulas contained the following vitamins: 5360 IU, vitamin A; 425 IU, vitamin D; 101 µg, vitamin K_1; 850 µg, folic acid; 32 mg, thiamine; 3.6 mg, riboflavin; 4.3 mg, vitamin B_6; 13 µg, vitamin B_{12}; 43 mg, niacin; 635 mg, choline; 635 µg, biotin; 22 mg, pantothenic acid. Each liter of both formulas contained the following trace minerals: 1310 mg, Na; 1960 mg, K; 1690 mg, Cl; 1060 mg, Ca; 1060 mg, P; 425 mg, Mg; 160 µg, I; 5.3 mg, Mn; 2.2 mg, Cu; 24 mg, Zn; 20 mg, Fe; 77 µg, Se; 130 µg, Cr; 160 µg, Mo.

Abbreviations: EPA, eicosapentaenoic acid; *GLA,* γ-linolenic acid; *IU,* international units; *MCT,* medium chain triglycerides.

(Courtesy of Gadek JE, and the Enteral Nutrition in ARDS Study Group: Effect of enteral feeding with eicosapentaenoic acid, γ-linolenic acid, and antioxidants in patients with acute respiratory distress syndrome. *Crit Care Med* 27[8]:1409-1430, 1999.)

test diet patients sustained new organ failure (Fig 3; Table 7). Although infection rates were similar for the 2 groups, the test diet group had a 17% reduction in the number of infections compared with the control diet group (79 vs 95). Patients receiving the test diet had fewer adverse events and a very low percentage of gastrointestinal complaints.

Conclusion.—The test diet is safe, effective, and well tolerated. It reduces pulmonary neutrophil recruitment and inflammation, improves oxygenation, and reduces ventilator time and ICU stays. The efficacy of the diet needs to be tested in patients with severe ARDS.

▶ Nutritional supplementation in critically ill patients has evolved from merely providing adequate caloric intake and promoting positive nitrogen balance to affecting immunomodulation by minimizing the production of inflammatory mediators. This multicenter study offers compelling evidence that diet rich in polyunsaturated long-chain fatty acids, as well as antioxidants, may reduce pulmonary inflammation. The improved clinical outcomes seen in this study, as well as other studies employing fish oil–based

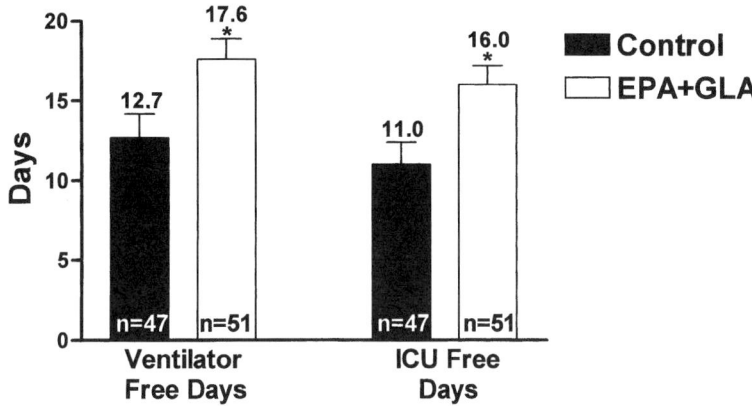

FIGURE 3.—Mean ± SE number of 30-day ventilator-free days and ICU-free days. The *asterisk* indicates that patients fed the eicosapentaenoic acid plus γ-linolenic acid (*EPA + GLA*) diet had 4.9 more ventilator-free days (*P* = .02) and 4.0 more ICU-free days (*P* = .01) compared with patients fed the control diet. (Courtesy of Gadek JE, and the Enteral Nutrition in ARDS Study Group: Effect of enteral feeding with eicosapentaenoic acid, γ-linolenic acid, and antioxidants in patients with acute respiratory distress syndrome. *Crit Care Med* 27[8]:1409-1420, 1999.)

formulas, suggest the need to reassess the manner by which we prescribe standard nutritional therapy. Cost-benefit analyses will be required to convince hospital administrators that "cutting the fat" from their budgets may not be fiscally or medically responsible.

D. M. Rothenberg, MD, FCCM

TABLE 7.—Summary of Outcome Variables

Viable	Intent to Treat			Evaluable		
	Control (n = 72)	EPA+GLA (n =70)	P Value	Control (n = 47)	EPA+GLA (n = 51)	P Value
Time on supplemental oxygen[a] (days)	17.1 ± 1.6	13.6 ± 1.2	.078	20.2 ± 2.1	15.8 ± 1.5	.053
Time on ventilator[a] (days)	13.2 ± 1.4	9.6 ± 0.9	.027	16.3 ± 1.9	11.0 ± 1.1	.011
Intensive care unit stay[a] (days)	14.8 ± 1.3	11.0 ± 0.9	.016	17.5 ± 1.7	12.8 ± 1.1	.016
Hospital stay[a] (days)	31.1 ± 2.4	27.9 ± 2.1	.278	34.6 ± 3.3	29.4 ± 2.6	.07
Mortality (%)	25 (19/76)	16 (11/70)	.165	19 (9/47)	12 (6/51)	.31
New organ failures[b] (%)						
Total	25 (19/76)	10 (7/70)	.018	28 (13/47)	8 (4/51)	.015
Cardiovascular	8 (6/76)	1 (1/70)		9 (4/47)	2 (1/51)	
Renal	9 (7/76)	4 (3/70)		9 (4/47)	2 (1/51)	
Hematologic	4 (3/76)	0 (0/70)		6 (3/47)	0 (0/51)	
Hepatic	4 (3/76)	0 (0/70)		2 (1/47)	0 (0/51)	
Neurologic	5 (4/76)			6 (3/47)	0 (0/51)	
Gastrointestinal	11 (8/76)	7 (5/70)		13 (6/47)	6 (3/51)	

*Values are mean ± SD.

†Percentage of patients, in each group, control or EPA+GLA, who have a new failure in any organ not present at baseline.
Abbreviation: EPA, eicosapentaenoic acid; *GLA*, γ-linolenic acid.

(Courtesy of Gadek JE, and the Enteral Nutrition in ARDS Study Group: Effect of enteral feeding with eicosapentaenoic acid, γ-linolenic acid, and antioxidants in patients with acute respiratory distress syndrome. *Crit Care Med* 27[8]:1409-1420, 1999.)

Increased Mortality Associated With Growth Hormone Treatment in Critically Ill Adults

Takala J, Ruokonen E, Webster NR, et al (Kuopio Univ, Finland; Aberdeen Royal Infirmary, Scotland; Southampton Gen Hosp, England; et al)
N Engl J Med 341:785-792, 1999   9–12

Background.—Essential organ function, tissue repair, wound healing, and immune function may be compromised during the increased protein turnover and negative nitrogen balance characteristic of critical illness. Although growth hormone can mitigate the catabolic process, the effect of high doses on hospital and ICU stay and outcome in critically ill patients has not been studied. The effect of treatment with high doses of growth hormone on clinical outcome was evaluated in 2 independent, prospective, multicenter, double-blind, randomized, placebo-controlled trials in parallel of adult patients who were hospitalized for a lengthy period.

Methods.—The 2 studies involved 247 patients in 6 hospitals in Finland (February 1994 to July 1997) and 285 patients in 12 hospitals in the United Kingdom, the Netherlands, Belgium, and Sweden (June 1994 to July 1997). Patients, aged 18 to 80 years, in intensive care and expected to stay there for at least 10 days because of cardiac surgery, abdominal surgery, multiple trauma, or acute respiratory failure, received subcutaneous injections of recombinant growth hormone, ranging from 0.07 to 0.13 mg/kg, or saline once daily in the morning for no longer than 21 days.

Results.—Baseline characteristics were similar for the 2 groups, and the average daily growth hormone dose was the same for survivors and nonsurvivors. In-hospital mortality was significantly higher for the growth-hormone groups in both studies (39% in the Finnish study and 44% in the multinational study) than for the placebo groups (20% and 18%, respectively). The pattern in mortality differences was the same at 6 months (43% and 52% for the respective growth hormone groups vs 23% and 25% for the placebo groups) with multiple-organ failure and septic shock or uncontrolled infection as the primary causes of death (Table 2).

Those treated with growth hormone who survived to discharge had longer periods of mechanical ventilation, intensive care, and hospitalization, and higher cumulative Therapeutic Intervention Scoring System scores than those who received placebo. Survivors receiving growth hormone in the multinational study had significantly poorer exercise tolerance than placebo-treated survivors. Nitrogen balance was significantly better in the growth hormone-treated patients than in the placebo patients in the Finnish study on days 7, 14, and 21.

Conclusion.—Administration of growth hormone to critically ill patients increases mortality and prolongs mechanical ventilation and length of hospital and ICU stays.

▶ For many years, clinicians have attempted to improve muscle strength in critically ill patients, particularly those who have difficulty in being weaned from mechanical ventilation. Results of previous data regarding the use of

TABLE 2.—In-Hospital Deaths and Causes of Death During Intensive Care

Deaths and Causes	Finnish Study			Multinational Study		
	Growth Hormone (N = 119)	Placebo (n = 123)	P Value	Growth Hormone (N = 139)	Placebo (N = 141)	P Value
Deaths						
Total—no. of patients (%)	47 (39)	25 (20)	<0.001	61 (44)	26 (18)	<0.001
Relative risk of death (95% CI)	1.9 (1.3–2.9)			2.4 (1.6–3.5)		
Diagnostic group—no. of patients/total no. (%)						
Cardiac surgery	10/24 (42)	6/25 (24)		21/40 (52)	8/47 (17)	
Abdominal surgery	17/33 (52)	11/36 (31)		12/25 (48)	10/25 (40)	
Trauma	2/7 (29)	1/8 (12)		4/20 (20)	1/25 (4)	
Acute respiratory failure	18/55 (33)	7/54 (13)		24/54 (44)	7/44 (16)	
APACHE II score during first 24 hr—no. of patients/total no. (%)						
≤20	30/79 (38)	12/83 (14)		42/100 (42)	13/92 (14)	
>20	17/40 (42)	13/40 (32)		19/39 (49)	13/49 (27)	
APACHE II score at enrollment—no. of patients/total no. (%)						
≤20	34/97 (35)	22/110 (20)		43/115 (37)	16/115 (14)	
>20	13/22 (59)	3/13 (23)		18/24 (75)	10/26 (38)	
Age—no. of patients/total no. (%)						
<55 yr	9/36 (25)	7/47 (15)		8/34 (24)	0/35	
55–70 yr	17/45 (38)	7/44 (16)		28/61 (46)	14/61 (23)	
>70 yr	21/38 (55)	11/32 (34)		25/44 (57)	12/45 (27)	
Causes of death during intensive care—no. of patients			0.66			0.71
Multiple-organ failure	12	6		22	11	
Septic shock or uncontrolled infection	15	4		16	4	
Cardiovascular cause	3	2		9	2	
Refractory respiratory failure	2	1		4	1	
Other	4	4		3	2	

Note: P values are for comparison between the treatment groups in each study.
Abbreviations: CI, confidence interval; APACHE, Acute Physiology and Chronic Health Evaluation.
(Reprinted by permission, from Takala J, Ruokonen E, Webster NR, et al: Increased mortality associated with growth hormone treatment in critically ill adults. N Engl J Med 341:785-792, 1999. Copyright 1999, Massachusetts Medical Society. All rights reserved.)

growth hormone in this context have been mixed. In this unique multicenter study, the use of subcutaneously injected recombinant growth hormone in a select group of critically ill patients showed a marked increase in morbidity and mortality, possibly reflecting the drug's complex mechanisms of action as they relate to immunomodulation.

An intriguing aspect of this study, which is unfortunately not specifically described, relates to the use of insulin-like growth factor for the treatment of acute renal failure. Clinical studies have alluded to the possible beneficial effect of insulin-like growth factor on the reparative phase of acute tubular necrosis. The ultimate mortality data from this study, however, may preclude any future studies involving the use of growth hormone analogues for the treatment of acute renal failure.

D. M. Rothenberg, MD, FCCM

A Randomized Clinical Trial of Continuous Aspiration of Subglottic Secretions in Cardiac Surgery Patients

Kollef MH, Skubas NJ, Sundt TM (Washington Univ, St Louis)
Chest 116:1339-1346, 1999   9–13

Background.—The incidence of ventilator-associated pneumonia (VAP) can be decreased by continuous aspiration of subglottic secretions (CASS) that pool above the endotracheal tube cuff. The incidence of VAP and other important clinical outcomes among patients receiving CASS was compared with outcomes in patients receiving routine postoperative medical care without CASS in a clinical trial.

Methods.—Patients older than 18 years undergoing cardiac surgery and requiring mechanical ventilation in the cardiothoracic ICU were randomly assigned to receive CASS (n = 160; 58 female) using a special endotracheal tube that creates a dorsal opening above the cuff, with a separate lumen for aspiration of subglottic secretions, or routine postoperative care (n = 183; 62 female). Subglottic suction was supplied continuously at 20 mm Hg or less with a standard wall unit.

Results.—There were no significant clinical or risk differences between groups at baseline. VAP developed, at an average of 3.8 days in 23 (6.7%) patients (39.7 episodes per 1000 ventilator days). These included 8 (5%) CASS patients (34.5 episodes per 1000 ventilator days) and 15 (8.2%) patients without CASS (43.2 episodes per 1000 ventilator days). VAP occurred significantly later in CASS patients than in patients without CASS (5.6 vs 2.9 days) (Fig 1). Multiple logistic regression analysis risk factors for development of CASS included supine positioning, duration of mechanical ventilation, and an acute Physiology and Chronic Health Evaluation II score. CASS was not associated with development of VAP, according to multivariate analysis. The average duration of mechanical ventilation, lengths of stay in the ICU and the hospital, and the number of organ derangements were similar for the 2 groups. Hospital mortality rates were also similar for the 2 groups.

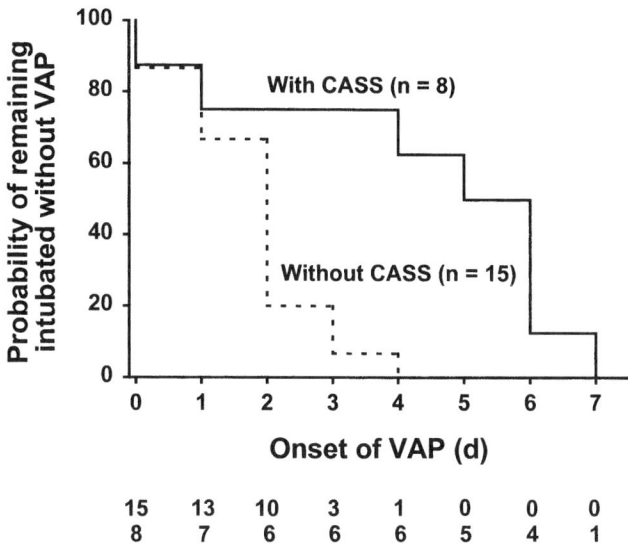

FIGURE 1.—Comparison of onset of ventilator-associated pneumonia (*VAP*), among patients in whom this nosocomial infection developed, according to the presence or absence of continuous aspiration of subglottic secretions (*CASS*). *Numbers at bottom* indicate intubated patients remaining without VAP (*upper row*, patients without CASS; *lower row*, patients receiving CASS). (Courtesy of Kollef MH, Skubas NJ, Sundt TM: A randomized clinical trial of continuous aspiration of subglottic secretions in cardiac surgery. *Chest* 116:1339-1346, 1999.)

Conclusion.—The rate of VAP was nonsignificantly lower and occurred significantly later in CASS patients than in patients without CASS.

▶ Although I do not see any benefit of this type of endotracheal tube for those patients undergoing fast track anesthesia for cardiac surgery, the additional cost of this device may be warranted for those patients in whom prolonged mechanical ventilation is anticipated. Patients with significant chronic obstructive pulmonary disease, obesity, low output syndrome, etc may benefit from CASS. A future study addressing patients specifically at risk of nosocomial pneumonia appears to be warranted.

D. M. Rothenberg, MD, FCCM

Significant Tracheal Obstruction Causing Failure to Wean in Patients Requiring Prolonged Mechanical Ventilation: A Forgotten Complication of Long-term Mechanical Ventilation
Rumbak MJ, Walsh FW, Anderson WMcD, et al (Univ of South Florida, Tampa)
Chest 115:1092-1095, 1999   9–14

Objective.—Despite the fact that most tracheostomy tubes have low-pressure, high-volume cuffs, tracheal injury still occurs with prolonged use. If the condition goes undetected in patients receiving long-term me-

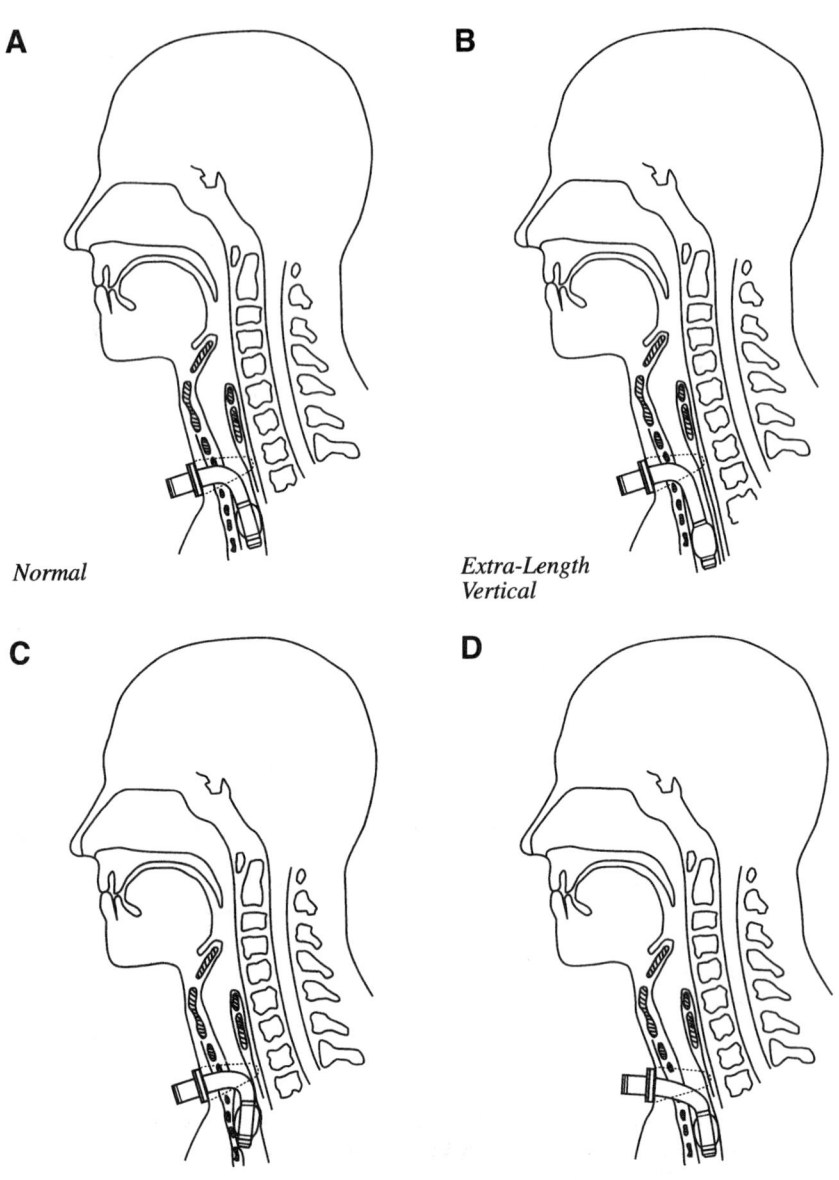

A Normal

B Extra-Length Vertical

C Extra-Length Horizontal Wrong Patient Selection

D Extra-Length Horizontal Obese Patient

FIGURE 2.—**A,** The normal tracheotomy tube in relation to the normal trachea. **D,** The "extra-long" tracheotomy tube for the obese patient. This is longer in the horizontal length. **C,** This reveals what happens to an extra-long tracheotomy tube if it is inserted into a normal trachea in an attempt to overcome an obstruction in the vertical length. **B,** This reveals the vertical extra-length placement of the correct tracheotomy tube that is usually custom made. A double-cuffed Portex can be used until the custom tube is available. Be aware that this cuff is a high-pressure, low-volume cuff. (Courtesy of Rumbak MJ, Walsh FW, Anderson WMcD, et al: Significant tracheal obstruction causing failure to wean in patients requiring prolonged mechanical ventilation: A forgotten complication of long-term mechanical ventilation. *Chest* 115:1092-1095, 1999.)

chanical ventilation, it may lead to failure to wean. Obstruction should be suspected when failure to wean is accompanied by rising peak airway pressures, difficulty in passing the tracheal suction catheter, difficulty in breathing, or sudden change in the weaning status (more than 30 breaths/min, pulse rate or blood pressure increase or decrease of 20% requiring reinstitution of mechanical ventilation).

Methods.—Between September 1994 and August 1997, records of 37 patients (14 men) requiring prolonged mechanical ventilation were retrospectively reviewed. Underlying conditions included chronic obstructive pulmonary disease, postcoronary artery bypass grafting, postpneumonectomy, severe pneumonia, acute lung injury, and ischemic heart disease. Fiberoptic bronchoscopy was performed after several failed weaning attempts.

Results.—Patients experienced difficulty in breathing or intermittent high peak airway pressures. Use of a longer tracheotomy tube relieved the obstruction and allowed weaning in 35 patients within 1 week (Fig 2). Three patients received tracheal stents. Two patients could not be weaned because of neurologic disease.

Conclusion.—Difficult-to-wean patients should undergo bronchoscopy to determine whether tracheal obstruction is the cause.

▶ Patients who require prolonged mechanical ventilation often fail to wean because of muscle fatigue, concurrent infection, or other organ system failure. Providing adequate nutrition, rest, and directive medical therapy maximizes the patient's chances to be successfully weaned and eventually liberated from mechanical ventilation. Upper airway obstruction distal to an endotracheal tube or tracheostomy should also be considered in those patients who have difficulty weaning. The authors state that by providing a longer tracheostomy tube this obstruction can be alleviated and patients successfully weaned. I can only assume that patients still require their tracheostomy although this is not mentioned in the article. Nonetheless, the authors raise a valid concern regarding patients who have difficulty weaning from mechanical ventilation.

D. M. Rothenberg, MD, FCCM

The Assessment of Four Different Methods to Verify Tracheal Tube Placement in the Critical Care Setting
Knapp S, Kofler J, Stoiser B, et al (Univ of Vienna)
Anesth Analg 88:766-770, 1999   9–15

Objective.—Unintended esophageal intubation is a leading cause of brain damage or death. Four different methods for detecting endotracheal tube position include auscultation, capnographic determination of end-tidal carbon dioxide concentration (ET_{CO_2}), esophageal detection method using a self-inflating bulb, and the transillumination method using a

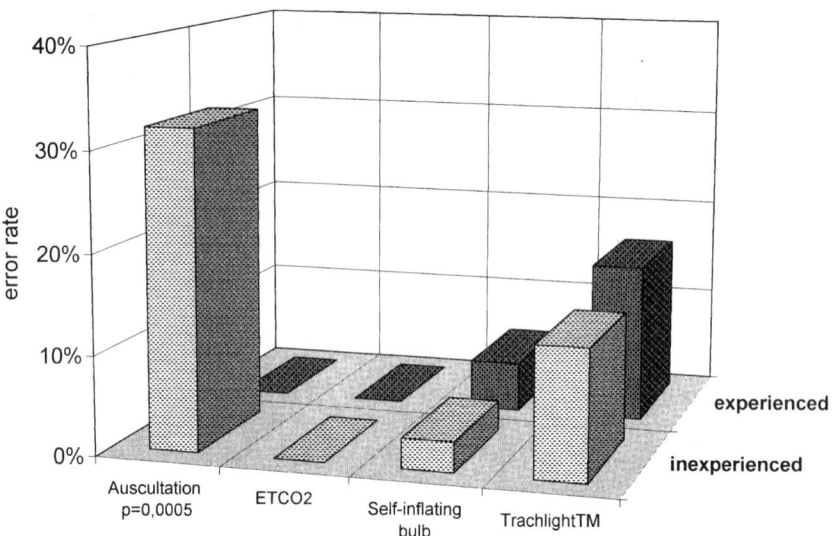

FIGURE 1.—Error rates of experienced and inexperienced examiners obtained by evaluating tube placement using one of four methods. (Courtesy of Knapp S, Kofler J, Stoiser B, et al: The assessment of four different methods to verify tracheal tube placement in the critical care setting. *Anesth Analg* 88[4]:766-770, 1999.)

lighted stylet. The reliability of these methods were compared, and the influence of examiner experience was assessed.

Methods.—Correct chest position of the endotracheal tube was verified by chest radiograph in 38 consecutive, intubated adult patients (16 women), with an average age 62 years, requiring prolonged mechanical ventilation. A second tube was inserted into the esophagus by the same investigator, both cuffs were inflated, the patient's head was covered so that only the tube ends were visible, and the tracheal tube was disconnected from the ventilator. A physician with 4 years' experience and a final year medical student with little experience in critical care determined the position of the tube using one of the four methods. During the test period, the patient received manual ventilation. The selection of the tube to be tested and the detection method were chosen randomly.

Results.—All patients were respiratorily and hemodynamically stable. Of the 152 tubes tested, 74 were in the tracheal position and 78 were in the esophageal position. Diagnosis of position was correct in 130 of 152 examinations by both examiners. In four cases, both examiners were wrong; in four cases, the experienced examiner was wrong; and in 14 cases, the inexperienced examiner was wrong. Using auscultation, the experienced examiner was right in all cases, but the inexperienced examiner was right in only 68% of cases ($P = .0005$). Using ET_{CO_2}, both examiners were right in all cases (Fig 1). Using the esophageal detection method, one experienced examiner and one experienced and inexperienced team was wrong. All results were false negative because the tube was placed in the trachea but the self-inflating bulb did not inflate. Using transillumination, the experienced examiner was wrong six times (16%; two false-positive, four false-negative findings) and the inexperienced examiner was wrong in five cases (13%; two false-positive, three false-negative findings).

Conclusion.—Use of capnography resulted in correct diagnoses of tube position in all patients, although examiner experience is important in performing auscultation procedure correctly. With the self-inflating bulb, results were accurate in 96% of cases, but transillumination was not reliable.

▶ It would seem that if ETco$_2$ is a standard monitor in the operating room to detect inadvertent esophageal intubation, then its use in the ICU would be that much more important, given the emergency and often tumultuous settings in which endotracheal intubation must be performed. This would seem even more critical in obese patients, in whom the use of self-inflating bulbs or syringe aspiration techniques may be inaccurate due to collapse of large airways under the influence of subatmospheric pressure.

D. M. Rothenberg, MD, FCCM

Complications of Emergency Intubation With and Without Paralysis
Li J, Murphy-Lavoie H, Bugas C, et al (Charity Hosp, New Orleans, La)
Am J Emerg Med 17:141-144, 1999   9–16

Objective.—Of 2 methods of endotracheal intubation — rapid-sequence intubation (RSI) and intubation minus paralysis ([IMP]—RSI is superior outside of the emergency setting. Because RSI represents an essential skill for emergency physicians, and little information about the safety and efficacy of RSI in the hands of emergency physicians is available, the complications of RSI and IMP were compared in emergency patients.

Methods.—During a 6-month period immediately after implementation of RSI protocols, data were gathered on 166 patients intubated with RSI that were similar to data gathered on 67 patients intubated with IMP in the

TABLE 1.—Complications Rapid-Sequence Intubation Versus
Intubation Minus Paralysis

	RSI		IMP		*P* Value
Total cases	166		67		
Cases with complications	46	28%	52	78%	<.0001
Multiple attempts (≤3)	41	25%	29	43%	<.0001
Multiple attempts (≥4)	3	2%	16	24%	<.0001
Esophageal intubation	5	3%	12	18%	<.0001
Unable to intubate	1	1%	12	18%	<.0001
Airway trauma	0	0%	19	28%	<.0001
Aspiration	0	0%	10	15%	<.0001
Death	0	0%	2	3%	.03

Note: Noninteger percentages have been rounded to the nearest integer value.
Abbreviations: RSI, rapid-sequence intubation; *IMP,* intubation minus paralysis.
(Courtesy of Li J, Murphy-Lavoie H, Bugas C, et al: Complications of emergency intubation with and without paralysis.
Am J Emerg Med 17:141-144, 1999.)

previous 3 months. Complications—including multiple attempts, esophageal intubation, aspiration, airway trauma, inability to intubate, and death—were recorded. The IMP group received a variety of sedatives but not neuromuscular block. The RSI group received succinyl choline or rocuronium.

Results.—IMP was performed by experienced third- and fourth-year residents and RSI by less-experienced second- through fourth-year residents. Where intubation was unsuccessful, emergency department personnel made additional attempts at their discretion. There was a significant increase in complications with RSI compared with IMP, mainly as a result of multiple attempts. Most RSI attempts were successful within 3 tries. Esophageal intubation occurred in 3% of patients and was corrected in all cases. There were no other complications. Both rate and severity of complications increased with IMP. Most IMP-associated complications were multiple combinations (Table 1).

Conclusion.—The use of RSI by emergency physicians improves patient care.

▶ It seems that each year I pick on our emergency medicine colleagues for their attempts to publish studies documenting the safety of using anesthetic agents, including muscle relaxants, for intubations in the emergency department. This year appears to be no exception. Although the authors attempt a prospective study, they themselves recognize the limitations of comparing endotracheal intubation techniques between different time periods and by different levels of trainees. In addition, the authors' definitions of aspiration and other complications are not clearly delineated.

Although information regarding the indication for intubation was collected, it was not reported in this manuscript and, thus, makes it difficult to determine which group of patients received these drugs in an appropriate fashion. I certainly hope that no patient received etomidate and succinylcholine to facilitate intubation in a setting of cardiopulmonary arrest. Nonetheless, this is not clearly delineated in the manuscript.

I am sure that our emergency room colleagues will continue to feel that these agents are appropriate to use for intubation. However, until larger, randomized, controlled studies are performed (with evidence that proper in-servicing and education have been done by anesthesiologists regarding the use of these drugs), I will remain skeptical of the authors' conclusion.

D. M. Rothenberg, MD, FCCM

Pneumothorax and Systemic Air Embolism During Positive-Pressure Ventilation
Ibrahim AE, Stanwood PL, Freund PR (Univ of Washington, Seattle)
Anesthesiology 90:1479-1481, 1999   9–17

Objective.—The mechanism of systemic air embolization, a complication of mechanical ventilation, is not known. A case was presented of a

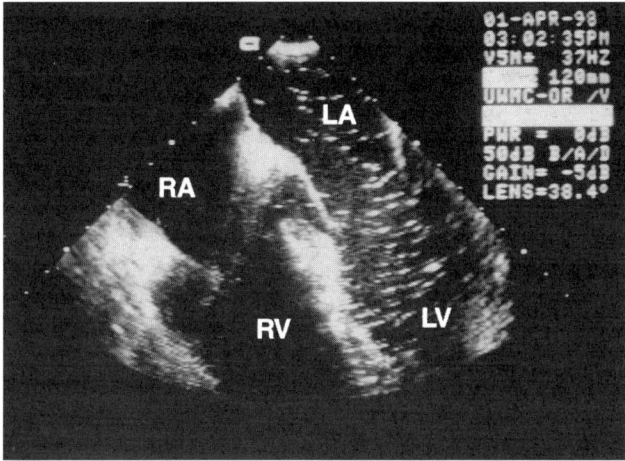

FIGURE 1.—The transesophageal 4-chamber view reveals numerous air bubbles in the left atrium (*LA*) and left ventricle (*LV*). No air bubbles are seen in the right atrium (*RA*) or right ventricle (*RV*). (Courtesy of Ibrahim AE, Stanwood PL, Freund PR: Pneumothorax and systemic air embolism during positive-pressure ventilation. *Anesthesiology* 90:1479-1481, 1999. Copyright American Society of Anesthesiologists, Inc. Used with permission of Lippincott-Raven Publishers.)

tension pneumothorax and systemic air emboli that developed during pancreatic debridement.

> *Case Report.*—Man, 58, with necrotizing pancreatitis of 3-weeks' duration, underwent operative pancreatic debridement. He had an IV line, right radial arterial line, and a right internal jugular triple-lumen central line. Anesthesia was induced with etomidate and fentanyl. He was given succinyl choline to facilitate intubation and intermittent boluses of pancuronium. He was mechanically ventilated and had a respiratory rate of 10 breaths/min.
>
> About 2 hours into the procedure, the patient had difficulty breathing, became cyanotic, and had high airway resistance. Tachycardia and hypotension developed. He had distant bilateral breath sounds. He was treated with 100% oxygen, chest compressions, crystalloid volume resuscitation, angiocatheters in the second thorocostal space, bilateral chest tube thoracostomies, and several boluses of epinephrine. Transesophageal echocardiography produced normal results. The patient had no intracardial septal defects, but a stream of bubbles, emanating from the tracheobronchial tree was observed in the left atrium and ventricle (Fig 1). When the endotracheal tube was advanced into the right mainstem bronchus to avoid left lung ventilation, the bubbles on transesophageal echocardiography disappeared (Fig 2). When the endotracheal tube was put back into the trachea, the bubbles reappeared. Bilateral chest thoracostomies were performed. Air escaped from

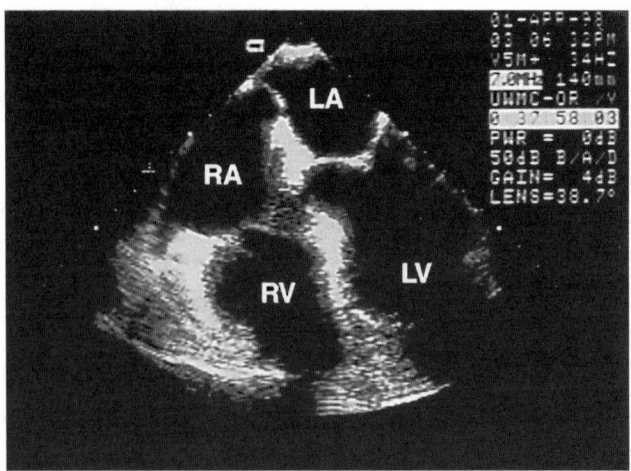

FIGURE 2.—Shown is the same 4-chamber view as in Figure 1 as the endotracheal tube is advanced into the right mainstem bronchus (occluding the left mainstem bronchus). Note the air bubbles in the left atrium (*LA*) and the left ventricle (*LV*) have disappeared. *Abbreviations: RA*, right atrium; *RV*, right ventricle. (Courtesy of Ibrahim AE, Stanwood PL, Freund PR: Pneumothorax and systemic air embolism during positive-pressure ventilation. *Anesthesiology* 90:1479-1481, 1999. Copyright American Society of Anesthesiologists, Inc. Used with permission of Lippincott-Raven Publishers.)

the left chest as the tube was placed. The patient improved immediately and the bubbles on the left side of the heart disappeared.

Discussion.—The pneumothorax was probably caused by barotrauma, although a surgical dissection cause cannot be ruled out. The pneumothorax that developed on the right side was caused by the right internal jugular central line placement. Probably an air embolism arose as a result of a bronchovenous connection from the left bronchial tree to the pulmonary veins, perhaps from rupture of an overdistended alveolus or subpleural cyst and laceration of a pulmonary vein creating a bronchopulmonary venous fistula.

Conclusion.—Systemic air embolism associated with mechanical ventilation should be suspected if there are mental status changes, seizures of unknown etiology, or myocardial injury.

▶ With the more frequent use of intraoperative transeophageal echocardiography, systemic air embolization may become more commonly described. The authors offer a unique theory as to why systemic air embolization developed in this patient.

D. M. Rothenberg, MD, FCCM

Hemodynamic Support and Maintenance of Perfusion

A Comparison of Standard Cardiopulmonary Resuscitation and Active Compression-Decompression Resuscitation for Out-of-Hospital Cardiac Arrest
Plaisance P, and the French Active Compression-Decompression Cardiopulmonary Resuscitation Study Group (Lariboisière Univ, Paris; et al)
N Engl J Med 341:569-575, 1999   9–18

Background.—Active compression-decompression CPR significantly improves survival when compared with standard CPR. Whether 1-year survival and neurologic outcome are also significantly improved when this technique is used during advanced life support was evaluated in patients with out-of-hospital cardiac arrest.

Methods.—Between November 1993 and May 1995, an evaluation was made of 1-year survival of all patients with cardiac arrest in metropolitan Paris or Thionville, France and receiving at-the-scene standard CPR (n = 377) or active compression-decompression CPR with a CardioPump (n = 373). Survival to hospital discharge without neurologic impairment and neurologic outcome were also assessed.

Results.—Although baseline characteristics of the 2 groups were similar, 1-year survival of patients receiving active compression-decompression CPR was significantly higher than for patients receiving standard CPR (Table 2). All 1-year survivors in both groups had cardiac arrests that were witnessed. Neurologic status had recovered in more 1-year survivors in the active compression-decompression group than in the standard CPR group

TABLE 2.—Short-term and Long-term Outcomes Among Patients Assigned to Standard CPR or Active Compression-Decompression CPR for Advanced Life Support

Outcome	Standard CPR (n = 377)	Active Compression-Decompression CPR (n = 373)	Odds Ratio (95% CI)*
	no. (%)		
Return of spontaneous circulation	111 (29)	146 (39)	1.5 (1.1-2.1)
Survival at 1 hr	88 (23)	117 (31)	1.5 (1.1-2.1)
Admission to intensive care unit	85 (23)	109 (29)	1.4 (1.02-1.97)
Survival at 24 hr	51 (14)	85 (23)	1.9 (1.3-2.8)
Survival at 7 days	20 (5)	38 (10)	2.0 (1.2-3.6)
Hospital discharge without neurologic impairment	7 (2)	21 (6)	3.2 (1.3-7.5)†
Survival at 1 yr	7 (2)	17 (5)	2.5 (1.03-6.16)

*Odds ratios are the odds of the outcome in question in the group that received active compression-decompression CPR compared with the odds in the standard CPR group.
†*P* = .01.

(71% vs 43%, $P = .34$). The duration of CPR was significantly shorter in the active compression-decompression group than in the standard CPR group (9.5 vs 22.3 min), despite the fact that the advanced life support unit arrived significantly more quickly for survivors in the standard CPR group than for patients in the active compression-decompression group (2.1 vs 14.1 min).

Conclusion.—The rate of survival at 1 year with active compression-decompression CPR is more than twice that with standard CPR and is higher than the hospital discharge rates associated with standard CPR in many metropolitan areas with trained emergency personnel.

▶ Asystole and pulseless electrical activity remain highly mortal events which, despite the use of alternative forms of CPR, still result in dismal survival rates. The ability to perform active compression-decompression resuscitation in the field will require a greater level of training for the lay population, who at this time have rudimentary skills in basic CPR. Improving overall survival appears to best be directed toward the management of out-of-hospital ventricular fibrillation with the use of automated external defibrillators.

D. M. Rothenberg, MD, FCCM

Amiodarone for Resuscitation After Out-of-Hospital Cardiac Arrest Due to Ventricular Fibrillation
Kudenchuk PJ, Cobb LA, Copass MK, et al (Univ of Washington, Seattle; Seattle Fire Dept)
N Engl J Med 341:871-878, 1999   9–19

Objective.—At least 250,000 persons die annually from sudden cardiac death. Whether antiarrhythmic drugs are helpful has not been convincingly demonstrated. Results of a randomized, placebo-controlled study to determine the efficacy of IV amiodarone in patients with out-of-hospital cardiac arrest from shock-refractory ventricular fibrillation or tachycardia were presented.

Methods.—Either amiodarone (300 mg) (n = 246; 76% male) or placebo (n = 258; 79% male) was randomly administered IV between November 1994 and February 1997 to patients with cardiac arrest who were unresponsive to 3 or more precordial shocks. The outcome measure was admission to the hospital with a spontaneous perfusing rhythm. Rates of survival were compared for the 2 groups.

Results.—The total average duration of resuscitation attempts was similar for both groups, lasting 42 minutes for the amiodarone group and 43 minutes for the placebo group. The average numbers of shocks delivered until spontaneous circulation returned were 4 and 6, respectively. The percentage of patients receiving antiarrhythmic drugs was similar in both groups, 80% and 82%, respectively. Resuscitated patients treated with amiodarone were significantly more likely than placebo patients to require treatment for hypotension (59% vs 48%) or bradycardia (41% vs 25%).

Amiodarone patients were significantly more likely than placebo patients to survive to hospital admission (44% vs 34%; odds ratio [OR], 1.6). Patients with ventricular fibrillation were significantly more likely than patients with asystole or pulseless electrical activity to survive to hospital admission (44% vs 14%; OR, 5.2). Patients with spontaneous return of circulation were significantly more likely than patients who remained pulseless to survive to hospital admission (53% vs 30%; OR, 2.7). More women than men survived to admission (43% vs 38%; OR, 1.6). The survival for women treated with amiodarone was significantly higher than for women receiving placebo (OR, 4.3). The study did not have sufficient statistical power to determine differences in survival to hospital discharge.

Conclusion.—Amiodarone-treated patients with refractory ventricular arrhythmias had significantly improved survival to hospital admission. Women treated with amiodarone had a significantly higher survival to hospital admission than did men. Additional studies need to be done to determine whether the survival difference extends to hospital discharge.

▶ Amiodarone appears to be the antiarrhythmic of the future, having supplanted many of the type I antiarrhythmic drugs for the treatment of chronic ventricular tachycardia and atrial fibrillation. Given the national shortage of bretylium, I would not be the least bit surprised to see amiodarone recommended as the second line of therapy (after lidocaine) for the treatment of ventricular tachycardia.

D. M. Rothenberg, MD, FCCM

Perioperative Resuscitation Knowledge Base
Porayko LD, Butler R (London Health Sciences Ctr, Ont)
Can J Anesth 46:529-535, 1999   9–20

Objective.—A survey was developed to assess the knowledge of Canadian anesthesiologists concerning special resuscitation measures during anesthesia and surgery for perioperative cardiac arrest. The relationship between the participant's score and the time elapsed since residency and since the last Advanced Cardiac Life Support course, the influence of the practice of cardiac anesthesia, and the perceived utility of current American Heart Association guidelines in anesthesia practice were analyzed.

Methods.—The survey was mailed to 200 randomly selected Canadian Anesthesia Society members. It included 10 clinical vignettes followed by scenarios from which anonymous participants were to select the best management intervention. Each correct answer contributed 1 point toward a maximum of 10. Each vignette was taken from a patient's chart. A passing score was 70% or greater.

Results.—A total of 124 responses were received. The average overall score was 5.1, the median score was 5, and the range was 0 to 9. Percentage scores ranged from 27% to 78% (Table 2). At least 1 "lethal error" was selected by 56% of participants. Although 25 (20.2%) respondents

TABLE 2.—Breakdown of Scoring by Question

Question	% Correct
1. Succinylcholine induced hyperkalemic arrest in a burn patient	71%
2. Ventricular fibrillation in patient with implantable defibrillator	30%
3. Rapid irregular wide complex rhythm in patient with Wolf-Parkinson-White syndrome undergoing cataract extraction . . .	41%
4. Bupivicaine induced cardiac arrest in parturient	39%
5. Pulseless electrical activity in a patient with chronic obstructive lung disease secondary to auto-PEEP	48%
6. Torsade des Pointes in patient with congenital prolonged QT interval	63%
7. Severe bradycardia and hypotension secondary to beta-blocker overdose	27%
8. Malignant Hyperthermia with rapid SVT and hypertension . . .	50%
9. Complete heart block in patient with LBBB induced by pulmonary artery catheter	78%
10. Bradycardia and hypotension in trauma victim with severe hypothermia	73%

(Courtesy of Porayko LD, Butler R: Perioperative resuscitation knowledge base. *Can J Anesth* 46:529-535, 1999.)

scored 70% or greater, only 17 scored 70% or greater and avoided a lethal error. Score and years of residency or time since last Advanced Cardiac Life Support course were unrelated. Participants who practiced cardiac anesthesia had significantly higher scores than those who did not.

Conclusion.—Because participants had lower scores and a higher lethal error rate than expected, research and education resources need to be committed to overcoming this knowledge deficit.

▶ To my knowledge, all residents in United States programs receive training in Advanced Cardiac Life Support as part of their initial house officer orientation. Unfortunately, unless these physicians remain active in American Heart Association–sponsored teaching programs at a provider level, studies have shown that most lose their skills and knowledge within 6 months of their initial training. This study corroborates these findings, but also points out the fact that the lack of knowledge may lead to potentially "lethal errors." The American Board of Anesthesiology is currently considering a mandate that requires all residents in accredited anesthesiology programs to have current Advanced Cardiac Life Support certification. Maintaining a knowledge base and skill level to appropriately manage crisis situations that commonly occur in the perioperative phase of care may be further enhanced by additional training with anesthesiology simulators.

D. M. Rothenberg, MD, FCCM

Facilitating Transthoracic Cardioversion of Atrial Fibrillation With Ibutilide Pretreatment
Oral H, Souza JJ, Michaud GF, et al (Univ of Michigan, Ann Arbor)
N Engl J Med 340:1849-1854, 1999   9–21

Objective.—It is not always possible to convert atrial fibrillation to sinus rhythm using electrical cardioversion. The class III antiarrhythmic

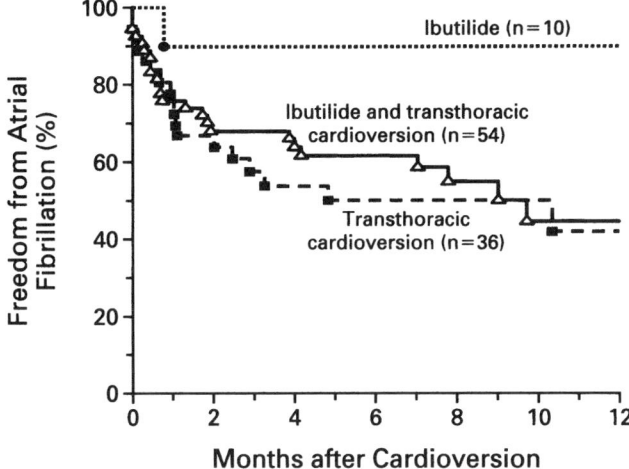

Months after Cardioversion

FIGURE 1.—Kaplan-Meier analysis of the percentage of patients remaining free of recurrent atrial fibrillation after the restoration of sinus rhythm with ibutilide, transthoracic cardioversion alone, or transthoracic with ibutilide pretreatment. There were no significant differences among the 3 groups ($P = .13$ by the log-rank test). The number of patients in each treatment group is shown in parentheses. (Reprinted by permission, from Oral H, Souza JJ, Michaud GF, et al: Facilitating transthoracic cardioversion of atrial fibrillation with ibutilide pretreatment. *N Engl J Med* 340:1849-1854, copyright 1999, Massachusetts Medical Society. All rights reserved.)

drug ibutilide can convert atrial fibrillation to sinus rhythm and reduce the energy requirement for ventricular defibrillation, though its effect on the energy requirement for atrial defibrillation is unknown. The ability of ibutilide to facilitate atrial fibrillation resistant to transthoracic electrical cardioversion was studied.

Methods.—One hundred consecutive patients referred for cardioversion of an episode of atrial fibrillation lasting more than 6 hours were included in the randomized trial. The mean duration of the episode was 117 days. All patients underwent transthoracic cardioversion. One group was pretreated with ibutilide, 1 mg; the other was not. For cardioversion, shocks were delivered in step-up fashion at 50, 100, 200, 300, and 360 J. If cardioversion could not be achieved in a patient who had not received ibutilide pretreatment, the drug was given and cardioversion was attempted again.

Results.—The rate of conversion to sinus rhythm was 100% among patients pretreated with ibutilide versus 72% in the control group. For the 14 patients in whom cardioversion failed, sinus rhythm was restored after ibutilide was given and cardioversion was attempted again. Mean energy required to achieve cardioversion was 166 J with ibutilide pretreatment and 228 J without ibutilide pretreatment. Of the total 64 patients who received ibutilide, 2 developed sustained polymorphic ventricular tachycardia; both of these patients had a left ventricular ejection fraction of 0.20 or less. At 6 months' follow-up, the 2 groups had comparable rates of freedom from atrial fibrillation (Fig 1).

Conclusions.—In patients with atrial fibrillation, treatment with ibutilide before transthoracic electrical cardioversion can facilitate cardioversion. Ibutilide should not be used in patients with very low ejection fractions. More research is needed to determine the most cost-effective use of ibutilide as an adjunct to transthoracic cardioversion.

▶ Atrial fibrillation occurs in approximately one third of patients undergoing cardiopulmonary bypass and results in increased morbidity in prolonged hospitalization. Given that ibutilide appears to be most effective when administered acutely, perhaps the combination of ibutilide and cardioversion will be the most optimal form of treatment for atrial fibrillation immediately following open-heart surgery.

Similar studies comparing cardioversion with or without low-dose amiodarone have also proved to be medically beneficial and cost-effective.[1]

D. M. Rothenberg, MD, FCCM

Reference

1. Catherwood E, Fitzpatrick WD, Greenberg ML, et al: Cost-effectiveness of cardioversion and antiarrhythmic therapy in nonvalvular atrial fibrillation. *Ann Intern Med* 130:625-636, 1999.

Preoperative Serum Potassium Levels and Perioperative Outcomes in Cardiac Surgery Patients
Wahr JA, for the Multicenter Study of Perioperative Ischemia Research Group (Univ of Michigan, Ann Arbor; et al)
JAMA 281:2203-2210, 1999   9–22

Background.—Preoperative serum potassium values of less than 3.5 mmol/L may be associated with perioperative mortality in patients with coronary artery disease. The recommendation to delay surgery in patients with hypokalemia is controversial because 2 studies have shown no difference in the incidence of intraoperative arrhythmias for patients with low or normal serum potassium levels. The prevalence of abnormal preoperative potassium levels and the incidence of adverse perioperative events was prospectively assessed in a multicenter observational study of patients undergoing elective coronary artery bypass graft surgery.

Methods.—Twelve-lead electrocardiograms were obtained within 1 week before surgery, within 3 days after surgery, and within 10 days after surgery in 2417 patients. Myocardial infarction was diagnosed by at least 2 of 3 blinded elecrocardiographers. Outcome measures included perioperative arrhythmias, death, cardiac death, and need for CPR.

Results.—Serum potassium levels of the 2402 (99.3%) eligible patients were normally distributed. Seventy (2.9%) patients had abnormally low serum potassium values (<3.5 mmol/L) and were more likely to be female and have a history of arrhythmias, hypertension, and diuretic use. There were perioperative arrhythmias in 1290 (53.7%) patients, with 238

(10.7%) having intraoperative arrhythmias, 329 (13.7%) having postoperative nonatrial arrhythmias, and 865 (36%) have postoperative atrial fibrillation or flutter. Hypokalemia was a significant predictor of serious preoperative arrhythmia (odds ratio [OR], 2.2), intraoperative arrythmia (OR, 2.0), and postoperative atrial fibrillation or flutter (OR, 1.7). The association between digoxin use and arrhythmia risk could not be determined because of the small number of digoxin users. There was a significant association between the need for CPR and potassium levels of less than 3.5 mmol/L (OR, 3.3) and greater than 5.2 mmol/L (OR, 3.0).

Conclusion.—Because preoperative hypokalemia (less than 3.5 mmol/L) significantly increases perioperative arrhythmia and the need for CPR, low-cost, low-risk preoperative potassium screening should be performed and potassium levels adjusted as appropriate for patients undergoing elective cardiac surgery.

▶ This study once again raises the question regarding the need for preoperative replacement of potassium in patients who are hypokalemic. Earlier studies have clearly shown the association of magnesium replacement and the diminishment of perioperative ventricular dysrhythmias. In a similar fashion it would seem prudent to correct hypokalemia in patients with underlying cardiac disease. In recognition of the fact that arrhythmias are usually associated with the rate of change of serum potassium and not necessarily the absolute value, future studies will need to determine the chronicity of the patient's hypokalemia, as well as how quickly serum potassium levels are to be corrected.

D. M. Rothenberg, MD, FCCM

▶ This study revisits the old question: How low should a preoperative potassium level be before surgery is canceled? They do answer the question—3.5 mmol/L. In cardiac patients, many are receiving β-adrenergic blockade therapy, and hence have high potassium levels so the significance of a low potassium level may be greater in a cardiac patient. The clinical implications of a low potassium level in predisposing to cardiac arrhythmias in a subset of patients who are already at greater risk for postoperative arrhythmia is clear and must be considered.

M. Wood, MD

Rapid Saline Infusion Produces Hyperchloremic Acidosis in Patients Undergoing Gynecologic Surgery
Scheingraber S, Rehm M, Sehmisch C, et al (Ludwig-Maximilians-Univ, Munich)
Anesthesiology 90:1265-1270, 1999   9–23

Objective.—Infusion of 0.9% saline during surgery results in acid-base changes. The influence of crystalloid infusion on acid-base changes was

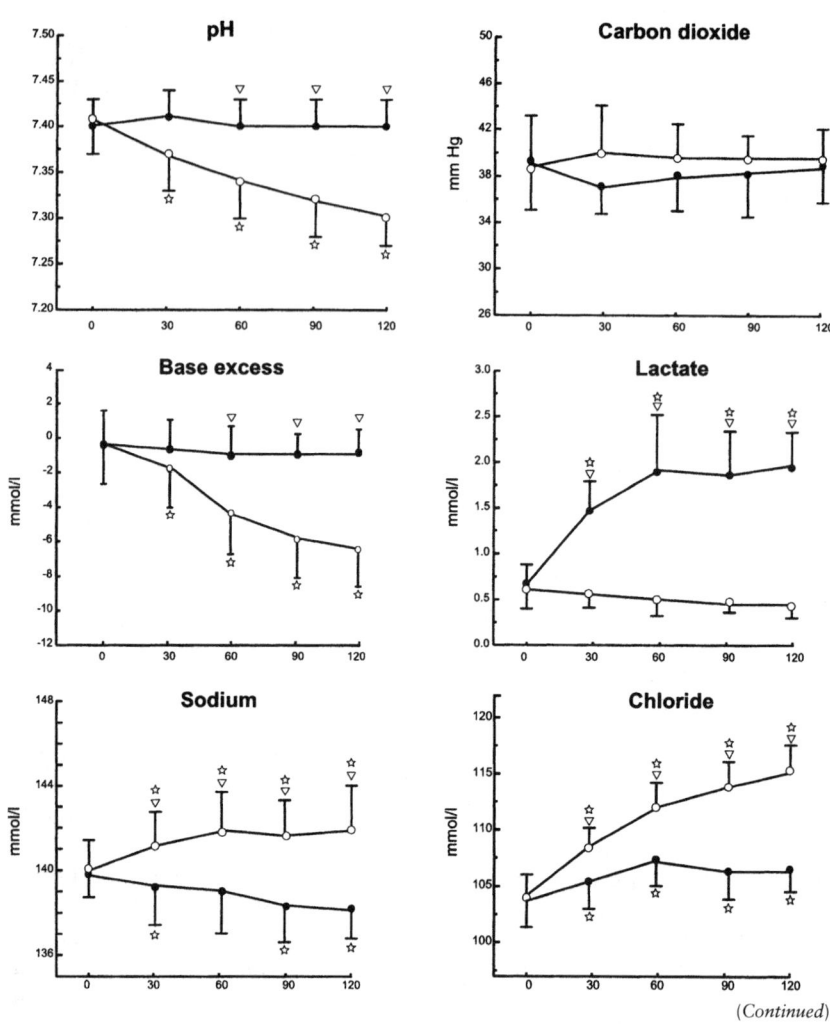

(*Continued*)

assessed by comparing patients who received 0.9% saline with patients who received lactated Ringer's solution.

Methods.—Either 0.9% saline (n = 12) or lactated Ringer's solution (n = 12) was administered to 24 women without cardiac, pulmonary, or renal diseases during elective lower abdominal gynecologic procedures. Beginning at the time of surgical incision and every 30 minutes thereafter, arterial blood was withdrawn to measure baseline values of partial pressure of arterial oxygen, pH, partial pressure of arterial carbon dioxide, and serum concentrations of sodium, potassium, chloride, lactate, and protein. Urine volume and temperature were measured, and blood loss was determined.

FIGURE 1 (cont.)

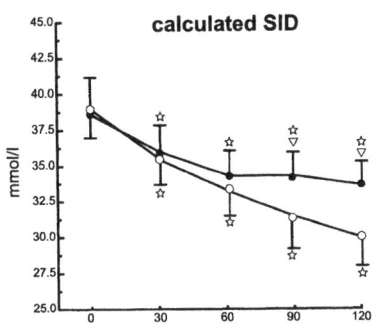
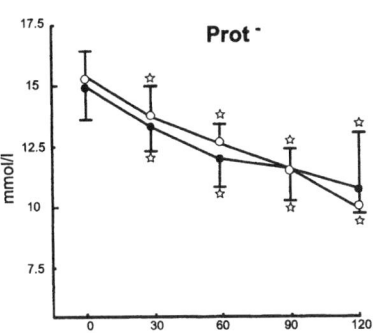

FIGURE 1.—Measured and calculated values (mean ± SD) at the different measuring points. Saline group is indicated by *white dots*, Ringer's group by *black dots. Star* indicates intragroup differences, $P < .05$. *Triangle* indicates intergroup differences, $P < .05$. *Abbreviations: SID*, strong ion difference; *Prot*, protein. (Courtesy of Scheingraber S, Rehm M, Sehmisch C, et al: Rapid saline infusion produces hyperchloremic acidosis in patients undergoing gynecologic surgery. *Anesthesiology* 90:1265-1270, 1999. Copyright American Society of Anesthesiologists, Inc. Used with permission of Lippincott-Raven Publishers.)

Potassium replacement was necessary in 8 patients in the saline group whose potassium ion concentration fell below 3.3 mmol. Bicarbonate concentration (Bic_{HH}) and base excess were calculated using the Henderson-Hasselbalch equation and the Siggaard-Andersen formula. Bic was also determined by subtracting the Prot⁻ from the strong ion differences using the Stewart model. The anion gap was defined as $Na^+ + K^+ - Cl^- - Bic_{HH}$.

Results.—In the saline group, pH decreased significantly from 7.41 to 7.28 (Fig 1). Administration of 0.9% saline resulted in hyperchloremic acidosis and a decrease in the strong ion difference.

Conclusion.—Infusion of 0.9% saline, but not lactated Ringer's solution, leads to hyperchloremic acidosis.

The Effect of Intravenous Lactated Ringer's Solution Versus 0.9% Sodium Chloride Solution on Serum Osmolality in Human Volunteers
Williams EL, Hildebrand KL, McCormick SA, et al (Allegheny Univ, Pittsburgh, Pa)
Anesth Analg 88:999-1003, 1999   9–24

Objective.—Because of the incomplete ionization of solutes in lactated Ringer's solution, the osmolalities of lactated Ringer's solution and 0.9% sodium chloride (NaCl) solution are not equal. Changes in osmolality associated with administration of large volumes of IV lactated Ringer's solution and NaCl solution were investigated in healthy human volunteers.

Methods.—NaCl solution or lactated Ringer's solution at 50 mL/kg were randomly administered in 1 hour to 20 volunteers on 1 occasion. On a second occasion, at least 3 days after the first, the groups were crossed over to the other regimen. Serum sodium, glucose, osmolality, and pH were measured in venous blood sampled before, immediately after, and 1 hour after each infusion.

Results.—Eighteen volunteers (6 women), aged 20 to 48 years, completed the study. Although serum osmolality changed nonsignificantly from baseline (T1) to infusion end (T2) after NaCl solution infusion, infusion of lactated Ringer's solution caused a significant decrease of 4 mOsm/kg. pH increased by 0.04 after lactated Ringer's solution infusion and decreased by 0.04 from T1 to T2 after NaCl solution infusion. The difference was significant. The pH at 1 hour after infusion end (T3) after NaCl solution infusion was unchanged. Serum glucose was unchanged at all time points for both regimens. All volunteers experienced head and neck swelling and discomfort associated with abdominal girth and extremities. Thirteen volunteers in the NaCl group reported lassitude and difficulty in abstract thinking. There was no correlation between abdominal discomfort and any other variable except pH at T2 for the NaCl group.

Conclusion.—Infusion of a large volume of lactated Ringer's solution, but not of NaCl solution, is associated with a decrease in serum osmolality. Infusion of a large volume of NaCl solution is associated with drowsiness and difficulty in abstract thinking, suggesting that the type of IV fluid administered may affect early recovery from anesthesia.

▶ Hypercholremic metabolic acidosis is a common complication after large-volume isotonic crystalloid infusions as was evidenced in both of these studies (Abstracts 9–23 and 9–24). Unfortunately, both studies failed to discuss why this occurs. Most anesthesiologists and surgeons assume that this acidosis is secondary to a "dilutional acidosis." However, this clearly has been shown *not* to be the mechanism of action. In physiologic terms, rapid administration of hyperchloremic solutions such as 0.9% NaCl solution leads to a preferential reabsorbtion of chloride and a subsequent bicarbonaturia. In essence, an iatrogenic renal tubular acidosis is created. Neither study documented urinary electrolytes, which most likely would have shown this change. Of additional interest was the lack of hyponatremia discussed in a previous study, in which a desalination effect was thought to induce hyponatremia, particularly in young healthy women.[1]

Finally, improving minute ventilation could easily have offset the degree of acidosis in the patients undergoing general anesthesia. By keeping minute ventilation fixed, the authors iatrogenically induced a respiratory acidosis, thus contributing to the marked degree in pH change. As the authors concluded, in a postoperative period in which narcotics induce respiratory acidosis and a hyperchloremic metabolic acidosis persists, detrimental changes in pH may occur. In addition, patients who are being weaned from mechanical ventilation will need to increase their minute ventilation to overcome a hyperchloremic metabolic acidosis.

Should isotonic solutions be required to maintain effective arterial blood volume, I recommend the following: 1 L of 0.45 normal saline with 1 to 2 ampoles of sodium bicarbonate added. This solution now contains 127 to 177 mEq/L of sodium, 50 to 100 mEq/L of bicarbonate, and 77 mEq/L of chloride. Once the pH has been corrected to an accepted level, preferably greater than 7.35, this solution may be changed to another standard isotonic solution.

D. M. Rothenberg, MD, FCCM

Reference

1. Steele A, Gowrishankar M, Abrahamson S, et al: Postoperative hyponatremia despite near-isotonic saline infusion: A phenomenon of desalination. *Ann Intern Med* 126:20-25, 1997. (1998 Year Book of Anesthesiology and Pain Management, pp 302-304.)

Cause of Metabolic Acidosis in Prolonged Surgery
Waters JH, Miller LR, Clack S, et al (Cleveland Clinic Found, Ohio; Orange Coast Mem Med Ctr; Univ of Calif, Irvine)
Crit Care Med 27:2142-2146, 1999   9–25

Objective.—Although metabolic acidosis develops in many patients undergoing extensive surgery—usually as a result of volume expansion after normal saline administration—the condition has manifested itself in patients with normovolemia. A study was made of the cause of acidosis in noncardiac, noninvasive surgery patients who were expected to have large blood loss and resuscitation needs. The relationship between volume expansion and acidosis development was also examined in this prospective observational study.

Methods.—Preoperative and postoperative plasma volumes were determined for 8 of 12 patients who underwent a variety of major surgical procedures lasting longer than 4 hours. Patients received preoperative fluid management. All patients required arterial and pulmonary artery catheter monitoring because of preexisting medical conditions or extensive fluid shifts inherent in the procedure. Patients with abnormal renal function or abnormal serum blood urea nitrogen and creatinine levels were excluded. Arterial blood gas parameters were determined and urinalysis was performed after anesthesia induction and after surgery.

Results.—The volume of normal saline–containing fluid was correlated with base excess change ($r^2 = 0.86$). Total chloride administered was also correlated with base excess change ($r^2 = 0.93$). Although acid-base changes suggested dilutional acidosis, there was no change in plasma volume.

Conclusion.—The change in base excess in these patients was related to chloride administration, probably from normal saline. Because perioperative acidosis may be the result of administering more fluid, chloride levels should be measured when acidosis occurs during prolonged surgical procedures.

▶ Although this study is flawed by the lack of a controlled group and the small number of patients assessed, it does attempt to address the mechanism by which saline-induced hyperchloremic acidosis occurs. Measurements of plasma volume failed to corroborate "dilution" as a cause of hypobicarbonatemia. Rather, a decrease in the so-called strong ion difference was seen, perhaps related to renal bicarbonate wasting.

D. M. Rothenberg, MD, FCCM

Sublingual Capnometry: A New Noninvasive Measurement for Diagnosis and Quantitation of Severity of Circulatory Shock
Weil MH, Nakagawa Y, Tang W, et al (Inst of Critical Care Med, Palm Springs, Calif; Univ of Southern California, Los Angeles; Desert Regional Med Ctr, Palm Springs, Calif)
Crit Care Med 27:1225-1229, 1999   9–26

Background.—Increases in tissue PCO_2 are characteristic of systemic perfusion failure. Animal studies have shown that sublingual PCO_2 ($PSLCO_2$) correspond to decreases in arterial pressure and cardiac index and increases in arterial blood lactate concentration that occur as a result of hemorrhage and sepsis. The feasibility and predictive value of $PSLCO_2$ measurements using comparisons with conventional blood pressure and arterial blood lactate measurements were investigated.

Methods.—Between November 1996 and September 1997, $PSLCO_2$ was measured at baseline and at 30-minute intervals for 6 hours using a microelectrode carbon dioxide sensor in 46 patients (15 females), aged 14 to 89 years, with acute circulatory failure. Arterial blood pressure, heart rate, and arterial blood lactate were also measured. Results were compared with those obtained in 5 healthy volunteers with $PSLCO_2$ ranging from 43 to 47 mm Hg after 8 minutes, and averaging 45.2 mm Hg.

Results.—The initial $PSLCO_2$ in 26 patients with arterial blood lactate values of more than 2.5 mmol/L (shock group) ranged from 48 to 135 mm Hg, significantly higher than the $PSLCO_2$ of 37 to 68 mm Hg found in the absence of shock. A $PSLCO_2$ threshold of 70 mm Hg predicted shock with a positive predictive value of 1. $PSLCO_2$ values ranged from 55 to 135 mm Hg, averaging 92.6 mm Hg, in patients who died. They ranged from 37 to 77 mm Hg, averaging 58.4 mm Hg, in patients who survived. A $PSLCO_2$ value of less than 70 mm Hg predicted survival with a positive predictive value of 0.93. Most patients who died had an admission $PSLCO_2$ value of less than 70 mm Hg.

Conclusion.—Measurement of $PSLCO_2$ is a simple, noninvasive technique for diagnosing the degree of circulatory shock.

▶ Although I am fascinated by the potential for a readily accessible device to measure tissue perfusion, the ability to achieve reliable calibration with this monitor will require larger prospective studies in critically ill patients. The bias and precision of such devices may be improved with the application of advanced optode technology. Dr Weil and his colleagues have given intensivists a brand new interpretation of what it means to say "Stick out your tongue and say ah."

D. M. Rothenberg, MD, FCCM

A Multicenter, Randomized, Controlled Clinical Trial of Transfusion Requirements in Critical Care
Hébert PC, for the Canadian Critical Care Trials Group (Univ of Ottawa, Ont; et al)
N Engl J Med 340:409-417, 1999   9–27

Background.—The optimal transfusion strategy for critically ill anemic patients has not been determined. To understand the potential risks and benefits of transfusions in critically ill patients, a randomized, controlled clinical trial compared a restrictive versus a liberal approach to red cell transfusions.

Methods.—The study group consisted of 838 critically ill patients who were admitted to 22 tertiary-level and 3 community ICUs in Canada from 1994 to 1997. Consecutive critically ill normovolemic patients were randomly assigned to either a restrictive strategy (transfusion when hemoglobin concentration decreased below 7.0 g/dL) or a liberal strategy (transfusion when hemoglobin concentration decreased below 10.0 g/dL). The primary outcome measure was 30-day death from all causes. Secondary outcomes included 60-day death from all causes, hospital mortality, and 30-day survival.

Results.—The overall 30-day mortality rate was not significantly different in these 2 study groups. Mortality rates were significantly lower in the restrictive transfusion strategy group among less acutely ill patients and younger patients. The mortality rate was not lower in the restrictive transfusion strategy group for patients with clinically significant cardiac disease. The mortality rate during hospitalization was significantly lower in the restrictive than in the liberal transfusion strategy group.

Conclusion.—A restrictive transfusion strategy, consisting of a threshold for red cell transfusion of 7.0 g/dL of hemoglobin, was at least as effective as, and in some cases superior to, a more liberal transfusion strategy in critically ill normovolemic patients. These results appear to be generalizable to most critically ill patients, with the exception of patients who have clinically significant cardiac disease.

▶ It is interesting to note that those patients who received liberal transfusion had a higher incidence of myocardial infarction, thus contradicting the authors' suggestion that there may be a benefit to increasing the hemoglobin concentration more than 10 g/dL in patients with coronary artery disease.

D. M. Rothenberg, MD, FCCM

Dopexamine Reduces the Incidence of Acute Inflammation in the Gut Mucosa After Abdominal Surgery in High-Risk Patients

Byers RJ, Eddleston JM, Pearson RC, et al (Univ of Manchester, England; Manchester Royal Infirmary, England)
Crit Care Med 27:1787-1793, 1999   9–28

Background.—About 20% of critically ill patients have acute inflammation in the stomach/duodenum. Dopexamine has dopaminergic receptor agonist properties but no α or direct β_1 effects. It may exhibit anti-inflammatory effects. Thus, a study was designed to examine histologically and endoscopically the effect of dopexamine on the gut mucosa. The study represented a side arm of a large prospective, randomized, controlled, multicenter European study (Effect of Dopexamine on Outcome after Major Abdominal Surgery).

Methods.—Patients (n = 38) with at least 1 high risk criterion, who were undergoing major abdominal surgery of at least 1.5 hours duration, submitted to endoscopy and biopsy of the upper gastrointestinal tract immediately after induction of anesthesia. After being stabilized, patients received placebo (n = 12, group A), 0.5 µg/kg per minute of dopexamine (n = 13, group B), or 2.0 µg/kg per minute of dopexamine (n = 13, group C). At 72 hours, endoscopy and biopsy were repeated in 27 patients. Upper gut blood flow was estimated using tonometry. pH was calculated at baseline; after surgery; and at 2, 6, 12, 24, and 30 to 36 hours after surgery.

Results.—Gastric pH decreased significantly and similarly in the 3 groups, with the greatest increase being recorded at the end of surgery. Erythema or hemorrhagic changes were found in 33.3% of group A, 38.5% of group B, and 15.4% of group C. Erosive disease was found in 25%, 7.7%, and 38.5%, respectively. At 72 hours, endoscopy revealed that the number of patients with no detectable abnormality had decreased to 25% in group A (2/8 patients), 20% in group B (2/10), and to 33.3% in group C (3/9). At 72 hours, 3 group A patients (37.5%), 2 group B patients (20%), and 1 group C patients (11.1%) had erosive disease. Polymorphonuclear neutrophil activation was found in 86%, 37.5%, and 37.5%, respectively. Endoscopic and histologic findings were not correlated.

Conclusion.—Even after critically ill patients have been stabilized, high-risk patients experience a reduction in gastric pH after abdominal surgery that is greatest right after surgery but persists for 30 to 36 hours. Although dopexamine protects against the inflammatory consequences of this decrease by an unknown mechanism, it does not prevent the decrease.

▶ I continue to be impressed with this drug, not so much related to its dopaminergic receptor agonist properties, but rather because of its anti-inflammatory effects. This is in direct contradistinction to low-dose dopamine, which may unfavorably affect immunomodulation by suppressing prolactin secretion, thus impairing lymphocyte function.

D. M. Rothenberg, MD, FCCM

Effects of Ibuprofen on the Physiology and Survival of Hypothermic Sepsis

Arons MM, for the Ibuprofen in Sepsis Study Group (Vanderbilt Univ, Nashville, Tenn)
Crit Care Med 27:699-707, 1999   9–29

Purpose.—Patients whose response to sepsis is hypothermic rather than febrile have a poor prognosis. It has been suggested that patients with hypothermic sepsis represent a clinically and biochemically distinct subgroup. This hypothesis was studied, along with the response to ibuprofen treatment in patients with hypothermic sepsis.

Methods.—The multicenter trial included 455 patients admitted to the ICU with severe sepsis and a known or suspected serious infection. Patients with hypothermic sepsis were identified, and their clinical and physiologic findings were compared with those of patients who had febrile sepsis. Plasma cytokines measured included tumor necrosis factor α (TNF-α) and interleukin (IL)-6, along with the lipid mediators thromboxane B_2 (TxB$_2$) and prostacyclin. Hypothermic patients were randomized to receive ibuprofen (10 mg/kg IV over 30 to 60 minutes every 6 hours for 8 doses, to a maximum of 800 mg) or to receive placebo.

Results.—Ten percent of the patients with sepsis were hypothermic, with a temperature of less than 35.5°C; the rest were febrile. The mortality rate was twice as high in the hypothermic group (70% vs 35%). Patients with septic hypothermia had significant baseline elevations of urinary TxB$_2$ metabolites, prostacyclin, and serum TNF-α and IL-6, compared with the febrile group.

Twenty-four patients with hypothermic sepsis were assigned to ibuprofen and 20 to placebo. The 30-day mortality rate was 54% in patients receiving ibuprofen versus 90% in those receiving placebo. Ibuprofen treatment was also associated with a trend toward increased number of days free from major organ system failures.

Conclusion.—About 10% of the patients with sepsis have a hypothermic rather than a febrile response. This condition is associated with increased levels of the cytokines TNF-α and IL-6 and of the lipid mediators TxB$_2$ and prostacyclin, as well as with increased mortality. Treatment with IV ibuprofen may reduce mortality in patients with hypothermic sepsis, although prospective confirmation of this finding is needed.

▶ A number of agents directed against inflammatory mediators such as cytokines (IL-6, TNF-α), bioactive lipids, (TxA$_2$, TxB$_2$), and endotoxin have been employed as "magic bullets" to treat or prevent systemic inflammatory response syndrome. Although the use of monoclonal antibodies directed against these inflammatory mediators has proved to be unsuccessful, recent data regarding the use of steroids or the nonsteroidal anti-inflammatory agent ibuprofen seem to be promising. Given the excessive mortality rate associated with hypothermic sepsis, a short course of IV ibuprofen seems justified.

D. M. Rothenberg, MD, FCCM

Infection Control

Compliance With Handwashing in a Teaching Hospital

Pittet D, and the Members of the Infection Control Program (Univ of Geneva, Switzerland; et al)
Ann Intern Med 130:126-130, 1999   9–30

Objective.—Nosocomial infections are responsible for 7% to 10% of in-hospital infectious complications. Transmission occurs primarily because of lack of compliance of health care workers with handwashing procedures. Factors associated with poor compliance with handwashing in a teaching hospital were investigated.

Methods.—In December 1994, 5 trained infection control nurses recorded potential opportunities for and actual performance of handwashing during 20-minute observation periods randomly distributed between day and night for 14 days in a sample of 48 wards. Compliance was defined as washing the hands with soap and water or with antiseptic solution. Noncompliance was defined as failure to wash, failure to remove gloves after patient contact, or touching a dirty and clean body site on the same patient. Handwashing was required whether or not gloves were worn.

Results.—A total of 2834 handwashing opportunities among 1043 health care workers were recorded. Compliance averaged 48%, with soap and water handwashing in 34% and hand antisepsis in 14%. Handwashing compliance was significantly lower in surgical wards and ICUs than in other locations, with the lowest compliance rate (36%) in ICUs, even though indications for hand washing were more frequent (43.4 opportunities/h). The highest compliance rate (59%) was in pediatric units where indications for hand washing were lower (24.4 opportunities/h). According to multivariate analysis, care in ICUs, higher-risk procedures, and a high activity index were risk factors for noncompliance. Compliance was highest among nurses. Compliance was only 11% for contact between clean and dirty body sites. Failure to change contaminated gloves was as common as failure to wash hands.

Conclusion.—Handwashing compliance was lowest with respect to activities that carried the highest risk for transmission. Compliance with handwashing requires 1 minute per opportunity. As the number of handwashing opportunities increases, the time involved in handwashing becomes prohibitive. Possibly, bedside hand antisepsis can be instituted to save time and increase compliance.

External Sources of Vancomycin-Resistant Enterococci for Intensive Care Units

Bonten MJM, Slaughter S, Hayden MK, et al (Cook County Hosp, Chicago; Rush Med College, Chicago)
Crit Care Med 26:2001-2004, 1998   9–31

Objective.—ICUs are frequently colonized with antibiotic-resistant bacteria, often vancomycin-resistant enterococci (VRE). The impact of previously colonized patients on the epidemiology of VRE colonization was evaluated in a prospective study.

Methods.—Rectal swabs were obtained from 301 patients consecutively admitted to the 16-bed medical ICU of a public teaching hospital. All swabs were inoculated and plated. Resistant genotypes were confirmed by polymerase chain reaction analysis and subjected to pulsed-field gel electrophoresis.

Results.—Fourteen strains of VRE colonization were found in 43 patients (14%). Of the 43 patients, 40 were in-hospital transfers or had been previously hospitalized within the previous year (Fig 2). Patients who had been hospitalized more than 3 days before transfer to the medical ICU had a significantly greater risk for VRE infection (odds ratio, 4.65) than did patients hospitalized for a shorter period. Eleven of 25 colonized patients (44%) had received antibiotics during their previous stay as compared with 15 of 137 noncolonized patients (11%). Four of the 14 strains were introduced from community patients and 10 strains from transfer or rehospitalized patients.

Conclusion.—VRE colonization appeared to have occurred on non–medical ICU wards. Three patients admitted directly from the community

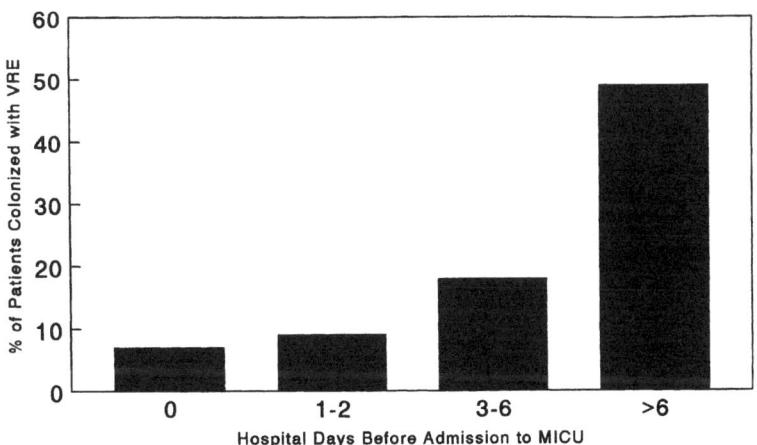

FIGURE 2.—Length of hospitalization before admission to the medical intensive care unit (*MICU*) and risk for colonization with vancomycin-resistant enterococci (*VRE*) on admission to the MICU. (Courtesy of Bonten MJM, Slaughter S, Hayden MK, et al: External sources of vancomycin-resistant enterococci for intensive care units. *Crit Care Med* 26[12]:2001-2004, 1998.)

were already colonized with VRE. Screening and isolation of VRE patients may be an effective infection control measure.

▶ VRE infections are a growing concern in ICUs throughout the world (Abstracts 9–30 and 9–31). Despite the knowledge that frequent handwashing can decrease the rate of VRE as well as other nosocomially acquired pathogens, compliance remains extremely poor. Although the use of gloves appears to be more prevalent, allergic reactions to latex and the failure to remove them when caring for a second patient limits the effectiveness of such protective measure. Strategies must be designed to improve access to sinks to decrease the amount of time required for handwashing for each type of patient care activity. Future studies must also address the question as to whether alcohol rinses or gels placed at the patient's bedside can decrease the incident of noscomial infection and improve compliance.

Finally, despite in-hospital techniques for minimizing nosocomial pathogen exposure, it appears that the VRE may be acquired by patients as outpatients and, as such, raises the question of whether patients should be routinely screened upon admission to ICUs. The reader is referred to a recent review article regarding the prevention of nosocomial infections in the ICU.[1]

D. M. Rothenberg, MD, FCCM

Reference

1. Weber DJ, Raasch R, Rutala WA: Nosocomial infections in the ICU: The growing importance of antibiotic-resistant pathogens. *Chest* 15:34S-41S, 1999.

A Comparison of Two Antimicrobial-Impregnated Central Venous Catheters
Darouiche RO, for the Catheter Study Group (Baylor College of Medicine, Houston; et al)
N Engl J Med 340:1-8, 1999   9–32

Introduction.—Previous studies have shown that rates of central venous catheter colonization and catheter-related bloodstream infection can be significantly reduced through the use of catheters impregnated with minocycline and rifampin or with chlorhexidine and silver sulfadiazine. However, no studies have directly compared the benefits of the 2 types of catheter. Minocycline/rifampin and chlorhexidine/silver sulfadiazine catheters were compared for their ability to prevent catheter colonization and catheter-related bloodstream infection.

Methods.—The prospective, multicenter trial included adult patients considered at high risk for catheter-related infection who were likely to require a central venous catheter for 3 days or longer. The patients were randomized to receive polyurethane triple-lumen catheters impregnated with minocycline/rifampin on the luminal and external surfaces or with chlorhexidine/silver sulfadiazine on the external surface only. Catheter tips and subcutaneous segments were cultured by both the roll-plate and

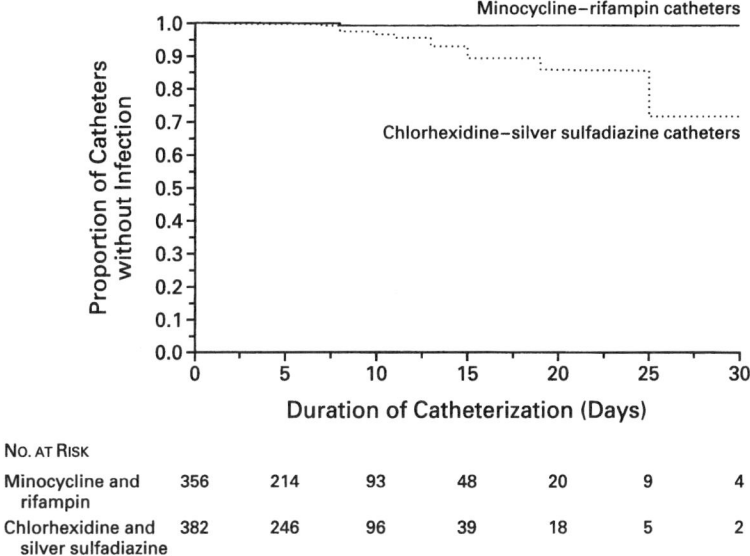

No. at Risk

Minocycline and rifampin	356	214	93	48	20	9	4
Chlorhexidine and silver sulfadiazine	382	246	96	39	18	5	2

FIGURE 1.—Kaplan-Meier curves for freedom from bloodstream infection with catheters impregnated with either minocycline and rifampin or chlorhexidine and silver sulfadiazine. The number of catheters in each group that were at risk for causing infection at various times are shown *below the figure.* The risk of bloodstream infection was significantly lower for catheters impregnated with minocycline and rifampin than for those impregnated with chlorhexidine and silver sulfadiazine ($P = .001$ by the log-rank test). (Reprinted by permission, from Darouiche RO, for the Catheter Study Group: A comparison of two antimicrobial-impregnated central venous catheters. *N Engl J Med* 340:1-8. Copyright 1999, Massachusetts Medical Society. All rights reserved.)

sonication methods after removal, with peripheral blood cultures performed as indicated. The analysis included a total of 738 catheters with evaluable culture results.

Results.—The 2 catheter groups were similar in their clinical characteristics and infection risk factors. The catheter colonization rate was 8.3% for minocycline/rifampin-impregnated catheters, compared with 22.8% for chlorhexidine/silver sulfadiazine-impregnated catheters. Catheters impregnated with minocycline and rifampin were also associated with a lower rate of catheter-related bloodstream infection (0.3% vs 3.4%) (Fig 1).

Conclusions.—This randomized trial suggests that anti-infective catheters impregnated with minocycline and rifampin carry a lower risk of colonization and infection than those impregnated with chlorhexidine and silver sulfadiazine. The authors emphasize that antimicrobial-impregnated catheters must complement, rather than replace, adequate aseptic technique.

Efficacy of Antiseptic-Impregnated Central Venous Catheters in Preventing Catheter-Related Bloodstream Infection: A Meta-Analysis
Veenstra DL, Saint S, Saha S, et al (Univ of Wash, Seattle)
JAMA 281:261-267, 1999   9–33

Objective.—Methods of lowering catheter-related bloodstream infection (CR-BSI), including aseptic techniques, proper catheter care, and coated catheters and catheter cuffs have reduced the incidence of CR-BSI. Although catheters coated with chlorhexidine-silver sulfadiazine may be less susceptible to antibiotic resistance, there are few studies of overall effectiveness. The efficacy of chlorhexidine-impregnated central venous catheters for the prevention of nosocomial catheter colonization and CR-BSI was quantitatively assessed in a meta-analysis.

Methods.—A MEDLINE search yielded 215 articles. Of these, 13 were randomized, controlled clinical trials reporting incidences of colonization or CR-BSI and sufficiently large to allow calculation of effect size.

Results.—Of the 13 studies selected and summarized, 10 examined catheter colonization and CR-BSI, 2 examined catheter colonization, and 1 examined CR-BSI. Of the 2830 catheters used, 2494 were triple-lumen, 306 were double-lumen, and 30 were single-lumen. Average catheter placement duration ranged from 5.1 to 11.2 days, and placement site was similar for treatment and control groups. Compared with the control group, the treatment group had significantly lower colonization and incidences of CR-BSI (odds ratio, 0.44 and 0.56, respectively).

Conclusion.—Compared with nonimpregnated catheters, impregnated catheters significantly reduced the incidence of colonization and CR-BSI. Effect size calculations showed that impregnated central venous catheters lowered bloodstream infection risk by 40%, thus potentially reducing associated mortality rate of 10% to 35% and associated costs as high as $30,000 per episode.

▶ In addition to routine hand-washing and meticulous attention to sterile insertion techniques, the use of second-generation central venous catheters bonded with antibacterial substances may decrease the incidence of nosocomial blood stream infections (Abstracts 9–32 and 9–33). The potential advantage of catheters impregnated with minocycline and rifampin versus those bonded with chlorhexidine and silver sulfadiazine may be related to the internal impregnation of these antibiotics versus the external bonding of the antibacterial agents, as well as to the more potent antibacterial effect of minocycline and rifampin over chlorhexidine and silver sulfadiazine. Despite the increase cost associated with routine use of these types of catheters, the ability to prevent CR-BSI should greatly outweigh the initial expense of these devices. A consensus seems to be building toward the use of these second-generation central venous catheters to prevent nosocomial infections.

D. M. Rothenberg, MD, FCCM

Emergence of Vancomycin Resistance in *Staphylococcus aureus*
Smith TL, for the Glycopeptide-Intermediate *Staphylococcus aureus* Working Group (Ctrs for Disease Control and Prevention, Atlanta, Ga; et al)
N Engl J Med 340:493-501, 1999   9–34

Objective.—The investigation of the first documented glycopeptide-intermediate *Staphylococcus aureus* infections in the United States and the clinical significance and public health implications of the emergence of these organisms were described.

> *Case 1.*—Man, 59, with diabetes mellitus, hypertension, metastatic small-cell carcinoma, and chronic renal failure requiring continuous peritoneal dialysis since 1992 was given a diagnosis of methicillin-resistant peritonitis and treated with IV vancomycin (1 g/72 h) for 2 weeks for this episode and the subsequent 4 recurrences over the next 5 months. His peritoneal catheter was not removed. Intermediate glycopeptide *S aureus* was cultured from his

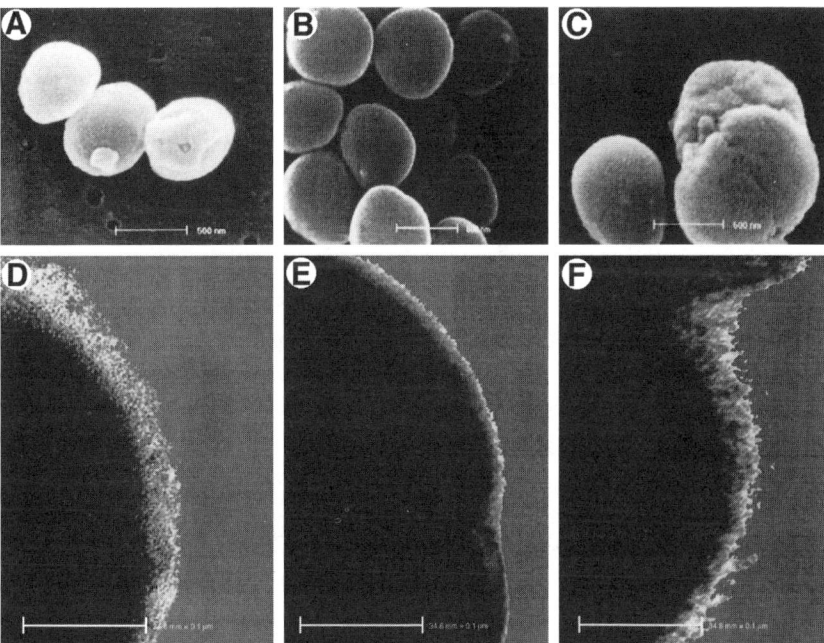

FIGURE 3.—Electron micrographs of *S aureus* isolates. **Top row** shows scanning electron micrographs magnified 50,000 times; **bottom row** shows transmission electron micrographs magnified 348,000 times. **Panels A** and **D** show a glycopeptide-intermediate *S aureus* isolate from 1 patient, in which increased extracellular material is evident. **Panels B** and **E** show methicillin-resistant *S aureus* from another patient showing a normal cell wall without increased extracellular material. **Panels C** and **F** show a glycopeptide-intermediate *S aureus* isolate from a third patient, with evidence of increased extracelluar material. (Reprinted by permission, from Smith TL, for the Glycopeptide-Intermediate *Staphylococcus aureus* Working Group: Emergence of vancomycin resistance in *Staphylococcus aureus*. *N Engl J Med* 340:493-501. Copyright 1999, Massachusetts Medical Society. All rights reserved.)

TABLE 1.—Situations in Which the Use of Vancomycin Should Be Discouraged

Routine prophylaxis
    Surgical patients without life-threatening allergy to beta-lactam antibiotics[34]
    Low-birth-weight infants[35]
    Patients on dialysis[36,37]
    Patients with neutropenia
    Patients with central venous catheters[36,38-43]
Empirical treatment
    Febrile patients with neutropenia who are not at high risk for resistant gram-positive infection[44-50]
    Febrile low-birth-weight infants
Decontamination of the digestive tract
Treatment based on indications
    Patients with single blood cultures positive for coagulase-negative staphylococci[51-53]
    Patients colonized with methicillin-resistant S. aureus[54,55]
    Patients with *Clostridium difficile* colitis (first-line therapy)[56]
    Patients on dialysis for whom convenience in treating infections is desirable[57-60]
    Patients with gram-positive infections not due to resistant organisms

Note: Data are from the Hospital Infection Control Practices Advisory Committee. (Recommendations for preventing the spread of vancomycin resistance: Recommendations of the Hospital Infection Control Practices Advisory Committee [HICPAC]. *MMWR Morb Mortal Wkly Rep* 44[RR-12]:1-13, 1995.)

(Reprinted by permission, from Smith TL, for the Glycopeptide-Intermediate *Staphylococcus aureus* Working Group: Emergence of vancomycin resistance in *Staphylococcus aureus*. N Engl J Med 340:493-501. Copyright 1999, Massachusetts Medical Society. All rights reserved.)

peritoneal fluid. Vancomycin treatment was unsuccessful, as was gentamicin therapy. The man was treated with oral trimethoprim-sulfamethoxazole and rifampicin. His peritoneal cultures became negative, and peritoneal dialysis was continued.

Case 2.—Man, 66, with congestive heart failure and diabetes mellitus was admitted for shortness of breath and was found to have a urinary tract infection with methicillin-resistant *S aureus*. Treatment with IV vancomycin and oral doxycycline was unsuccessful. Renal failure developed and required peritoneal dialysis. A methicillin-resistant *S aureus* infection developed and was treated unsuccessfully with IV vancomycin. A blood culture grew *S aureus* with intermediate resistance to glycopeptides. The man's infection was eradicated with IV gentamicin. After pedal and pulmonary edema developed, he was treated with oral rifampicin. Renal insufficiency developed. Blood cultures grew *Candida glabrata* and *Candida parapsilosis*. Peritoneal fluid cultures grew *Staphylococcus epidermidis*. No *S aureus* was cultured. The man was treated with oral doxycycline and ciprofloxacin but died 34 days after admission.

Results.—An investigation of contacts found no carriage of *S aureus* with intermediate resistance to glycopeptides. Pulsed field gel electrophoresis found a difference of 2 bands between the 2 *S aureus* isolates with intermediate resistance to glycopeptides, and scanning and electron microscopy revealed a layer of extracellular material of unknown composition that was thicker in the isolates resistant to vancomycin than in isolates resistant to methicillin (Fig 3).

TABLE 2.—Recommendations for Preventing the Spread of
Glycopeptide-Resistant Staphylococci

Laboratory
Ensure presence of pure *S. aureus* isolate
Use one of the following quantitative methods to determine the minimal inhibitory concentration with
    24-hour incubation
    Broth microdilution
    Agar dilution
    Agar-gradient diffusion
Retest isolates associated with minimal inhibitory concentrations ≥4 μg per milliliter and those from
    patients whose condition does not improve with glycopeptide therapy
Report all *S. aureus* isolates associated with minimal inhibitory concentrations ≥4 μg per milliliter of
    glycopeptide to the state health department and the CDC
Immediately notify infection-control personnel, the clinical care unit, and attending physician when
    an *S. aureus* isolate associated with a minimal inhibitory concentration ≥4 μg per milliliter is
    recognized
Infection control
Isolate the patient in a private room
    Minimize the number of persons caring for the patient
    Begin one-on-one care by specified personnel
Initiate epidemiologic and laboratory investigations with the assistance of the state health department
    and the CDC
Educate all health care personnel about the epidemiology of *S. aureus* with intermediate resistance to
    glycopeptides and about appropriate infection-control precautions
Monitor and strictly enforce compliance with contact precautions[62]
Determine whether transmission has already occurred by performing baseline cultures of specimens
    from hands and nares of the following:
    Those with physical contact with the patient
    The patient's health care providers
    The patient's roommates
Use contact precautions (gown, mask, gloves, and antibacterial soap for hand washing)[62]
Assess efficacy of precautions by monitoring personnel for acquisition of the isolate
Consult with the state health department and CDC before transferring the patient (for emergencies
    only) or discharging him or her
Inform the following appropriate personnel about the presence of a patient with glycopeptide-
    intermediate *S aureus*:
    Patient's accepting physician
    Admitting or emergency room personnel
    Personnel admitting patients to unit

Note: Recommendations were modified from Centers for Disease Control guidelines. (Interim guidelines for prevention
and control of Staphylococcal infection associated with reduced susceptibility to vancomycin. *MMWR Morb Mortal Wkly
Rep* 46:626-628, 635, 1997.
(Reprinted by permission, from Smith TL, for the Glycopeptide-Intermediate *Staphylococcus aureus* Working Group:
Emergence of vancomycin resistance in *Staphylococcus aureus*. *N Engl J Med* 340:493-501. Copyright 1999, Massachu-
setts Medical Society. All rights reserved.)

Conclusion.—The finding of vancomycin resistance in *S aureus* calls for recommendations to reduce the development and spread of these strains (Tables 1 and 2).

▶ If you thought that vancomycin-resistant enterococcus was a scary situation, imagine the emergence of bacteria with no known form of therapy! The initial reports of resistant *S aureus* should not come as too much of a surprise to those of us who have witnessed the routine use of vancomycin as surgical prophylaxis for patients seen with a remote or unsubstantiated allergy to penicillin or to β-lactam antibiotics. This report should empower hospital epidemiologists to take control of antibiotic ordering so as to prevent the spread of other resistant organisms. I am afraid, however, that this course of action may be too late to help the spread of resistant *S aureus.*

D. M. Rothenberg, MD, FCCM

Insulin Infusion Improves Neutrophil Function in Diabetic Cardiac Surgery Patients
Rassias AJ, Marrin CAS, Arruda J, et al (Dartmouth-Hitchcock Med Ctr, Lebanon, NH)
Anesth Analg 88:1011-1016, 1999   9–35

Objective.—Diabetic patients are at increased risk of infection after surgery, probably because of a number of factors that impair the immune system. Because hyperglycemia may alter leukocyte function and the function of polymorphonuclear neutrophils, the effect of aggressive insulin therapy on polymorphonuclear neutrophil function was evaluated during cardiac surgery in diabetic patients.

Methods.—Between March 1996 and June 1997, elective cardiac surgery with cardiopulmonary bypass (CPB) was performed on 26 diabetic patients who were prospectively randomly allocated to receive standard

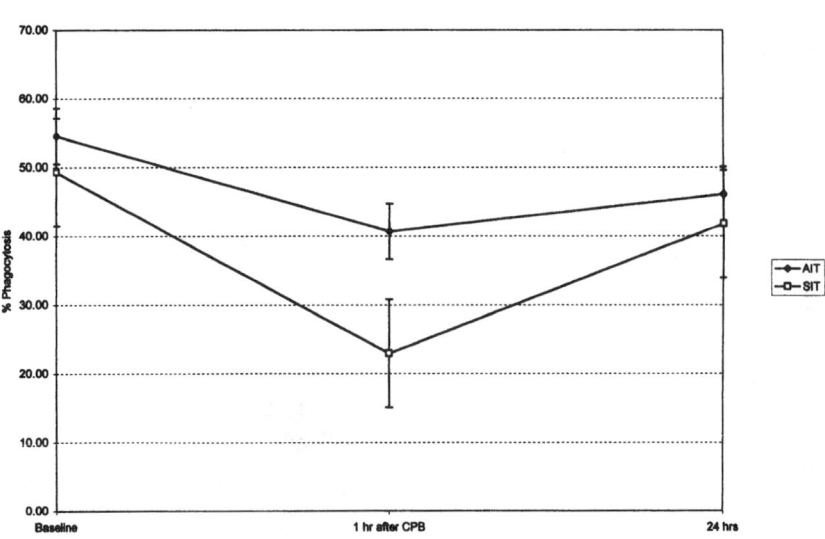

FIGURE 3.—Percentage of phagocytic activity of peripheral blood polymorphonuclear neutrophils (PMNs) at baseline, 1 hour after cardiopulmonary bypass (*CPB*), and 24 hours postoperatively. One hour after CPB, the difference in phagocytic activity between the aggressive insulin therapy (*AIT*) group and the standard insulin therapy (*SIT*) group was statistically significant (*P* < .02). (Courtesy of Rassias AJ, Marrin CAS, Arruda J, et al: Insulin infusion improves neutrophil function in diabetic cardiac surgery patients. *Anesth Analg* 88[5]:1011-1016, 1999.)

insulin therapy (SIT) (n = 13) or aggressive insulin therapy (AIT) (n = 13). Oral hypoglycemic medications were not administered the morning of surgery. Neutrophil levels were determined at baseline, at 1 hour after cardiopulmonary bypass, and on the first postoperative day. High glucose levels (>450 mg/dL) were achieved by starting with an infusion of insulin (4 U/h) after an IV bolus of 13 U. Insulin concentration was measured hourly.

Results.—Compared with that of the SIT group, the average glucose level in the AIT group was significantly reduced. Polymorphonuclear neutrophil phagocytosis activity was significantly reduced in the SIT group 1 hour after CPB. The reduction in the AIT group was less pronounced (Fig 3). The respective decreases from baseline were 25% and 54%. On postoperative day 1, phagocytic activity had returned to 85% of baseline levels in both groups. Two major infections and 1 minor infection were observed in the SIT group. There were no infections in the AIT group.

Conclusion.—Diabetic patients receiving aggressive insulin therapy had improved phagocytic activity after CPB, indicating that impaired polymorphonuclear neutrophil function is partially reversible. Only nonspecific neutrophil function was affected. Immune function returned essentially to baseline by postoperative day 1.

▶ Although neutrophil phagocytic activity decreased in both the AIT and the SIT groups, this effect was far more pronounced in patients receiving SIT. Two patients in the SIT group were observed to have major infections. However, the small number of patients studied precludes any direct clinical ramifications. Nonetheless, there seems to be little support for nonaggressive glucose control in the perioperative period of care in patients undergoing CPB, and studies such as this should help convince anesthesiologists and surgeons alike that normoglycemia should be the goal for all patients.

D. M. Rothenberg, MD, FCCM

Continuous Intravenous Insulin Infusion Reduces the Incidence of Deep Sternal Wound Infection in Diabetic Patients After Cardiac Surgical Procedures
Furnary AP, Zerr KJ, Grunkemeier GL, et al (Providence St Vincent Med Ctr, Portland, Ore)
Ann Thorac Surg 67:352-362, 1999   9–36

Purpose.—Deep sternal wound infection (DSWI) is a very serious complication of cardiac surgery, and diabetes is an important risk factor. A new protocol to prevent DSWI in patients with diabetes mellitus—focusing on aggressive control of postoperative blood glucose levels by continuous insulin infusion (CII)—was evaluated.

Methods.—The prospective study included 2 consecutive groups of diabetic patients undergoing open heart surgery. The first group included 968 patients treated between 1987 and 1991. In this group, postoperative

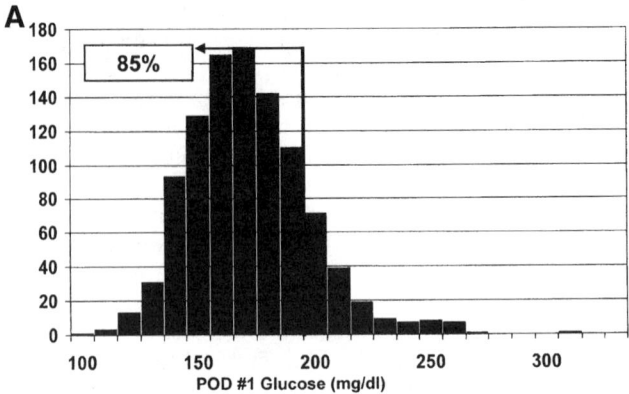

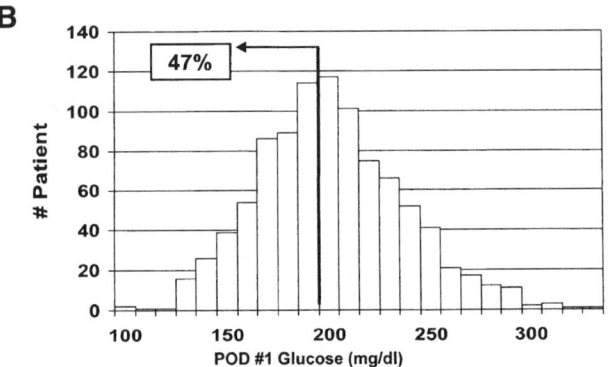

FIGURE 1.—Distribution curves of mean glucose levels on postoperative day 1 in patients in the continuous insulin infusion (CII) study group (A) and control (intermittent subcutaneous insulin injections) group (B). *Vertical line* represents the desired goal of 200 mg/dL. Tighter glucose control with CII is reflected by the fact that 85% of the CII study group successfully achieved levels below 200 mg/dL. In the control group, in contrast, there is only a 47% compliance with target levels. (Reprinted with permission from the Society of Thoracic Surgeons, from Furnary AP, Zerr KJ, Grunkemeier GL, et al: Continuous intravenous insulin infusion reduces the incidence of deep sternal wound infection in diabetic patients after cardiac surgical procedures. *Ann Thorac Surg* 67:352-362, 1999.)

glucose control was achieved by using intermittent subcutaneous insulin injections, individualized according to a sliding scale. Injections were given every 4 hours to maintain a target blood glucose level of less than 200 mg/dL. The second group included 1499 patients operated on from 1991 to 1997. These patients received postoperative CII, titrated to the patient's most recent fingerstick glucose measurement, to maintain blood glucose level between 150 and 200 mg/dL. The incidences of DSWI were compared between the 2 groups.

Findings.—The 2 groups were similar in their preoperative and intraoperative characteristics. A total of 2117 bypass grafting procedures were performed, 68% of which used at least 1 internal thoracic artery. Thirty-six percent of patients were insulin dependent. At admission, 48% had their blood glucose levels controlled by oral agents and 10% by diet only,

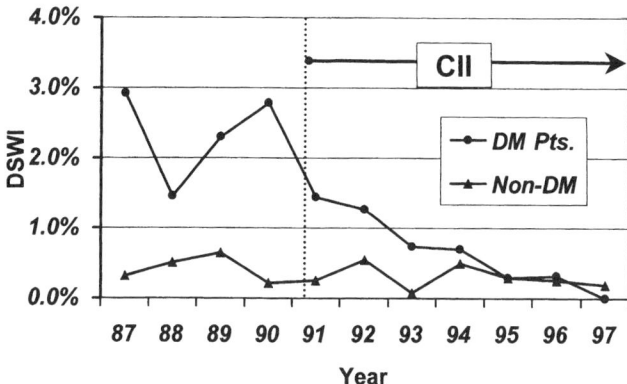

FIGURE 3.—Annual rates of deep sternal wound infection (*DSWI*) in diabetic and nondiabetic patients after cardiac surgical procedures from 1987 through 1997. Note the significant downward trend (slope, −0.52%/y, P = .03) since the implementation of the continuous insulin infusion (*CII*) protocol. Diabetic DSWI rates since 1995 appear to have normalized to that of the nondiabetic population. *Abbreviations: DM*, diabetes mellitus; *Pts.*, patients. (Reprinted by permission from the Society of Thoracic Surgeons, from Furnary AP, Zerr KJ, Grunkemeier GL, et al: Continuous intravenous insulin infusion reduces the incidence of deep sternal wound infection in diabetic patients after cardiac surgical procedures. *Ann Thorac Surg* 67:352-362, 1999.)

with 6% having no glucose control. The overall incidence of DSWI was 1.3%. Three fourths of the DSWIs occurred after discharge, thus requiring a second hospitalization. Analysis of daily mean blood glucose levels showed significantly improved postoperative glucose control with CII. From the operative day through the third postoperative day, mean blood glucose levels were significantly lower in the patients receiving CII (Fig 1) The rate of DSWI decreased from 1.9% in the control group to 0.8% in the CII group, a 2.5-fold reduction. On multivariate analysis, CII reduced the risk of DSWI by one third. Factors increasing the risk of DSWI included obesity and use of an internal thoracic artery pedicle; both factors were more common in the CII group. Implementation of the CII protocol was followed by a significant downward trend in the rate of DSWI in patients with diabetes, such that the condition was no different from that in nondiabetic patients (Fig 3).

Conclusion.—A policy of aggressive glucose control using postoperative CII can significantly reduce the risk of DSWI wound infection in diabetic patients undergoing open heart surgery. This policy seems to work by reducing hyperglycemia on the first and second postoperative day, the time that represents the major risk factor for DSWI in diabetic patients. Aggressive postoperative glucose control has the potential to reduce the high costs and mortality associated with DSWI in patients with diabetes.

▶ If one looks beyond the fact that no informed consent or institutional review board approval was obtained for this study, that the data were collected prospectively and analyzed retrospectively, and that blood glucose levels of 150 to 200 mg/dL were considered acceptable, the results are still compelling! The authors identified obesity and the use of an internal mammary artery graft as risk factors for development of DSWI. Despite the fact that the CII group had both an increased number of obese patients and more patients receiving internal mammary artery grafts, this group had a significant decrease in the incidence of DSWI. I would not be the least bit surprised if, by the use of a more appropriate insulin protocol and tighter control of serum glucose levels, there could be an even greater reduction in DSWIs.

D. M. Rothenberg, MD, FCCM

Management of Sympathetic Overactivity in Tetanus With Epidural Bupivacaine and Sufentanil: Experience With 11 Patients
Bhagwanjee S, Bösenberg AT, Muckart DJJ (King Edward VIII Hosp, Congella, South Africa)
Crit Care Med 27:1721-1725, 1999   9–37

Background.—There is no uniformly effective method for controlling or preventing the sympathetic overactivity that commonly occurs in severe tetanus. The benefits and risks of continuous epidural infusion of a local anesthetic agent (bupivacaine) and a synthetic opioid (sufentanil) for management of sympathetic overactivity were retrospectively described.

Methods.—Between January 1991 and March 1996, 11 patients (4 females), with an average age of 42 years and with tetanus and sympathetic overactivity, were treated with a continuous epidural infusion of bupivacaine and sufentanil (100 mg and 50 µg, respectively, diluted to 50 mL with normal saline) at 0.1 mL/kg per hour at an infusion rate of 15 mL/h. If the desired clinical response was not achieved, the dosage was changed to 50 mg bupivacaine and 100 µg sufentanil diluted to 50 mL with normal saline. All patients received midazolam.

Results.—Patients averaged 29 days in the ICU and 23 days receiving ventilatory support. All patients were intubated and ventilated within 24 hours of admission. Sympathetic overactivity developed in all patients at an average of 19 days. The reduction in sympathetic overactivity was clinically and statistically significant, as evidenced by significant decreases in maximum systolic and diastolic blood pressures and maximum heart rate and significant increases in minimum blood pressures and heart rate. The respective differences between pre-epidural and postepidural blood pressure and heart rate changes were 40 and 20 mm Hg and 28 beats/min. Complications included nosocomial pneumonia in 9 patients, acalculous cholecystitis in 1, *Candida albicans* sepsis in 1, and epidural sepsis in 2.

Conclusion.—Continuous epidural infusion of bupivacaine and sufentanil for management of sympathetic overactivity in patients with tetanus is effective. Careful attention must be paid to the catheter site to prevent epidural sepsis.

▶ I reviewed this study because of its uniqueness in the use of prolonged infusions of epidural analgesics. Epidurally administered local anesthetics have been used successfully in the past to treat the sympathetic overactivity of tetanus. Of interest in this study however is the number of patients who received epidural anesthesia, presumably through the same catheter for upwards of 39 days! One has to wonder about the risk-benefit ratio of this form of therapy given the difficulty in diagnosing an epidural abscess in patients already prone to nosocomial infection, and who are heavily sedated and often pharmacologically paralyzed.

D. M. Rothenberg, MD, FCCM

The Effect of Midazolam and Propofol on Interleukin-8 From Human Polymorphonuclear Leukocytes
Galley HF, Dubbels AM, Webster NR (Univ of Aberdeen, Scotland)
Anesth Analg 86:1289-1293, 1998   9–38

Objective.—Anesthetics and sedatives can lead to postoperative immune suppression. Interleukin (IL)-8 levels increase in response to infection or stress. An examination was made of the effect of 2 IV anesthetics often used as sedatives in ICU patients on both IL-8 release and IL-8 messenger RNA expression in isolated healthy human polymorphonuclear leukocytes (PMNs).

Methods.—Normal PMNs were isolated from healthy volunteers by the single-layer gradient method. Cultured PMNs were stimulated with lipopolysaccharide and incubated with varying concentrations of midazolam or propofol for 4 to 20 hours. IL-8 levels in cells and supernatant were determined by Northern blotting and phosphorimaging. Differences between groups were analyzed by the Mann-Whitney U-test.

Results.—Lipopolysaccharide increased and midazolam and propofol decreased extracellular IL-8 levels (Fig 1). Lipopolysaccharide increased intracellular IL-8 levels, which increased further in the presence of midazolam and propofol.

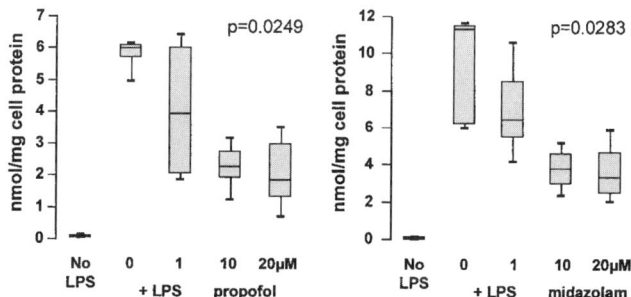

FIGURE 1.—Extracellular IL-8 accumulation from isolated human PMNs. Cells were exposed to propofol or midazolam with and without lipopolysaccharide (*LPS*) for 20 hours, and IL-8 was measured in the culture medium. Box and whisker plots indicate median, 25th, and 75th percentiles, with ranges as *vertical lines*. Data represent 6 to 8 separate experiments and were assessed by the Mann-Whitney *U*-test or Kruskal-Wallis 1-way analysis of variance as appropriate. (Courtesy of Galley HF, Dubbels AM, Webster NR: The effect of midazolam and propofol on interleukin-8 from human polymorphonuclear leukocytes. *Anesth Analg* 86[6]:1289-1293, 1998.)

Conclusion.—Anesthetics apparently slow or suppress transport or secretion of cellular IL-8 and may predispose ICU or surgery patients to infection.

▶ The immunomodulating effects of anesthetic agents are not often considered when instituting sedative therapy in critically ill patients. I am uncertain about the clinical applicability of this study, as 1 of these 2 agents is often necessary to provide anxiolytic therapy for these patients. Future studies examining lorazepam or diazepam may be of interest in the event that either of these 2 agents is shown to have less suppressant effects on white cell function.

D. M. Rothenberg, MD, FCCM

Growth of *Staphylococcus aureus* in Diprivan and Intralipid: Implications on the Pathogenesis of Infections
Langevin PB, Gravenstein N, Doyle TJ, et al (Univ of Florida, Gainesville)
Anesthesiology 91:1394-1400, 1999   9–39

Objective.—Both Diprivan and Intralipid increase the risk of bacterial and fungal infections. Intralipid apparently suppresses reticuloendothelial function and depresses the immune system, and Diprivan appears to support bacterial growth. To determine whether bacterial replication alone could account for the increased risk of infection, the ability of *Staphylococcus aureus* to grow into clinically significant numbers in Intralipid or Diprivan was tested in rabbits.

Methods.—The effects of temperature (16°C, 22.5°C, and 30°C) on the 24-hour growth of *S aureus* was tested in Intralipid and Diprivan cultures or in Intralipid containing 0.005% EDTA. *S aureus*, with and without Intralipid, was injected intravenously into New Zealand white rabbits. Blood samples were obtained 1, 5, 10, 20, 60, and 120 minutes after inoculation. After 24 hours, biopsy specimens of liver, kidney, lung, and spleen were obtained and analyzed for bacterial growth.

Results.—Although there was no growth in cultures containing EDTA, slow bacterial growth did occur in Intralipid at all temperatures tested. All biopsy samples from rabbits not given Intralipid contained equal amounts of bacteria. Kidney samples from rabbits given Intralipid contained significantly more bacteria than other biopsy samples.

Conclusion.—Diprivan and Intralipid do not appear to be good media for promoting bacterial growth. The increased risk of infection after administration of Diprivan or Intralipid apparently results from another mechanism.

▶ This article leaps to an unjustified speculation. The authors' actual experimental results indicate that Diprivan is not a particularly good, bacterial friendly, growth medium. This is not at all surprising. The authors could not resist jumping to the completely unjustified conclusion that somehow, by some mysterious unidentified means, the drug might somehow promote infection some other way. First, no evidence is presented that it does, indeed, promote infection. They should have quit while they were ahead.

J. H. Tinker, MD

Neurologic Critical Care

Sufentanil, Fentanyl, and Alfentanil in Head Trauma Patients: A Study on Cerebral Hemodynamics

Albanèse J, Viviand X, Potie F, et al (Marseilles Univ, France)
Crit Care Med 27:407-411, 1999   9–40

Objective.—In head-injured patients, opioids and hypnotic drugs are used to prevent a decrease in cerebral perfusion pressure (CPP) and an increase in intracranial pressure (ICP); however, their use is controversial. The effects of bolus injection and infusion of sufentanil, alfentanil, and fentanyl on cerebral hemodynamics and electroencephalogram (EEG) activity in patients with increased intracranial pressure after severe head trauma were examined in a randomized, unblended, crossover study.

Methods.—Subjects were 6 male head trauma patients with Glasgow Coma Scores of 8 or less. A continuous infusion of propofol (3 mg/kg per hour) was used to control ICP between 15 and 25 mm Hg, and neuromuscular blockade was achieved with a continuous infusion of vecuronium bromide (8 mg/h). At 24-hour intervals in a crossover fashion, patients were randomly administered equipotent doses of either sufentanil (6 minute injection of 1 mg/kg), alfentanil (100 mg/kg) or fentanyl (10 mg/kg) followed by an infusion of 0.005, 0.75, and 0.075 mg/kg per minute, respectively. Mean arterial pressure (MAP), ICP, CPP, and jugular bulb oxygen saturation were monitored throughout the 60-minute study and recorded every minute.

Results.—Sufentanil, fentanyl, and alfentanil increased ICP significantly by 9, 8, and 5.5 mm Hg, respectively. Maximum increases over baseline occurred at 5 minutes after sufentanil injection (47%), 6 minutes after fentanyl injection (47%), and 3 minutes after alfentanil injection (31%). MAP concomitantly decreased by 21, 24, and 26 mm Hg, respectively, and CPP by 30, 31, and 34 mm Hg, respectively. Although MAP and CPP gradually increased over the next 5 minutes, they remained significantly depressed throughout the study. The ischemia index was unchanged. After opioid injection, EEG fast activity decreased and background activity improved in all but 1 patient. EEG tracings gradually returned to baseline during infusion.

Conclusion.—Continuous infusion rather than bolus injection should be used for sedation of head-injured patients. ICP increase is probably the result of vasodilation, which leads to an increase in cerebral blood volume and, thus, to an increase in brain volume.

▶ This study would have been more interesting if the authors had (1) measured cerebral blood volume and/or cerebral blood flow, or (2) maintained MAP with, for example, phenylephrine. In this fashion perhaps, it would have been possible to better determine how these narcotics affect ICP.

D. M. Rothenberg, MD, FCCM

Measuring Brain Tissue Oxygenation Compared With Jugular Venous Oxygen Saturation for Monitoring Cerebral Oxygenation After Traumatic Brain Injury
Gupta AK, Hutchinson PJ, Al-Rawi P, et al (Univ of Cambridge, England)
Anesth Analg 88:549-553, 1999   9–41

Objective.—Although continuous monitoring of jugular venous oxygen saturation ($SjVO_2$) is an accepted method for evaluating cerebral perfusion to avoid tissue anoxia in patients with severe head injury, the procedure may not be practical in a clinical setting because of the presence of artifacts. Sensors measuring the partial pressure of oxygen (PO_2), carbon dioxide, and brain pH may be able to monitor regional changes in tissue oxygenation without introducing as many artifactual data. PO_2 was measured during hyperventilation in head-injured patients. Changes in PO_2 (ΔPO_2) and $SjVO_2$ ($\Delta SjVO_2$) in areas with and without focal pathology were compared.

Methods.—The partial pressure of oxygen, carbon dioxide, brain pH, and temperature were measured in 13 mechanically ventilated head-injured patients (5 women) aged 26 to 78 years. Two sensors were inserted into each patient, 1 into the femoral artery and 1 into brain tissue. A CT scan identified whether the sensor had been placed in brain tissue with or without focal pathology. After a 30-minute baseline reading, patients were hyperventilated by decreasing the partial pressure of carbon dioxide in 4-mm increments to 22 mm Hg. Hyperventilation was discontinued if $SjVO_2$ dropped below 50%.

Results.—There were no complications associated with insertion of the brain sensor. There was no difference in PO_2 values at different partial pressure of carbon dioxide levels between normal brains and brains with lesions (Fig 1). There were no differences between groups with respect to PO_2 after hyperventilation (Fig 2). Although there was little correlation between $\Delta SjVO_2$ and ΔPO_2 in the group with focal pathology, there was a significant correlation between the 2 variables in the group without focal pathology (Fig 4).

Conclusion.—There was a significant difference in response to hyperventilation for brain tissue with and without focal pathology. Changes in $SjVO_2$ were not correlated with changes in PO_2, suggesting that measurement of oxygenation in brain tissue may be a more accurate measure of regional oxygenation than jugular venous oxygen saturation.

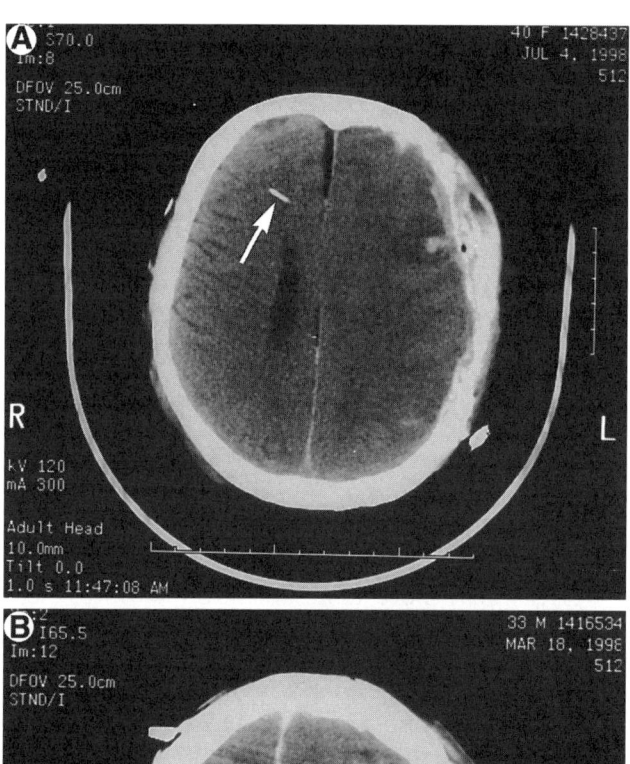

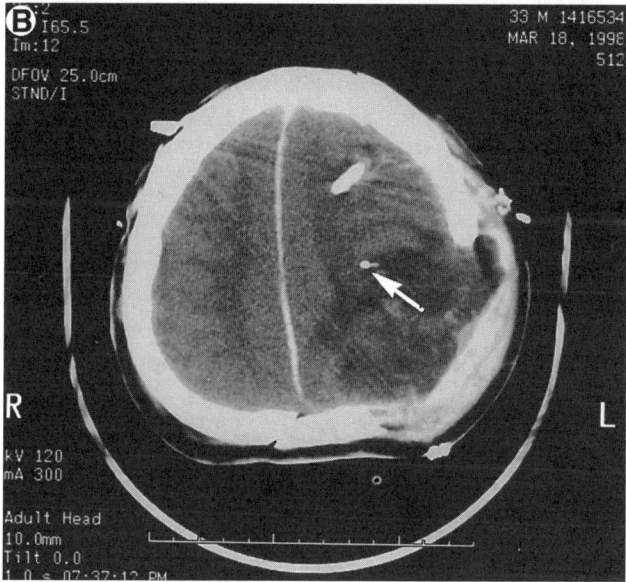

FIGURE 1.—A, CT scan of tissue sensor in area of no focal injury. **B,** CT scan of tissue sensor in area of focal pathology (*arrow* denotes tip of sensor). (Courtesy of Gupta AK, Hutchinson PJ, Al-Rawi P, et al: Measuring brain tissue oxygenation compared with jugular venous oxygen saturation for monitoring cerebral oxygenation after traumatic brain injury. *Anesth Analg* 88[3]:549-553, 1999.)

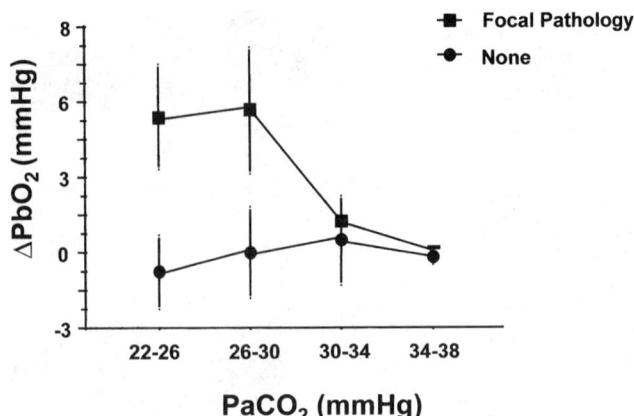

FIGURE 2.—Effect of decreasing partial pressure of carbon dioxide ($PaCO_2$) on the change in tissue oxygen partial pressure (ΔPbO_2) in the groups with focal pathology and with no focal pathology. (Courtesy of Gupta AK, Hutchinson PJ, Al-Rawi P, et al: Measuring brain tissue oxygenation compared with jugular venous oxygen saturation for monitoring cerebral oxygenation after traumatic brain injury. *Anesth Analg* 88[3]:549-553, 1999.)

▶ Tissue PO_2 levels may prove to be a simple method of monitoring for cerebral ischemia, especially during therapeutic maneuvers. Conceivably, tissue probes in both focal and nonfocal areas of pathology may help direct therapy so as to avoid regional hypoperfusion. Future clinical studies will need to be performed to validate this technique.

D. M. Rothenberg, MD, FCCM

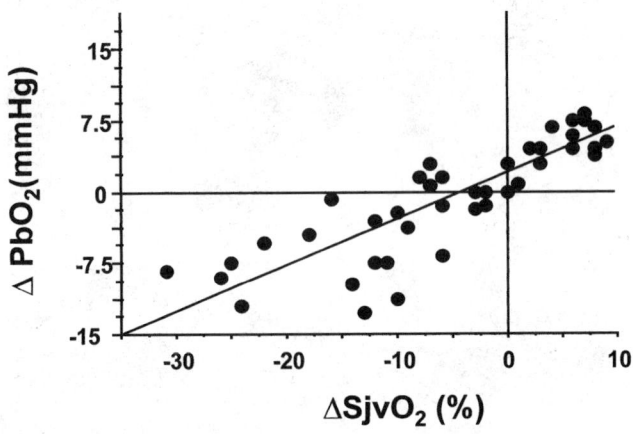

FIGURE 4.—Change in jugular venous oxygen saturation ($\Delta SjvO_2$) plotted against change in tissue oxygen partial pressure (ΔPbO_2) with the sensor not in an area of focal pathology ($r^2 = 0.69$, $P = .0001$). (Courtesy of Gupta AK, Hutchinson PJ, Al-Rawi P, et al: Measuring brain tissue oxygenation compared with jugular venous oxygen saturation for monitoring cerebral oxygenation after traumatic brain injury. *Anesth Analg* 88[3]:549-553, 1999.)

Safety of Intrathecal Sodium Nitroprusside for the Treatment and Prevention of Refractory Cerebral Vasospasm and Ischemia in Humans

Thomas JE, Rosenwasser RH, Armonda RA, et al (Wills Eye Hosp and Neurosensory Inst, Philadelphia)
Stroke 30:1409-1416, 1999   9–42

Background.—The cause of the delayed type of cerebral vasoconstriction (DCV) that occurs after subarachnoid hemorrhage is not known. Patients who do not respond to treatment are at increased risk for stroke, congestive heart failure, and death. Administration of intrathecal sodium nitroprusside (ITSNP) has been suggested as a remedy for suspected deficiencies in the vasodilatory influence of nitric oxide and as a means of reversing DCV and salvaging neurologic function. Results of 171 treatments were presented.

Methods.—Patients (n = 21) with cerebral aneurysms and subarachnoid hemorrhage of grade 3 or higher received ITSNP (1-4 mg/mL in the patient's CSF) by intraventricular or subdural catheter or direct infusion. Twelve (57%) patients did not respond to conventional therapy, and 10 patients received prophylactic ITSNP. Outcome measures were lasting angiographic reversal of vasoconstriction at day 10; treatment failure within 30 minutes, at which time cerebral angioplasty was performed if appropriate; and adverse events. Twice daily transcranial Doppler recordings were performed by a single operator.

Results.—There were 3 brief episodes of hypotension associated with high doses of ITSNP in patients who were treated successfully. Six patients treated prophylactically experienced nausea. No patient had cyanate toxicity or detectable serum cyanate levels. There were no treatment-related adverse events. All treated patients were discharged, 16 with good or excellent outcome who had clinical grade 3 or lower subarachnoid hemorrhage and 5 with a less than good outcome 4 of whom had clinical grade 4 subarachnoid hemorrhage. A grade 4 patient discharged to rehabilitation has since made an excellent recovery. All patients with DCV receiving at least 30 mg of ITSNP had complete and rapid reversal of cerebral vasoconstriction without angioplasty. One patient with a delayed response had improved transcranial Doppler in anterior circulation vessels not treated by angioplasty and achieved an excellent outcome. Patients receiving intraoperative ITSNP required much smaller amounts to effect dilatation.

Conclusion.—ITSNP appears to be a safe and effective acute and prophylactic treatment for DCV refractory to conventional therapy in patients with subarachnoid hemorrhage of grade 3 or higher.

▶ Cerebral artery vasospasm in patients suffering from aneurysmal subarachnoid hemorrhage continues to be a clinical dilemma. The use of the calcium channel antagonist nimodipine has decreased the morbidity and mortality of subarachnoid hemorrhage; however, data suggest that the mechanism of action of such therapy is unrelated to the relief of vasospasm.

In addition, despite the use of so called "HHH" therapy (hypervolemia, hypertension, and hemodilution), there are few controlled studies documenting its efficacy. These preliminary data suggest a target organ approach to relieving cerebral artery vasospasm. In a manner similar to the ability to administer nitric oxide directly to the alveoli, thus mitigating the hypotensive effects of such therapy, so, too, may we be able to administer nitroprusside intrathecally, thus avoiding the deleterious effects of this agent when administered systemically. A randomized, controlled, blinded study is certainly necessary to establish ITSNP as standard therapy for cerebral artery vasospasm.

D. M. Rothenberg, MD, FCCM

10 Pain Management

Acute Pain

Antinociceptive Effect Induced by the Combined Administration of Spinal Morphine and Systemic Buprenorphine

Niv D, Nemirovsky A, Metzner J, et al (Tel-Aviv Univ, Israel; Univ of Southern California, Los Angeles; Universitat des Saarlandes, Homburg, Germany)
Anesth Analg 87:583-586, 1998
10–1

Objective.—Spinal and systemic administration of morphine produces a synergistic analgesic effect. The antinociceptive effect of spinal morphine and systemic buprenorphine was tested.

Methods.—Morphine (1-5 µg) was injected intrathecally via a catheter in the lumbar subarachnoid space, and buprenorphine (50-500 µg/kg) was injected intraperitoneally into male Wistar rats. Nociception was tested by tail immersion 3 times at 5-minute intervals before drug administration, at 5, 10, 15, 20, 30, 45, and 60 minutes, and at half-hour intervals thereafter until tail withdrawal latencies returned to baseline values.

Results.—Equivalent and significant effects were achieved at 2 µg of intrathecal morphine and 50 µg/kg of intraperitoneal buprenorphine,

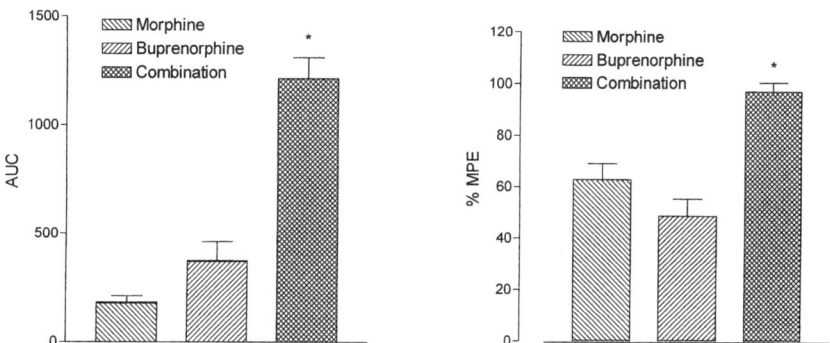

FIGURE 3.—Area under the curve (*AUC*) and percentage of maximal possible effect (*%MPE*) of 4 µg of intrathecal morphine, 100 µg/kg of intraperitoneal buprenorphine (expected effect of the combination), and a combination of 2 µg of intrathecal morphine with 50 µg/kg intraperitoneal buprenorphine (observed effect of the combination). All bars represent the mean AUC or %MPE of 6 to 16 animals. Error bars denote SEM. *$P < .01$. (Courtesy of Niv D, Nemirovsky A, Metzner J, et al: Antinociceptive effect induced by the combined administration of spinal morphine and systemic buprenorphine. *Anesth Analg* 87[3]:583-586, 1998.)

which produced a percent maximal possible effect (%MPE) increase of 97.1% and a significant increase in withdrawal latencies. The %MPE increased in a dose-dependent fashion for both drugs. The maximal effect, achieved with 4 μg intrathecal morphine and 100 μg/kg intraperitoneal buprenorphine, produced a %MPE of 62.9% and 48.8%, respectively (Fig 3).

Conclusion.—The combination of 2 μg of intrathecal morphine and 50 μg/kg intraperitoneal buprenorphine produced a maximal supra-additive antinociceptive effect that maintains a significant level of analgesia with the minimum doses of opioids.

▶ While these data are encouraging, the supra-additive effect of this drug combination needs to be confirmed in a human postoperative pain model. Many drug combinations have been shown to be synergistic in animal models of experimental pain but not in clinical situations involving acute or chronic pain. In addition, the test for supra-additivity utilized in this study is not very rigorous. An isobolographic analysis, using several doses at the same dose ratios, provides much better evidence of synergy. Nevertheless, this drug combination makes sense and may, as the authors suggest, be less likely to produce respiratory depression than epidural plus systemic morphine.

S. E. Abram, MD

Efficacy and Costs of Patient-Controlled Analgesia Versus Regularly Administered Intramuscular Opioid Therapy
Choinière M, Rittenhouse BE, Perreault S, et al (Univ of Montreal; McGill Univ, Montreal)
Anesthesiology 89:1377-1388, 1998   10–2

Objective.—The clinical and cost benefits of patient-controlled analgesia (PCA) were compared in a prospective study with those of regularly administered intramuscular (IM) injections of opioids after hysterectomy.

Methods.—Women undergoing abdominal hysterectomy were randomly allocated to receive PCA (n = 63) or regular injections (n = 63) of IM morphine for 48 hours after surgery. Patient satisfaction was assessed with a visual analog scale and by asking if the patient would select the same analgesia treatment again. Side effects and cost of drug treatment were determined.

Results.—There were no significant differences between groups with respect to nausea and vomiting, pruritus, urinary retention, and respiratory depression (Table 3). With respect to patient satisfaction, 83% of the IM group and 94% of the PCA group would select the same analgesia treatment again. Time to sit in a chair without assistance was significantly longer for the PCA group than for the IM group. Side effects occurred in all patients; analgesia treatment was discontinued in 10% of the PCA group and 11% of the IM group because of side effects. Total costs (labor,

TABLE 3.—Mean Ratings Obtained on the Various Pain Measures in the PCA and IM Groups

	PCA Group (N = 51)	IM Group (N = 54)	P	95% CI of the Mean Difference	1-β
VAS pain scales					
At rest	1.8 ± 1.0	1.7 ± 1.1	0.73	(−0.4, 0.4)	0.94
When changing position	4.1 ± 2.4	3.7 ± 1.9	0.34	(−0.5, 1.2)	0.84
When walking	4.0 ± 2.5	2.9 ± 1.9	0.03 (NS)*	(−0.3, 2.1)	0.03
VAS pain relief scale	7.9 ± 1.4	8.3 ± 1.5	0.28	(−1.0, 0.1)	0.91
McGill Pain Questionnaire	21 ± 12	21 ± 13	0.89	(−4.7, 5.4)	—

*Bonferroni's corrected α level: 0.05/5 tests→P value = 0.01.
Abbreviation: VAS, Visual Analogue Scale.
(Courtesy of Choinière M, Rittenhouse BE, Perreault S, et al: Efficacy and costs of patient-controlled analgesia versus regularly administered intramuscular opioid therapy. *Anesthesiology* 89:1377-1388, 1998. Copyright American Society of Anesthesiologists, Inc. Used with permission of Lippincott-Raven Publishers.)

nonlabor, drug, and treatment of side effects) were higher for the PCA group than for the IM group.

Conclusion.—PCA is more expensive than IM analgesia and is not more effective with respect to pain relief, side effects, and patient satisfaction.

▶ It is surprising that this study was undertaken at all, given the large body of evidence demonstrating better analgesia and lower costs associated with PCA when compared with IM analgesics. Undoubtedly, the good clinical outcome with IM morphine is related to close attention on the part of the nursing staff. One might argue that under normal circumstances (ie, over-worked, understaffed nursing) IM opioids might not be as effective as PCA, which is not dependent on nursing availability or motivation. On the other hand, the cost savings generally attributed to PCA were not evident even though nursing labor costs were higher. This study provides motivation to look at other low-technology drug administration options as alternatives to PCA.

S. E. Abram, MD

Adrenaline Markedly Improves Thoracic Epidural Analgesia Produced by a Low-Dose Infusion of Bupivacaine, Fentanyl and Adrenaline After Major Surgery: A Randomised, Double-blind, Cross-over Study With and Without Adrenaline
Niemi G, Breivik H (Natl Hosp, Oslo, Norway)
Acta Anaesthesiol Scand 42:897-909, 1998   10–3

Objective.—The combination of adrenaline, fentanyl, and bupivacaine given epidurally after surgery exerts a synergistic effect. The effects of removing adrenaline from this combination on postoperative pain intensity, pain relief, and side effects were investigated in a prospective, randomized, double-blind, crossover study.

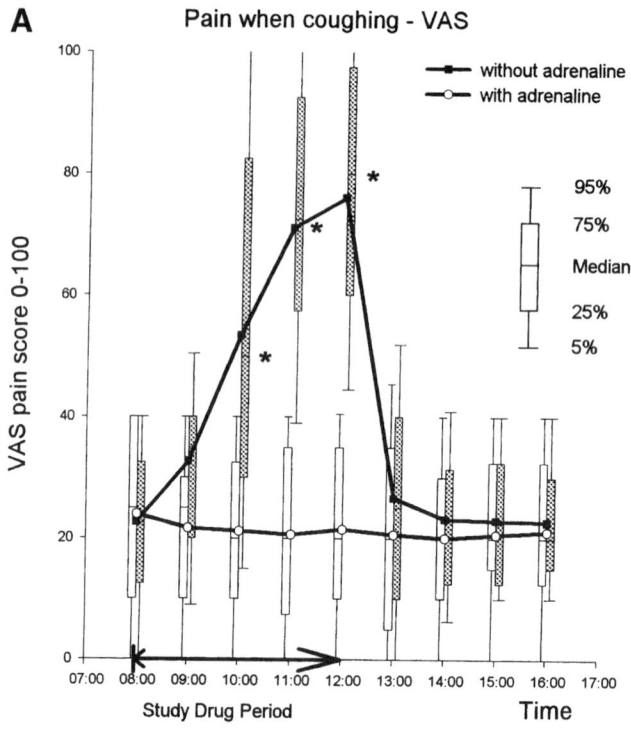

A Pain when coughing - VAS

(Legend)
- ■ without adrenaline
- ○ with adrenaline

- 95%
- 75%
- Median
- 25%
- 5%

VAS pain score 0-100

Study Drug Period

Time

(Continued)

Methods.—After thoracotomy or laparotomy, 12 patients received an epidural infusion (10 mL/h) of bupivacaine (1 mg/mL)–fentanyl (2 µg/mL)–adrenaline (2 µg/mL) (EDA) and 12 received EDA without adrenaline, on the first postoperative day for 4 hours. After an overnight period during which both groups received EDA, the groups were switched to the other arm of the study on the second postoperative day for 4 hours, followed by a control period of 4 hours during which both groups again received EDA. Sensory and motor blockade, pain at rest and when coughing, need for rescue analgesia, and study dry consumption were recorded.

Results.—The sensory block regressed significantly without adrenaline and was quickly reestablished when adrenaline was added back to the infusion. There was a significant difference between the 2 groups in pain intensity with and without adrenaline (Fig 3). The need for rescue analgesia was greater and systolic blood pressure was significantly higher in those receiving EDA without adrenaline. The quality of pain relief was significantly better in patients receiving EDA with adrenaline. Patients receiving EDA with adrenaline tended to be out of bed more often than those receiving EDA without adrenaline. Serum fentanyl requirements were significantly higher in patients receiving EDA without adrenaline than in patients receiving EDA with adrenaline (Fig 6).

FIGURE 3 (cont.)

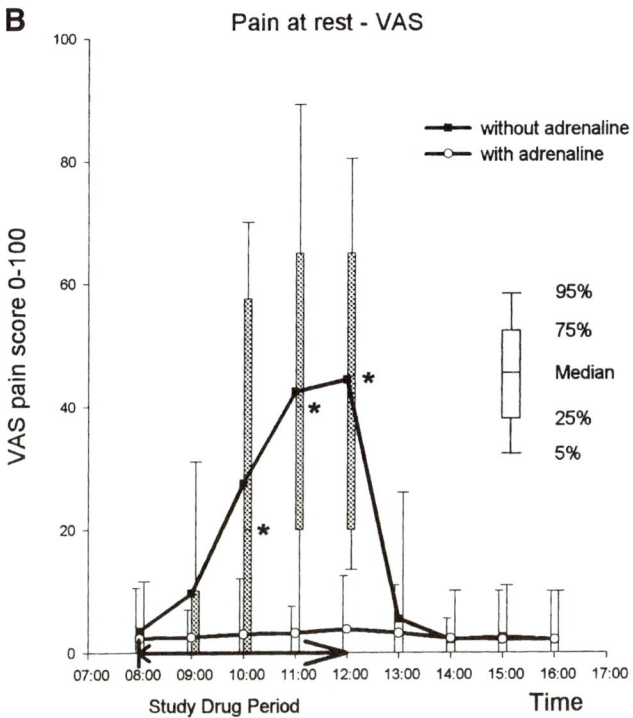

B

Pain at rest - VAS

—■— without adrenaline
—○— with adrenaline

VAS pain score 0-100

95%
75%
Median
25%
5%

Study Drug Period   Time

FIGURE 3.—Pain scores (Visual Analogue Scale, [VAS] 0-100) while coughing (A) and at rest (B) during continuous epidural analgesia with our triple epidural mixture with fentanyl and bupivacaine with or without adrenaline. The line scatter plot shows the mean VAS values. In the box-whisker plot the box contains 50% of the data (interquartile range) and is crossed with a thin bar at the median. The whiskers are the 5th and 95th percentiles. *Significantly different from the standard mixture with adrenaline (Wilcoxon Signed Ranks test; $P < .001$). (Courtesy of Niemi G, Breivik H: Adrenaline markedly improves thoracic epidural analgesia produced by a low-dose infusion of bupivacaine, fentanyl and adrenaline after major surgery: A randomised, double-blind, cross-over study with and without adrenaline. *Acta Anaesthesiol Scand* 42:897-909, 1998.)

Conclusion.—The presence of adrenaline in EDA potentiates sensory blockade and pain relief, and decreases the requirement for fentanyl.

▶ It is surprising that there has been so little investigation of the addition of epinephrine to spinal and epidural opioids and local anesthetics for the treatment of postoperative pain. The antinociceptive effect of spinal and epidural epinephrine administration has been demonstrated in both animal and human models, and there is evidence that the addition of epinephrine to epidurally administered opioids and local anesthetics improves analgesia and reduces systemic blood levels. The authors provide historical evidence for the safety of epinephrine infusions containing up to 5 µg/mL, and found that a concentration as low as 2 µg/mL was effective at improving analgesia and reducing fentanyl blood levels.

S. E. Abram, MD

Serum Fentanyl concentration

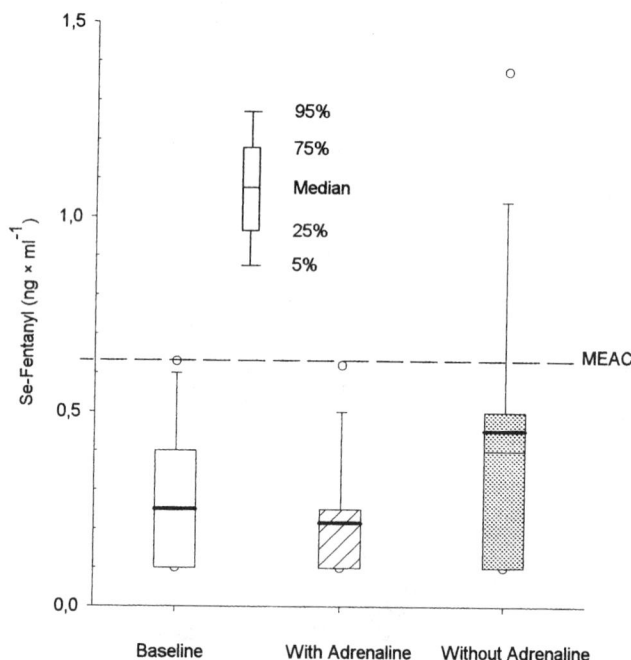

FIGURE 6.—Mean serum fentanyl concentration was 0.25 ng/mL during epidural infusion of the adrenaline-containing epidural mixture at baseline. At the end of the 4-hour infusion without adrenaline, the mean serum fentanyl concentration had doubled to 0.45 ng/mL (paired t test; P < .01). In comparison, at the end of the 4-hour infusion with adrenaline, the mean serum fentanyl concentration was unaltered from baseline (0.22 ng/mL). The mean minimum effective analgesic concentration (MEAC) for fentanyl in serum has been determined as 0.63 ng/mL. (From Niemi G, Breivik H: Adrenaline markedly improves thoracic epidural analgesia produced by a low-dose infusion of bupivacaine, fentanyl and adrenaline after major surgery: A randomised, double-blind, cross-over study with and without adrenaline. *Acta Anaesthesiol Scand* 42:897-909, 1998. Courtesy of Gourlay GK, Kowalski SR, Plummer JL, et al: Fentanyl blood concentration–analgesic response relationship in the treatment of postoperative pain. *Anesth Analg* 67:329-337, 1998.)

Postoperative Analgesic Effects of Three Demand-Dose Sizes of Fentanyl Administered by Patient-Controlled Analgesia

Camu F, Van Aken H, Bovill JG (Vrije Universiteit Brussel, Belgium; Klinik und Poliklinik für Anaesthesiologie und Operative Intensivmedizin der Westf, Münster, Germany; Univ of Leiden, The Netherlands)
Anesth Analg 87:890-895, 1998   10–4

Objective.—Although patient-controlled analgesia (PCA) is commonly used to control postoperative pain, demand-dose sizes have not been examined to determine the optimal dose combining the benefits of significant pain relief with the least amount of respiratory depression, oxygen desaturation, or adverse events. The safety and efficacy of 20-, 40-, and 60-µg demand doses of fentanyl delivered over 24 hours period as short continuous infusion by PCA to patients with moderate to severe postoperative pain was investigated in a randomized, double-blind study.

Methods.—Patients who had undergone major abdominal surgery received titrated doses of IV fentanyl (10 µg every 1-5 minutes) until their visual analog scale scores were less than 2. Then they were randomly allocated to receive on-demand PCA fentanyl (20, 40, or 60 µg/L or 2 mL infused at a constant rate over 10 minutes). Oxygenation, respiratory rate, blood pressure, and heart rate were monitored before and after titration with fentanyl.

Results.—Patients in the 40-µg group required significantly more fentanyl during the titration period than did patients in the 60-µg group. Overall patient global assessments scores were high, and serious adverse events were absent in 42%, 52%, and 68% of the 20-, 40-, and 60-µg dose groups, respectively. Corresponding physician pain relief assessments were 42%, 67%, and 72%. The response rate and dose-dependent decrease in pain intensity at rest and during movement in the 60-µg group was significantly higher than in the 20-µg group. Adverse events were reported by 31 patients in the 20-µg group, 38 in the 40-µg group, and 32 in the 60-µg group, with the most common adverse events being nausea and vomiting. The mean respiratory rate was significantly slower in the 60-µg group than in the 20-µg group and significantly lower than in the 40-µg group. Oxygen saturation, heart rate, and blood pressure were similar in all 3 groups.

Conclusion.—Fentanyl is safe and effective for moderate to severe postoperative pain. The optimal PCA demand dose appears to be 40 µg.

▶ There are theoretical reasons that fentanyl may be more effective and may have fewer side effects than less potent drugs such as morphine or meperidine when used postoperatively. This may be particularly true for patients who received opioids preoperatively. It is important, therefore, that the optimal PCA dose be determined.

S. E. Abram, MD

Intravenous Administration of Caffeine Sodium Benzoate for Postdural Puncture Headache
Yücel A, Özyalçin S, Talu GK, et al (Med Faculty of Istanbul, Turkey)
Reg Anesth Pain Med 24:51-54, 1999   10–5

Objective.—Caffeine relieves postdural puncture headache (PDPH). The safety and efficacy of prophylactic administration of intravenous caffeine sodium benzoate in reducing PDPH in patients receiving spinal anesthesia was evaluated in a randomized, double-blind, placebo-controlled study.

Methods.—Either 1000 mL normal saline solution with 500 mg caffeine sodium benzoate (group C, n = 30) or 1000 mL normal saline solution (group S, n = 30) was administered to patients undergoing lower abdom-

TABLE 3.—Incidence of Headache

	No + Mild Headache	Moderate + Severe Headache	X^2	P
Group C	27 (19 + 8)	3 (1 + 2)		
				.03*
Group S	19 (14 + 5)	11 (4 + 7)	5.96 (df:1)	

*Significant.
Abbreviations: C, caffeine; *S,* saline solution.
(Courtesy of Yücel A, Özyalçin S, Talu GK, et al: Intravenous administration of caffeine sodium benzoate for postdural puncture headache. *Reg Anesth Pain Med* 24:51-54, 1999.)

inal or lower extremity surgery during the first 20 minutes after spinal anesthesia administration. Electrocardiography, noninvasive blood pressure monitoring, and pulse oximetry monitoring were performed every 15 minutes for 2 hours. Headache pain was assessed on a Visual Analogue Scale (VAS) every 4 hours for 48 hours. Patients assessed headache symptoms on day 5 and were followed up for side effects for 5 days.

Results.—VAS headache scores were significantly lower in group C than in group S for the first 4 days; scores on day 5 were similar. Group S patients had significantly more moderate and severe headaches than did group C patients (Table 3). Two group S patients required an epidural blood patch for intractable headache. Analgesic requirements were significantly lower in group C than in group S. No side effects were reported.

Conclusion.—Prophylactic administration of caffeine sodium benzoate is a safe and effective measure for minimizing PDPH.

▶ In a population expected to have a fairly high headache incidence (young patients, use of 22-gauge cutting needles) prophylactic caffeine appeared to reduce the incidence of PDPH. Such prophylactic use of the drug is probably not indicated when small-gauge pencil-point needles are used. It would be useful to determine whether this technique would be helpful after wet taps with epidural needles.

S. E. Abram, MD

Pre-Incision Infiltration With Lidocaine Reduces Pain and Opioid Consumption After Reduction Mammoplasty
Rosaeg OP, Bell M, Cicutti NJ, et al (Univ of Ottawa, Ont)
Reg Anesth Pain Med 23:575-579, 1998   10–6

Background.—Before surgical closure, infiltration of the wound with local anesthetic agents may reduce discomfort and the need for postoperative opioids. The analgesic efficacy of preoperative tumescent infiltration with lidocaine for reduction mammoplasty was investigated in a randomized, double-blind clinical study.

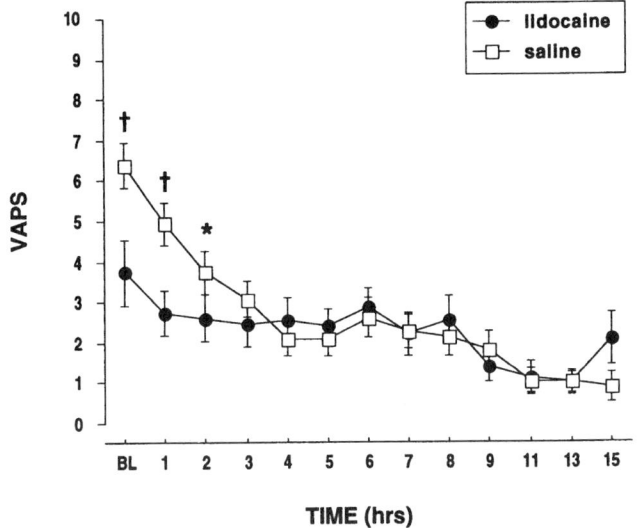

FIGURE 1.—Visual analogue pain scores after surgery in patients receiving lidocaine (group 1) and saline solution (group 2). Values indicate mean ± 95% confidence limits. *P < .05; †P < .001. (Courtesy of Rosaeg OP, Bell M, Cicutti NJ, et al: Pre-incision infiltration with lidocaine reduces pain and opioid consumption after reduction mammoplasty. *Reg Anesth Pain Med* 23:575-579, 1998.)

Methods.—Women with mammary hypertrophy were assigned to pre-incision infiltration with 5 mL/kg of 0.35% lidocaine with 1:1,000,000 epinephrine into each breast after induction of general anesthesia (group 1) or to similar injections of saline solution with 1:1,000,000 epinephrine (group 2). Each group consisted of 15 patients.

Findings.—Group 2 patients had higher visual analogue pain scores up until 3.5 hours after surgery. Recipients of saline solution also had a greater consumption of IV morphine during all 1-hour postoperative intervals, although these differences were statistically significant only until 4.5 hours after surgery. In group 1, total IV morphine intake in the first 9.5 hours postoperatively was 16.9 mg, compared with 31.1 mg in group 2. Postoperative nausea and vomiting occurred in 87% of both groups. The groups did not differ in the time it took to achieve fitness for discharge with postanesthesia discharge scores of 9 or greater (Fig 1).

Conclusions.—Tumescent infiltration with lidocaine before reduction mammoplasty improves pain relief in the early postoperative period. It also decreases the need for opioid analgesic medication.

▶ Although some studies demonstrate prolonged (several days or more) reduction of postoperative pain after preoperative tissue infiltration of local anesthetic, the effects seen in this study were very transient. This suggests a residual local anesthetic effect rather than a preemptive blockade of spinally mediated hyperalgesia. Most previous studies that assessed the effect of preoperative versus postoperative tissue infiltration have failed to demonstrate a preemptive effect.

S. E. Abram, MD

Effects of Prophylactic Nalmefene on the Incidence of Morphine-Related Side Effects in Patients Receiving Intravenous Patient-controlled Analgesia
Joshi GP, Duffy L, Chehade J, et al (Univ of Texas, Dallas)
Anesthesiology 90:1007-1011, 1999   10–7

Background.—IV patient-controlled analgesia (PCA) is a common technique used in the treatment of postoperative pain. Patients using this system, however, can have opioid-related side effects, such as nausea, vomiting, and pruritus. A low-dose naloxone infusion can reduce these effects. Nalmefene is a new, pure opioid antagonist with a longer duration of action than naloxone. Its effect on opioid-related side effects has not been evaluated. The dose-response of nalmefene for preventing morphine-related side effects in IV PCA was determined, as was the effect of nalmefene on the quality of analgesia.

Methods.—One hundred twenty women who underwent lower abdominal surgery were included in the study. General anesthesia was induced with IV thiopental and rocuronium and was maintained with desflurane, nitrous oxide, and fentanyl or sufentanil. Neostigmine and glycopyrrolate were used to reverse neuromuscular blockade. No prophylactic antiemetic drugs were used. After surgery, patients were randomly assigned to receive nalmefene 15 µg, nalmefene 25 µg, or saline. The need for antiemetic and antipruritic drugs and total use of morphine were recorded for 24 hours. The incidence of postoperative nausea, vomiting, pruritus, and pain was recorded 30 minutes after patients arrived in the postanesthesia unit. At 24 hours, patients were asked what they remembered about these side effects.

Results.—Patients receiving nalmefene had significantly less need for antiemetic and antipruritic drugs than did patients given placebo. The need to treat side effects was similar in both groups given nalmefene. Prophylactic nalmefene decreased patients' remembrance of nausea and itching as reported at 24 hours. Total consumption of morphine was similar in both groups, but patients who had nalmefene retrospectively described their pain as less severe than did patients given placebo.

Discussion.—These results indicate that prophylactic nalmefene can significantly decrease the need for antiemetic and antipruritic drugs in patients using IV PCA with morphine. The use of nalmefene does not appear to affect the quality of analgesia.

▶ The authors did not offer an explanation of why a systemic opioid antagonist reduced the side effects of systemic morphine. Low-dose opioid antagonists have been analgesic in certain animal models, as well as in postoperative pain studies. Blockade of the hyperalgesic effect of dynorphin has been proposed as a possible mechanism.

S. E. Abram, MD

Analgesic and Adverse Effects of a Low Dose of Intrathecally Administered Hyperbaric Neostigmine Alone or Combined With Morphine in Patients Submitted to Spinal Anaesthesia: Pilot Studies
Klamt JG, Garcia LV, Prado WA (Faculty of Medicine of Ribeirão Preto, Brazil)
Anaesthesia 54:27-31, 1999
10–8

Background.—Intrathecal (IT) neostigmine has produced long-lasting analgesia postoperatively and improved opioid analgesia. IT neostigmine produces dose-dependent analgesia, but can also cause nausea, vomiting, and fecal incontinence.

Methods.—The analgesic and adverse effects of IT hyperbaric neostigmine alone or with morphine were determined in 2 patients with severe lower limb ischemic pain, 5 patients who had cesarean section, and 19 patients who had orthopedic surgery with spinal anesthesia.

Results.—In the 2 patients with severe lower limb ischemic pain, hyperbaric neostigmine (50 µg in glucose 8%) produced analgesia that lasted for more than 6 hours, but patients also experienced vomiting. Among the 5 patients who had cesarean section, 2 patients received neostigmine 25 µg alone, 1 patient received neostigmine 25 µg plus morphine 50 µg, and 2 patients received morphine 100 µg alone. In the 3 patients who received neostigmine alone or with morphine, neostigmine produced no discernible analgesic effect, and the patients experienced severe nausea and vomiting within 15 minutes of IT injection of neostigmine. The 2 patients given morphine 100 µg alone had analgesia for more than 24 hours and mild pruritus. In the 19 patients who had orthopedic surgery with spinal anesthesia, neostigmine 25 µg alone produced analgesia that did not last as long as neostigmine 25 µg plus morphine 50 µg, or as long as morphine 100 µg alone.

Discussion.—In these patients, hyperbaric neostigmine alone or combined with morphine produced nausea, vomiting, anxiety, somnolence, and involuntary defecation. In some patients, the nausea and vomiting lasted from 9 to 12 hours. Most patients given neostigmine and morphine had more severe nausea, vomiting, and somnolence. The low clinical efficacy of this drug may impair the design of double-blind studies and restrict its clinical use.

▶ Previous studies have shown consistent potentiation of IT morphine analgesia by doses of neostigmine that fail to produce nausea. This study suggests that the therapeutic window for intrathecal neostigmine is quite narrow.

S. E. Abram, MD

Use of Continuous Retropleural Bupivacaine in Postoperative Pain Management for Pediatric Thoracotomy

Gibson MP, Vetter T, Crow JP (Children's Hosp Med Ctr, Akron, Ohio)
J Pediatr Surg 34:199-201, 1999   10–9

Background.—Managing postoperative pain in patients who have had thoracotomy is often difficult and can be even more difficult in children because of their inability to effectively express what they are feeling. Although various methods of pain management have been investigated, there is little information on postoperative pain management after thoracotomy in pediatric patients.

Methods.—In a retrospective study, the medical records of 13 pediatric patients (aged 7-18 years) who had thoracotomy during a 3-year period were reviewed. In 7 patients, a retropleural catheter was inserted before closure of the thoracotomy by placing an epidural catheter posterior to the parietal pleura. The space was entered 2 intercostal levels below the incision and advanced superiorly 4 intercostal spaces. Bupivacaine (0.125% or 0.25%) at 0.5 mL/kg per hour was administered. The postoperative need for morphine of the 7 study patients and 6 control patients was compared. The separate Student's *t* test was used for analysis.

Results.—Among the 13 patients, 7 had anterior spinal release and fusion, 5 had mediastinal operations, and 1 had lobectomy. The study and control groups were similar in age, weight, and type of surgery. Patients had infusion through the retropleural catheter for an average of 3.8 days. The total mean postoperative use of morphine was 0.88 mg/kg in patients with a retropleural catheter and 2.32 mg/kg in control patients.

Discussion.—These results show that a continuous infusion of bupivacaine using a unique retropleural technique decreased the postoperative need for morphine in children who had thoracotomy. The use of this catheter may be useful in managing postoperative pain in children who undergo thoracotomy.

▶ The placement of thoracic epidural catheters in anesthetized patients remains controversial. The technique of thoracic paravertebral analgesia, with intra-operative catheter placement, provides a reasonable alternative that avoids the risk of spinal cord or nerve root injury. As the authors point out, the use of 0.25% bupivacaine administered at a rate of 0.5 mL/kg per hour may produce higher than acceptable blood levels.

S. E. Abram, MD

The Safety and Efficacy of Intrathecal Opioid Analgesia for Acute Post-operative Pain: Seven Years' Experience With 5969 Surgical Patients at Indiana University Hospital
Gwirtz KH, Young JV, Byers RS, et al (Indiana Univ, Indianapolis)
Anesth Analg 88:599-604, 1999   10–10

Objective.—One institution's 7-year experience with the efficacy and side effects of intrathecal (IT) opioid analgesia for acute postoperative pain was prospectively evaluated.

Methods.—Patient satisfaction, side effects, complications, and naloxone use were assessed on postoperative day 1 with the use of daily quality assurance data in 5969 adult patients receiving IT opioid analgesia after major urologic, orthopedic, general, vascular, thoracic, and nonobstetric gynecologic surgery according to dosing guidelines.

Results.—Data were available for 5705 patients (95.6%).

Conclusion.—Single-dose IT opioid administration after major surgery effectively controlled acute pain without producing significant side effects or complications.

▶ Although the safety and efficacy of IT opioids are well documented, it is useful to examine the experience of a single institution, using specific doses and protocols. The low incidence of respiratory depression and the absence of respiratory arrest are reassuring.

S. E. Abram, MD

Transdermal Nitroglycerine Enhances Spinal Sufentanil Postoperative Analgesia Following Orthopedic Surgery
Lauretti GR, de Oliveira R, Reis MP, et al (Univ of São Paulo, Brazil)
Anesthesiology 90:734-739, 1999   10–11

Objective.—It has been suggested that high-dose nitroglycerine patches enhance the effect of analgesia. The influence of transdermal nitroglycerine patches on the analgesic effect of intrathecal (IT) sufentanil was evaluated in patients undergoing orthopedic surgery.

Methods.—Patients (n = 56), premedicated with 0.05 to 0.1 mg/kg IV midazolam before undergoing orthopedic surgery, were randomly allocated to receive 15 mg bupivacaine and either IT saline solution and placebo transdermal test drug (n = 13), 10 µg IT sufentanil and placebo transdermal test drug (n = 15), IT saline solution and 5 mg per 24 hours nitroglycerine transdermal patch (n = 13), or 10 µg IT sufentanil and 5 mg per 24 hours nitroglycerine transdermal patch (n = 15). Patients rated pain and nausea on a 0 to 10 Visual Analogue Scale. Outcome was time to first rescue medication.

Results.—Times to first rescue medication were 231 minutes for the control group, 325 for the saline solution group, 269 for the nitroglycerine group, and 785 for the sufentanil/nitroglycerine group. The number of IM diclofenac rescue injections in 24 hours averaged 2.5, 2.3, 2, and 1, respectively. The corresponding overall 24-hour Visual Analogue Scale pain and nausea/vomiting scores were 1.7 and 0.5, 1 and 0.4, 1 and 0.5, and 0.3 and 0.7, respectively. All differences were significant.

Conclusion.—The transdermal nitroglycerine patch appears to enhance the antinociceptive effects of postoperative IT sufentanil.

▶ Nitric oxide has been shown to play a role in the development of "wind-up," or spinal sensitization, and spinally administered nitric oxide synthase inhibitors can reduce hyperalgesia associated with formalin injection or nerve injury. It is unlikely, therefore, that the effect of nitroglycerine, a nitric oxide donor, on prolongation of spinal opioid analgesia is mediated at the spinal level.

S. E. Abram, MD

Continuous Interscalene Brachial Plexus Block for Postoperative Analgesia Following Shoulder Surgery
Lehtipalo S, Koskinen L-OD, Johansson G, et al (Umeå Univ Hosp, Sweden)
Acta Anaesthesiol Scand 43:258-264, 1999   10–12

Objective.—The efficacy of continuous interscalene brachial plexus block, patient-controlled analgesia (PCA), and morphine (IV and intramuscular) for postoperative analgesia in the control of postoperative shoulder pain was compared. In addition, postoperative correlations between degree of pain and respiratory and circulatory variables and "stress metabolites" in microdialysates from subcutaneous tissue were compared and evaluated.

Methods.—Thirty patients (10 women), aged 18 to 71 years, scheduled for acromioplasty and premedicated with oral lorazepam (2.0-2.5 mg) were randomly allocated to receive intramuscular and IV morphine (MO, n = 10), continuous interscalene brachial plexus block with bupivacaine (PL, n = 10), or PCA (n = 10). Visual Analogue Scale pain score, heart rate, blood pressure, respiratory rate, and SpO_2 were recorded 0, 2, 4, 6, 8, 12, 16, 20, and 24 hours postoperatively. Glucose, lactate, and glycerol levels were monitored every 30 minutes. The degree of sensory and motor block was assessed 2 hours after surgery in 8 PL patients.

Results.—Postoperative pain was significantly lower in the PL group than in the MO and PCA groups at all time points except at 16 and 20 hours. Lactate level in the PL group increased significantly over time but was not significantly higher than lactate values in the MO and PCA groups. Glucose level was significantly increased in all groups at all time points. Respiratory rates decreased significantly in the first 4 hours in the PCA (16.9 vs 13.5 breaths/min) and MO groups (18.4 vs 15.5 breaths/min), but changes in heart rate and systolic blood pressure were not significant. Side effects were similar in all groups. Visual Analogue Scale scores were low.

Conclusion.—Continuous interscalene plexus block is effective for pain management after shoulder surgery and has fewer side effects than PCA and morphine.

▶ Because patients were followed up for only 24 hours, it is not clear whether the improved analgesia was related to the initial bolus injection or to the continuous infusion. Catheter displacement is a problem with this technique, because the interscalene space is narrow and neck movement can cause catheter migration.

S. E. Abram, MD

Percutaneous Electrical Nerve Stimulation: An Alternative to Antiviral Drugs for Acute Herpes Zoster
Ahmed HE, Craig WF, White PF, et al (Univ of Texas Southwestern Med Ctr, Dallas)
Anesth Analg 87:911-914, 1998   10–13

Objective.—Whether antiviral drugs decrease the pain of postherpetic neuralgia is controversial. Percutaneous electrical nerve stimulation (PENS) therapy was compared with standard antiviral therapy with respect to pain, impact on the patient's physical activity and quality of sleep, resolution of the herpes lesions, and incidence and severity of postherpetic neuralgia in a randomized, single-blind study.

Methods.—Fifty patients with recent acute-onset herpes zoster lesions were given 500 mg famciclovir 3 times a day for 1 week (control group) or PENS therapy for 30 minutes 3 times a week for 2 weeks. The severity of postherpetic neuralgic pain was rated on a 0 to 100 Visual Analogue Scale.

Results.—The PENS group healed significantly faster than the control group (4.6 vs 5.6 days). The decrease in pain scores was significantly greater in the PENS group than in the control group at 2 weeks (67% vs 45%). The amount of physical activity improved significantly more in the PENS group than in the control group (78% vs 60%). Quality-of-sleep scores were significantly higher in the PENS group than in the control group (55% vs 37%). PENS therapy was significantly associated with a decrease in pain severity at 3 and 6 months in patients age 50 years and older.

Conclusion.—PENS therapy effectively treats the pain of acute herpes zoster infection as effectively as antiviral therapy, and it promotes healing and improves quality of sleep in infected individuals.

▶ This study raises more questions than it answers. If this modality is indeed effective, we have little information with which to direct our therapy. We are not told which frequencies are optimal, how long each treatment lasts, how often treatments are given, or what stimulation parameters were used (pulse shape, width, amplitude). We are not told whether there was immediate pain relief or, as is often seen with transcutaneous electrical nerve stimulation, increased pain during stimulation. The term used to describe the technique is misleading, as there is no direct stimulation of the intercostal nerve. Although this technique deserves further assessment, I hope that it will not be widely adopted without better scientific scrutiny.

S. E. Abram, MD

Intra-articular Morphine for Pain Relief After Knee Arthroscopy
Rosseland LA, Stubhaug A, Skoglund A, et al (Univ Hosp, Oslo, Norway; Gjøvik Gen Hosp, Norway)
Acta Anaesthesiol Scand 43:252-257, 1999   10–14

Objective.—Some studies have questioned the efficacy of intra-articular morphine after arthroscopy. The analgesic effect of 1- and 2-mg intra-articular morphine injections in day care patients who underwent diagnostic and minor interventional knee arthroscopy during local infiltration anesthesia was evaluated in a parallel-group, double-blind, randomized study.

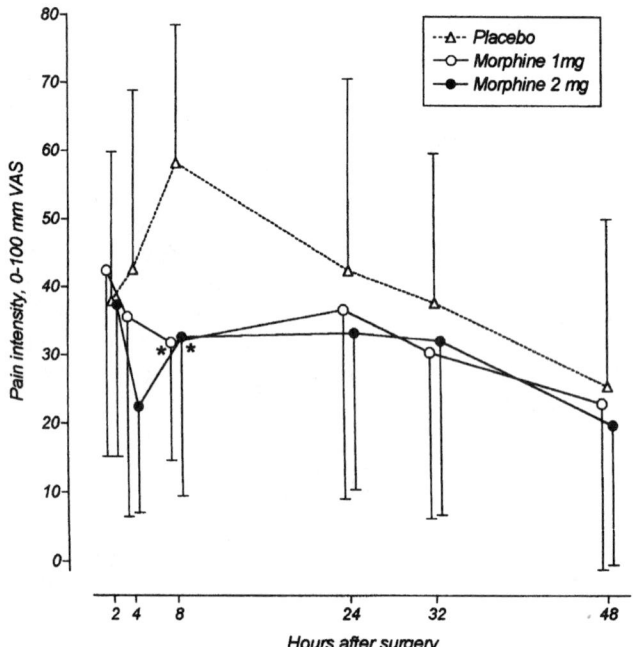

FIGURE 3.—Mean pain intensity (with SD) for a subgroup (n = 28) having Visual Analogue Scale (*VAS*) pain score of 10 mm or more 2 hours after surgery. Results for patients receiving morphine 1 mg (*open circles, solid line,* n = 10), morphine 2 mg (*closed circles, solid line,* n = 9), and placebo (*open triangles, broken line,* n = 9). *Significantly different from placebo; Kruskal-Wallis test, *P* < .05. (Courtesy of Rosseland LA, Stubhaug A, Skoglund A, et al: Intra-articular morphine for pain relief after knee arthroscopy. *Acta Anaesthesiol Scand* 43:252-257, 1999.)

Methods.—Ninety patients, all older than 18 years of age, were randomly allocated to receive 0, 1, or 2 mg morphine hydrochloride in 5 mL isotonic saline solution administered into the knee joint at the end of surgery. Patients evaluated pain on a 100-mm Visual Analogue Scale 2, 4, 8, 24, 32, and 48 hours after surgery, rated pain on a 5-point global scale, and recorded side effects at 48 hours. Paracetamol requirements were recorded.

Results.—Eighty-six patients completed the study. There were no significant differences between groups with respect to postoperative pain intensity or analgesic requirements. Most patients had mild pain throughout the study. In the subgroup with higher pain intensity, there was a significant difference between the treatment and placebo groups at 8 hours (Fig 3). Patients in this subgroup who received 2 mg morphine used less paracetamol than patients in the placebo group. Side effects were similar among groups and were mild.

Conclusion.—Intra-articular morphine effectively relieved pain only in a subgroup of patients with higher pain intensity.

▶ There are several messages that one can take away from this study. An important message is that peripheral opioid receptors become active after inflammation and therefore are not likely to play a role in noninflammatory types of pain. Another message concerns the variability in pain after a given surgical intervention. The low incidence of postoperative pain in this study may be related to the anesthetic technique (local anesthetic infiltration plus intra-articular local anesthetic). Local anesthetics block the humoral components to inflammation and hyperalgesia, such as migration of lymphocytes and release of cytokines. As the authors point out, the analgesic effect of intra-articular opioid may be better demonstrated with general anesthesia alone.

S. E. Abram, MD

Optimization of the Dose of Intrathecal Morphine in Total Hip Surgery: A Dose-Finding Study
Slappendel R, Weber EWG, Dirksen R, et al (Sint Maartenskliniek, Nijmegen, The Netherlands; Univ Hosp Nijmegen, The Netherlands)
Anesth Analg 88:822-826, 1999   10–15

Objective.—Although intrathecal (IT) morphine provides excellent analgesia, it can be accompanied by unpleasant side effects. Because smaller doses of morphine might minimize those side effects, the optimum dose of IT morphine that relieves pain and minimizes side effects after total hip surgery was studied in a randomized, double-blind trial.

Methods.—Total hip surgery patients, premedicated with midazolam, were randomly allocated to receive bupivacaine and either 0.025 (group 1, n = 35), 0.05 (group 2, n = 37), 0.1 (group 3, n = 37), or 0.2 mg (group 4, n = 34) of IT morphine. Pain scores, the amount of morphine administered by patient-controlled analgesia, side effects, and postoperative nausea and vomiting were recorded for 24 hours.

Results.—All Visual Analogue Scale scores were less than 3. Side effects were similar among the groups. Women had a significantly higher incidence of postoperative nausea and vomiting than men in all groups (77% vs 44%). Itching side effects were dose related. Heart rates, which decreased by 6% to 16% in all groups, normalized within 12 hours. The incidence of hypotension was 48.6% in group 1, 56.8% in group 2, 54.0% in group 3, and 73.5% in group 4. The difference between groups 3 and 4 was significant.

Conclusion.—IT morphine at a dose of 0.1 mg provides effective analgesia for total hip surgery patients without producing unpleasant side effects.

▶ Fifteen years after the introduction of neuraxial opioids into clinical practice, we are still fine tuning techniques. Studies, such as this one, are very helpful in the development of care maps, which optimize treatment outcomes and minimize costs.

S. E. Abram, MD

A Comparison of Epidural Ropivacaine Infusion Alone and in Combination With 1, 2, and 4 µg/mL Fentanyl for Seventy-Two Hours of Postoperative Analgesia After Major Abdominal Surgery
Scott DA, and the Ropivacaine Investigation Group (St Vincent's Hosp, Melbourne, Australia; et al)
Anesth Analg 88:857-864, 1999   10–16

Objective.—Although epidural ropivacaine is less toxic than bupivacaine, its analgesic effectiveness and side effects in combination with an opioid have not been studied. The safety and effectiveness of ropivacaine (2 mg/mL) in combination with 1, 2, or 4 µg/mL of fentanyl for pain management after abdominal surgery were investigated in a prospective, randomized, double-blind trial.

Methods.—Patients were randomly allocated to receive ropivacaine alone (group R, 60 patients), or with 1 µg/mL fentanyl (group R1F, 59 patients), 2 µg/mL fentanyl (group R2F, 62 patients), or 4 µg/mL fentanyl (group R4F, 63 patients). Vital signs and Visual Analogue Scale (VAS) pain scores were monitored for as long as 72 hours after surgery.

Results.—The average length of infusion was significantly longer in group R4F than in group R. Technical infusion failures occurred in 9% of patients, and efficacy failures occurred in 38% of group R patients, 39% of group R1F, 34% of group R2F, and 16% of group R4F. VAS pain scores were significantly lower for group R4F than for groups R and R1F. Coughing VAS scores were all less than 20 mm and were significantly lower for group R4F than for group R. More than 80% of patients on all 3 days rated the quality of analgesia as good or excellent. No motor block was detected in more than 80% of patients during the study. By day 3, 97% of patients were walking with average VAS scores of less than 25 mm. The primary reasons for failure to walk were nausea (14%), dizziness (18%), tiredness or drowsiness (14%), pain (12%), motor block (10%), and hypotension (8%). Hypotension was significantly more common in the R4F group than in the other 3 groups (52% vs 31% to 34%). The incidence of pruritus tended to increase with the increasing dose of fentanyl. Two patients experienced a high block that resolved within 30 minutes after the infusion was stopped.

Conclusion.—Epidural ropivacaine after major abdominal surgery provides effective analgesia. The addition of fentanyl significantly improves the quality and duration of analgesia but increases the incidence of side effects.

▶ The optimal dose of fentanyl (4 mg/mL) used in conjunction with ropivacaine is not surprising and is in the range of doses commonly used. One should keep in mind the fact that fentanyl is not acting spinally and could just as well be administered via another route (IV, transmucosal, or transdermal).

S. E. Abram, MD

Preoperative Oral Dextromethorphan Does Not Reduce Pain or Analgesic Consumption in Children After Adenotonsillectomy

Rose JB, Cuy R, Cohen DE, et al (Children's Hosp of Philadelphia; Univ of Pennsylvania, Philadelphia)
Anesth Analg 88:749-753, 1999

10–17

Objective.—Better postoperative analgesia for children after adenotonsillectomy is needed. Dextromethorphan administered before surgery has been shown to reduce pain in adults after tonsillectomy. The analgesic effectiveness of dextromethorphan administered before adenotonsillectomy in children was investigated in a randomized, double-blind, placebo-controlled, prospective study.

Methods.—Placebo (n = 19), 0.5 mg/kg of dextromethorphan (n = 19), or 1.0 mg/kg of dextromethorphan (n = 19) were administered to 57 children (28 girls), aged 6 to 12 years, 60 minutes before surgery. Morphine (0.075 mg/kg IV) and oral acetaminophen (25-35 mg/kg) were administered before incision. Pain scores were measured every 15 minutes using the Children's Hospital of Eastern Ontario Pain Scale (CHEOPS) until the patient was released from the postanesthesia care unit. Patients rated pain on a Visual Analogue Scale (VAS) every 30 minutes until they were discharged. The VAS at 24 hours was obtained by telephone. Children with pain scores greater than 6 were given morphine. The morphine requirement was recorded. Postoperative behavior was rated on a 4-point scale (1, asleep; 2, awake and calm; 3, awake and crying; and 4, thrashing). Parental satisfaction was recorded.

Results.—Three of the original 60 patients were excluded from the study for protocol violations. There was no difference between groups with respect to morphine consumption, CHEOPS scores, VAS scores, or parental satisfaction.

Conclusion.—Preoperative medication with dextromethorphan does not improved postoperative analgesia in children after adenotonsillectomy.

▶ Although *N*-methyl-D-aspartate antagonists inhibit spinal sensitization in certain animal models, there is, so far, little evidence that preoperative administration affects postoperative pain or opioid requirements.

S. E. Abram, MD

Effects of Perioperative Analgesic Technique on the Surgical Outcome and Duration of Rehabilitation After Major Knee Surgery

Capdevila X, Barthelet Y, Biboulet P, et al (Lapeyronie Univ Hosp, Montpellier, France)

Anesthesiology 91:8-15, 1999   10–18

Objective.—Although early functional recuperation after major knee surgery is important, it can cause severe pain. Few studies have examined the role of analgesia in the rehabilitation process. The influence of continuous epidural infusion (CEI), continuous femoral block (CFB), and intravenous patient-controlled analgesia with morphine (PCA) on the functional outcome and duration of hospitalization after major knee surgery were prospectively evaluated.

Methods.—Before surgery, 56 knee surgery patients (28 women), aged 18 to 75 years, were randomly allocated to receive postoperative CFB (n = 20), CEI (n = 17) (1% lidocaine, 2 γg/mL clonidine, and 0.03 mg/mL morphine administered at 0.1 mL/kg per hour), or PCA (n = 19) (1 mg doses of morphine with a 7-minute lockout and a maximum dose of 30 mg in 4 hours). Pain and function were measured on a Visual Analogue Scale (VAS) at rest at 1, 6, 12, 24, and 48 hours after the onset of analgesia and during early maximal amplitude of knee flexion at 24 and 48 hours, 5 and 7 days, and 1 and 3 months. Side effects were recorded.

Results.—CEI resting VAS scores were significantly lower than those of the PCA group at all time points and significantly lower than the CFB group 6 to 12 hours after analgesia (Fig 1). Two CEI patients and 6 CFB patients required 1 dose of rescue medication on day 1. Serious side effects, most apparent in the CEI group, included urinary retention, dysesthesia, and arterial hypotension. CEI and CFB groups achieved their target mobilization levels at 24 and 48 hours more frequently and consistently than did the PCA group (Table 4). Similar results were observed for maximal amplitude of knee flexion (Table 5). At 1 and 3 months, all 3 groups had similar results. The duration of rehabilitation was significantly longer for the PCA group (50 days) than for the CEI (37 days) and CFB (40 days) groups.

Panel A

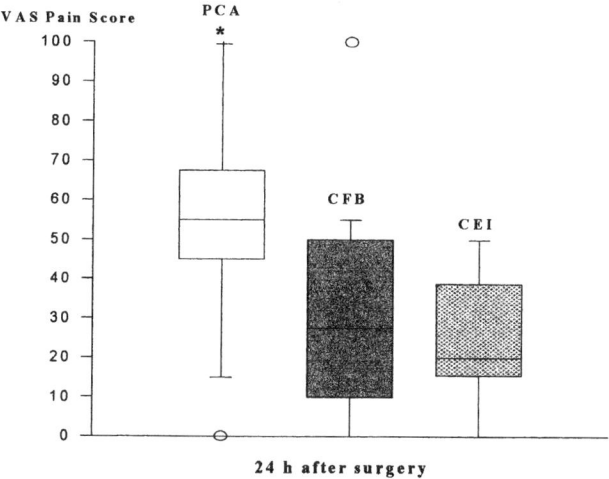

24 h after surgery

Panel B

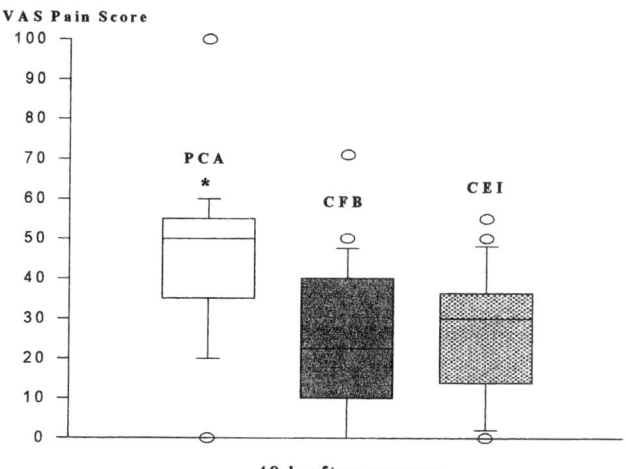

48 h after surgery

FIGURE 1.—Comparison of the visual analogue scale values during continuous passive motion (CPM) of the 3 groups at **Panel A** 24 h and **Panel B** 48 h. The box represents the 25th through 75th percentiles; the dark line is the median; the extended bars represent the 10th through 90th percentiles, and the circles represent values outside this range. *$P < .01$ versus continuous femoral block (CFB) and continuous epidural infusion (CEI). (Courtesy of Capdevila X, Barthelet Y, Biboulet P, et al: Effects of perioperative analgesic technique on the surgical outcome and duration of rehabilitation after major knee surgery. *Anesthesiology* 91:8-15, 1999. Copyright American Society of Anesthesiologists, Inc. Used with permission of Lippincott-Raven Publisher.)

TABLE 4.—Quality of Early Rehabilitation (Degrees)

	PCA		CFB		CEI	
Postoperative Hours	24 h	48 h	24 h	48 h	24 h	48 h
Surgeon's mobilization target	40	50	40	50	40	50
Achieved mobilization	30* (10-40)	40* (32-40)	40 (34-40)	50 (48-50)	40 (40-40)	50 (45-50)
Deferred mobilization (number of patients)	5	3	2	0	1	0

Note: Values of achieved mobilization are median (25th–75th percentiles).
*$P < .05$ versus continuous femoral block (CFB) and continuous epidural infusion (CEI).
(Courtesy of Capdevila X, Barthelet Y, Biboulet P, et al: Effects of perioperative analgesic technique on the surgical outcome and duration of rehabilitation after major knee surgery. *Anesthesiology* 91:8-15, 1999. Copyright American Society of Anesthesiologists, Inc. Used with permission of Lippincott-Raven Publishers.)

Conclusion.—Compared with the use of PCA, use of CEI and CFB shortened the overall hospital stay and improved functional recuperation. Because CEI use resulted in serious side effects, the regional analgesia technique of choice is CFB.

▶ This study focuses on an important end point: functional recovery. The authors provide evidence that a short-term intervention can produce long-term benefits, namely accelerated rehabilitation as measured over 1 month postoperatively. In this case, the improved early postoperative analgesia allows patients to tolerate more-rigorous early physical rehabilitation. Capdevila et al show that there are measurable benefits to be gained from continuous regional analgesia in groups other than critically ill thoracotomy and laparotomy patients. The lower incidence of side effects and the absence of the risk of epidural hemorrhage make continuous peripheral block a reasonable first choice.

S. E. Abram, MD

TABLE 5.—Functional Outcome: Knee Flexion (Degrees) at Day 5, Upon Discharge From the Surgical Ward (Day 7), and at 1- and 3-month Follow-ups

	PCA	CFB	CEI
Day 5	60 (50-70)*	80 (65-85)	85 (75-100)
Discharge	80 (65-90)*	90 (70-95)	90 (77.5-100)
1 month	90 (85-100)	95 (95-100)	105 (100-120)
3 month	125 (100-125)	125 (105-125)	130 (115-130)

Note: Values are median (25th–75th percentiles).
*$P < .05$ versus continuous femoral block (CFB) and continuous epidural infusion (CEI).
(Courtesy of Capdevila X, Barthelet Y, Biboulet P, et al: Effects of perioperative analgesic technique on the surgical outcome and duration of rehabilitation after major knee surgery. *Anesthesiology* 91:8-15, 1999. Copyright American Society of Anesthesiologists, Inc. Used with permission of Lippincott-Raven Publishers.)

Clinical Experience With Oral Ketamine

Enarson MC, Hays H, Woodroffe MA (Univ of Alberta, Edmonton)
J Pain Symptom Manage 17:384-386, 1999   10–19

Objective.—Ketamine, a short-term general anesthetic, has been studied as an analgesic agent in patients with chronic nonmalignant pain. Use of oral ketamine as an adjunct to ongoing therapy with individualized combinations of opioids, anticonvulsants, and antidepressants is described in a retrospective review.

Methods.—Oral ketamine (100 mg/d, titrated every 2 days by 40 mg/d) was prescribed for 21 patients (13 women), aged 29 to 81 years, with central and peripheral chronic neuropathic pain syndromes.

Results.—Final doses ranged from 40 to 500 mg/d with a median dose of 22 mg/d. Five patients were discontinued from the study because of psychomimetric symptoms, 4 for intolerable side effects, and 4 for lack of efficacy. Response was equivocal in 4 patients. Three patients (2 women) benefited from ketamine therapy ranging from 100 to 240 mg/d, reporting improvements in mood, energy, activity, and sleep.

Conclusion.—Certain selected patients with chronic pain may benefit from ketamine treatment.

▶ It would help if we knew more about the pain mechanisms of those patients who responded well to this therapy. I would anticipate that ketamine would be most valuable for opioid-unresponsive patients with neuropathic pain. It would also be encouraging to see some long-term benefit after a temporary course of treatment, but this was apparently not encountered. The patient who continued ketamine use despite a lack of analgesia is disturbing. One wonders if this constitutes a substance abuse issue. I would question the wisdom of allowing that patient to continue treatment. It is analogous to letting a patient continue long-term opioids in the absence of pain relief.

S. E. Abram, MD

Pleural Bupivacaine for Pain Treatment After Nephrectomy

Greif R, Wasinger T, Reiter K, et al (Univ of California, San Francisco; Donauspital, Vienna)
Anesth Analg 89:440-443, 1999   10–20

Background.—The role of pleural analgesia after nephrectomy is debated. IV opioid requirements in patients with and without pleural bupivacaine were investigated.

Methods.—Thirty-seven patients undergoing elective nephrectomy were assigned randomly to postoperative IV piritramid alone or combined with pleural bupivacaine. The latter consisted of 20 mL boluses of 0.25% bupivacaine administered every 6 hours through a pleural catheter inserted

TABLE 2.—Postoperative Opioid Use

	Pleural Bupivacaine (n = 19)	IV Piritramid (n = 18)
Time to first opioid request (h)	4.7 ± 1.0	2.8 ± 1.0*
Piritramid (mg)		
Postoperative Day 1	23 ± 3	45 ± 6*
Postoperative Day 2	9 ± 2	23 ± 4*

Note: Values are mean plus or minus SD.
*Statistically significant differences.
(Courtesy of Greif R, Wasinger T, Reiter K, et al: Pleural bupivacaine for pain treatment after nephrectomy. *Anesth Analg* 89[2]:440-443, 1999.)

in the medial axillary line at the sixth intercostal space. The catheter was removed 48 hours after placement.

Findings.—Although pain scores were comparable in the 2 groups, the piritramid requirement was significantly lower in patients receiving pleural bupivacaine than in those given piritramid alone (Table 2). Time from surgery completion to the first opioid request was significantly longer in patients given bupivacaine. In 1 patient, a small pneumothorax developed but resolved spontaneously.

Conclusions.—Pleural analgesia is effective and has a significant opioid-sparing effect. It significantly prolongs the time to the first request for postoperative opioid administration and decreases the total dose needed by half.

▶ There has been relatively little recent literature regarding the use of interpleural analgesia. This study serves as a reminder that there are effective alternatives to epidural analgesia for patients undergoing thoracic, upper abdominal, or flank surgery. Interpleural analgesia may be a safer alternative in patients whose coagulation function is borderline. Although the consequences of hemothorax are not trivial, they are probably less devastating and easier to treat than an epidural hematoma.

S. E. Abram, MD

Chronic and Cancer Pain

Widespread Musculoskeletal Chronic Pain Associated With Smoking: An Epidemiological Study in a General Rural Population
Andersson HI, Ejlertsson G, Leden I (Bromölla Health Centre, Sweden; Lund Univ, Sweden; Kristianstad College for Health Professions, Sweden; et al)
Scand J Rehabil Med 30:185-191, 1998   10–21

Objective.—Whereas a number of studies have established an association between smoking and low-back pain, there have not been studies of the relationship, if any, of smoking and widespread musculoskeletal pain. The associations between smoking and chronic pain were investigated in a cross-sectional study.

Methods.—A questionnaire was mailed to 1806 randomly selected individuals, aged 25 to 74 years, asking about chronic pain in different locations, other symptoms, socioeconomic and educational level, and nicotine habits. Pain prevalence and tobacco habits were compared statistically, and correlations were tested using multiple logistic regression.

Results.—Smoking was reported by 28.5% of respondents. More young women than young men smoked, and smoking decreased with age for both sexes. Smoking was more prevalent among blue collar workers than among white collar workers and farmers (31.5% vs 22.8% and 18.8%). Only men (18.8%) used oral snuff. Current smokers of both sexes reported more chronic pain in neck, low back, and multiple locations, compared with never smokers. Chronic pain in concurrent snuff users occurred in 56.7% of current smokers, 56.5% in former smokers, and 35.9% in never smokers. The corresponding prevalences in those who did not use snuff were 53.6%, 52.5%, and 43.8%, respectively. Current and former smokers had similar prevalences of low back and widespread pain that were higher than those of never smokers. According to multiple regression analysis, current smoking increased the risk of low back pain (odds ratio [OR], 1.58) and widespread pain (1.60), compared with never smokers. The corresponding risk factors for former smokers were similar (OR, 1.66 and OR, 1.59, respectively). Neck and shoulder pain were not correlated with smoking. Widespread pain was also correlated with depression (OR, 1.93), difficulties in relaxing (OR, 1.97), sleep disturbances (OR, 1.60), and fatigue (OR, 1.63).

Conclusion.—Both current and former smokers had increased low back and chronic widespread pain compared with never smokers. The reasons for this pain syndrome need to be elucidated in prospective studies.

▶ Smoking has been identified as a risk factor for the development of chronic pain, especially low back and cervical pain, and is associated with an increased risk of failure in the treatment of low back pain. Nevertheless, few physicians counsel their patients about the influence of smoking on the development and persistence of chronic painful conditions. Studies on the influence of smoking cessation on established pain problems are needed in order to provide honest and effective advice to our patients who smoke.

S. E. Abram, MD

Gabapentin for the Treatment of Postherpetic Neuralgia: A Randomized Controlled Trial
Rowbotham M, for the Gabapentin Postherpetic Neuralgia Study Group (Univ of California, San Francisco; et al)
JAMA 280:1837-1842, 1998   10–22

Background.—Postherpetic neuralgia, a syndrome of often intractable neuropathic pain after herpes zoster, is very difficult to treat in many patients. The safety and efficacy of gabapentin, an anticonvulsant drug, for reducing postherpetic neuralgia pain were investigated.

Methods.—Two hundred twenty-nine patients were enrolled in the multicenter, randomized, double-blind, placebo-controlled trial. The 8-week treatment consisted of a 4-week titration to a maximum dosage of 3600 mg/day of gabapentin or matching placebo and a 4-week maintenance at the maximum tolerated dose. Concomitant tricyclic antidepressants, narcotics, or both were continued if treatment was stabilized before study entry and remained constant during the study.

Findings.—In an intent-to-treat analysis, patients given gabapentin had a significant reduction in their mean daily pain score, from 6.3 to 4.2 points, compared with a 6.5 to 6.0 decline in patients given placebo. The gabapentin recipients also had improvement in secondary pain measures and changes in pain and sleep intereference. Scores on the Quality of Life Questionnaire and Profile of Mood States favored the active treatment group. Withdrawals because of toxicity were similar in the 2 groups, although the gabapentin group more commonly had somnolence, dizziness, ataxia, peripheral edema, and infection.

Conclusion.—Gabapentin is an effective treatment for pain and sleep interference associated with postherpetic neuralgia. In addition, mood and quality of life were improved with this agent.

▶ Gabapentin has been a valuable addition to our list of therapies for postherpetic neuralgia and other peripheral neuropathies. It is not clear whether it is more efficacious than older anticonvulsants, but it is clearly better tolerated. There are few serious drug interactions and there is little potential for bone marrow, hepatic, or renal dysfunction. There is considerable variation in dose requirement and it is common to find that doses of 3600 mg/d, the maximum used in this study, or higher are required to optimize analgesia. Cost of this therapy is a real concern.

S. E. Abram, MD

Bedside Implantation of a Trial Spinal Cord Stimulator for Intractable Anginal Pain

Janfaza DR, Michna E, Pisini JV, et al (Brigham & Women's Hosp, Boston)
Anesth Analg 87:1242-1244, 1998   10–23

Objective.—Spinal cord stimulation relieves intractable anginal pain. A novel approach to placement of a temporary spinal cord stimulator at the bedside, thus eliminating the need to move a critically ill patient from the coronary care unit to the radiology department, is described.

> *Case Report.*—Woman, 64, with refractory intractable angina, coronary artery disease, congestive heart failure, severe peripheral vascular disease, a history of stroke, noninsulin-dependent diabetes mellitus, chronic renal insufficiency, and steroid-requiring chronic

obstructive lung disease was bed fast as a result of pain and was not considered a candidate for coronary revascularization. Thoracic epidural analgesia was rejected because of concerns about the patient's ability to care for an indwelling catheter. A percutaneous catheter was not considered because of the risk of infection. Spinal cord stimulation was selected as the best option, with the trial stimulator inserted close to the dermatomal level of her pain and the permanent electrode placed from a lumbar approach and directed cephalad to the appropriate level under fluoroscopy. Because of the patient's critical condition, the trial spinal cord stimulator was placed at the bedside with fluoroscopic guidance. The temporary leads were inserted at the T4-5 interspace. The electrode was inserted until temporary paresthesia was elicited at the level of the patient's self-reported anginal pain. The electrode was attached to a pulse generator, stimulation was begun, and pain relief was immediate. IV nitroglycerine was discontinued over 24 hours. Three days later the patient did not need pain medication, and she was discharged on day 7. Her angina was controlled, and her functional ability improved.

Conclusion.—The novel bedside placement of a spinal cord stimulator under fluoroscopic guidance safely and effective mediated acute intractable anginal pain.

▶ Although this patient did well, I suspect that placement of the epidural electrode without fluoroscopy involved a measure of luck. A better alternative might be to transport the patient to the fluoroscopy suite with appropriate monitoring, tunnel and externalize the electrode leads if the patient experiences immediate relief, and implant the pulse generator after 2 to 3 days if benefit persists.

There is considerable experience with dorsal column stimulation for the treatment of angina, and evidence is growing that there is a beneficial effect on ischemia as well as reproducible pain relief. In addition to the expense, the relatively low use of this technique may be related to the fact that it is not performed by cardiologists.

S. E. Abram, MD

Oral Transmucosal Fentanyl Citrate (OTFC) for the Treatment of Breakthrough Pain in Cancer Patients: A Controlled Dose Titration Study
Portenoy RK, Payne R, Coluzzi P, et al (Mem Sloan-Kettering Cancer Ctr, New York; MD Anderson Cancer Ctr, Houston; City of Hope Med Ctr, Duarte, Calif; et al)
Pain 79:303-312, 1999   10–24

Objective.—Treating breakthrough pain in cancer patients is a challenge. The safety and efficacy of escalating doses of a new formulation, oral transmucosal fentanyl citrate (OTFC), were tested as specific therapy for breakthrough pain in cancer patients receiving varied scheduled oral opioid regimens for chronic cancer-related pain in a randomized, double-blind, multicenter study.

Methods.—Adult cancer patients receiving 60 to 1000 mg oral morphine per day, who had experienced at least 1 episode/d of breakthrough pain for the 3 days prior to screening, and who had achieved at least partial relief from oral opioid rescue drugs were eligible for the study. Patients (n = 65, 28 male), aged 26 to 74 years, were randomly assigned to receive either 200 or 400 µg OTFC unit doses in a double-blind fashion after 2 days of opioid dose stabilization and baseline data gathering. Patients were allowed to use up to 4 unit doses, containing 200, 400, 600, 800, 1200, or 1600 µg of fentanyl citrate, for as many as 2 breakthrough pain periods per day.

The size of the unit dose was increased or decreased until each patient could treat breakthrough pain with 1 dose on 2 consecutive days, or a dose of 1600 µg was ineffective, or the 2-day study period had ended. The request to increase the dosage was ignored randomly one third of the time to create uncertainty about the actual dose administered. Patients completed a questionnaire regarding their pain and kept a daily diary. Adverse events were recorded.

Results.—Among the 32 patients receiving the 200 µg dose and the 33 patients receiving the 400 µg dose, 78% and 70%, respectively, were successfully titrated. The higher doses provided significantly more pain relief and a greater average pain intensity difference than the lower doses. The higher doses received a significantly better global rating. Patients receiving the 200 µg dose required more dose increases than patients receiving the 400 µg dose. Analysis of pain scores did not show any difference between the 200 and 400 µg doses. There was no relationship between doses of fentanyl citrate required to control breakthrough pain and the scheduled opioids that patients were already taking. Most adverse effects of fentanyl citrate were not serious and included sleepiness, nausea, and dizziness.

Conclusion.—OTFC is a safe and effective treatment for cancer patients with breakthrough pain. The effective breakthrough dose can be found by dose titration.

▶ Several factors make this opioid preparation particularly effective. First, the drug itself has a high intrinsic activity, and it is likely that it may be more efficacious and produce fewer side effects at effective doses than other commonly used drugs such as morphine or meperidine. Second, it has an extremely rapid onset. Third, the route of administration is convenient, is under patient control, and can be used in any setting. Fourth, the drug is already available as a long-acting preparation (transdermal). Fifth, there is at least theoretical evidence that tolerance develops less readily with more potent, efficacious drugs such as fentanyl.

The dose titration of OTFC is still being optimized. The safest method of dose titration is to use lower doses, allowing patients to use multiple unit doses per episode. In this way, the dose may be optimized within 2 or 3 days.

S. E. Abram, MD

Epidemiology of Complex Regional Pain Syndrome: A Retrospective Chart Review of 134 Patients
Allen G, Galer BS, Schwartz L (Univ of Washington, Seattle)
Pain 80:539-544, 1999   10–25

Objective.—Complex regional pain syndrome (CRPS) and its effect on the health care, legal, and workers' compensation systems is poorly understood. A retrospective chart analysis of patients with CRPS referred to a United States university–based tertiary chronic pain clinic examined the demographics, health care utilizations, and prevalence of workers' compensation and legal issues in this population, as well as the history of immobilization and evidence of myofascial dysfunction.

Methods.—Data from the 1992 to 1997 medical records of 134 patients (30% male, 79% white), aged 18 to 71 years, with reflex sympathetic dystrophy or CRPS were reviewed.

Results.—The average age at the time of injury was 14 to 64 years, and the average duration of pain before seeking pain center evaluation was 30 months. The initial injuries were sprain/strain (29%); postsurgical (24%); fractures (16%); contusions or crush injuries (8%); venipuncture, lacerations, and spinal cord injuries (11%); and unspecified (6%). Most were extremity injuries about equally divided between upper and lower extremities. About 56% were occupational injuries. Approximately 23% of patients were involved in a lawsuit over the CRPS. Patients saw an average of 4.8 physicians before seeking help from the pain center. Of the 38% of patients who had a bone scan, 53% of the scans were interpreted as being consistent with reflex sympathetic dystrophy.

Most of the patients had received antidepressants (78%), 60% had received anticonvulsants, and 70% had received opiates. Most (88%) had received physical therapy, 45% had received occupational therapy, and 50% had received psychotherapy. Forty-seven percent of patients had previously been immobilized as a result of injury for an average of 3 weeks. Documented myofascial components were present in 56% of the charts. The longer the duration of CRPS, the more likely the patient was to have myofascial dysfunction. Symptoms lasted for an average of 35.4 months in patients with myofascial pain and 22.8 months in patients without myofascial pain.

Conclusion.—Patients with CRPS typically seek multiple consultations and treatments for their symptoms. A significant percentage of these patients have a history of immobilization and myofascial dysfunction.

▶ It is reassuring to find a lack of correlation between "typical reflex sympathetic dystrophy findings" on bone scan and a clinical diagnosis of

CRPS or reflex sympathetic dystrophy. I was involved in a medicolegal case in which a patient with classic and severe signs and symptoms of reflex sympathetic dystrophy was denied compensation in a personal injury case because he had a negative bone scan. It is distressing to find that many patients with typical findings are prescribed physician-imposed immobilization. The coexistence of myofascial pain, particularly in patients with upper extremity CRPS, is an important message.

S. E. Abram, MD

The Natural History of Pain in Alcoholic Chronic Pancreatitis

Ammann RW, and Zurich Pancreatitis Study Group (Univ Hosp, Zurich, Switzerland)
Gastroenterology 116:1132-1140, 1999   10–26

Objective.—The progression and treatment of pain in chronic pancreatitis is poorly understood. Types of pain in chronic pancreatitis were characterized and classified in a prospective study of a large mixed medical-surgical patient series followed for as long as 35 years to assess the relationship of different types of pain to local complications and early and late stage of alcoholic chronic pancreatitis, and to characterize the pain profile in patients with and without surgery.

Methods.—There were 207 patients. Patients with acute relapsing pancreatitis (type A) and patients with prolonged periods of persistent daily pain and/or clusters of recurrent severe pain exacerbations (type B) were prospectively evaluated during early-stage chronic pancreatitis (no calcification and only minor or no exocrine insufficiency) and late-stage chronic pancreatitis (with calcification or persistent exocrine insufficiency). Surgery for pain was performed on 116 patients (13 women), and 91 (5 women) were treated nonsurgically. There were 56 patients in the first group and 54 in second group who died and 6 patients and 4 patients, respectively, who were lost to follow-up. A staging system was developed for characterizing the evolution of pain from the early through late stages of the disease.

Results.—Patients had had alcoholic chronic pancreatitis for an average of 17 years. The frequency of hospitalization for type A pain was similar for the surgical and nonsurgical groups. The number of hospitalizations for type A and B pain in the surgical patients was significantly higher than for nonsurgical patients (0.85 vs 0.39 per year). Recurrent pain was more common in early alcoholic chronic pancreatitis, whereas chronic pain was associated with local complications. Indications at first surgery were pseudocysts in 77 patients, high ductal pressure in 16, and cholestasis in 19. A second surgery was performed in 39 patients with type B pain. Pain was caused by pseudocysts in 7 patients, abscess in 5, high ductal pressure in 5, and cholestasis in 18.

Pain was relieved by cyst drainage in about 67% of patients. Complete and permanent pain relief was achieved for an average of 11 years in the nonsurgical group, for 10.9 years after the first surgery, and for 6.8 years after the second surgery. In both groups, about 55% of patients had exocrine insufficiency after 6 years, and 80% had exocrine insufficiency at 10 years. Continued, unchanged alcohol consumption was reported by 75% of patients.

Conclusion.—Complete and permanent pain relief was achieved in most patients in late-stage alcoholic chronic pancreatitis either as the result of surgical intervention to treat complications or spontaneously where no complications occurred.

▶ I was initially puzzled by the discrepancy between the authors' treatment success for patients with alcoholic chronic pancreatitis and my own. In my experience, it has been rare for any patient with pain from this condition to respond to any treatment, surgical or medical. It is our experience that patients who continue to drink have an especially poor prognosis. Part of this discrepancy might be explained by the fact that the authors excluded all patients using opioids, whereas essentially all of my patients have been receiving opioids for a considerable length of time. This study, therefore, may have selected patients with less severe pain and certainly avoided many of the drug-dependence issues that complicate treatment for this group of patients.

S. E. Abram, MD

Prolonged Analgesic Effect of Ketamine, an *N*-Methyl-D-Aspartate Receptor Inhibitor, in Patients With Chronic Pain
Rabben T, Skjelbred P, Øye I (Ullevål Hosp, Oslo, Norway; Univ of Oslo, Norway)
J Pharmacol Exp Ther 289:1060-1066, 1999   10–27

Objective.—The role of N-methyl-D-aspartate receptor–related mechanisms in patients with chronic pain by using ketamine as a pharmacologic probe was examined in a randomized, double-blind, crossover study.

Methods.—A dose of 1.0 mg/kg of pethidine (control) or 0.4 mg/kg of ketamine and 0.05 mg/kg of midazolam were administered IM to 30 patients (4 men), aged 29 to 89 years, with trigeminal neuropathic pain. One week later, 26 patients were crossed over to the other arm. One week after IM challenge, patients received a dose of oral ketamine (4 mg/kg) or placebo at bedtime for 3 successive nights. Pain was assessed on a Visual Analogue Scale scale in the morning and evening 3 days before and 3 days after IM challenge.

Results.—Nine patients had no reduction in pain. Eight patients had many hours of pain relief after ketamine injection. Nine patients had short-term relief from ketamine injection. Four patients were withdrawn because of adverse events. Both pethidine and ketamine produced side effects that included dizziness, sedation, and dry mouth, but ketamine caused more complaints of sensory disturbances and feelings of insobriety, most lasting less than 1 hour. One of 9 nonresponders and 6 of 8 responders preferred ketamine. On oral ketamine or placebo administration, 5 of 8 of the original responders reported pain relief after taking ketamine. None of the nonresponders reported pain relief after oral ketamine.

Conclusion.—Response to ketamine in patients with chronic trigeminal pain appears to depend on whether the pain is caused by N-methyl-D-aspartate receptor–dependent or receptor-independent mechanisms.

Oral Ketamine Is Antinociceptive in the Rat Formalin Test: Role of the Metabolite, Norketamine

Shimoyama M, Shimoyama N, Gorman AL, et al (Cornell Univ, New York; Mem Sloan-Kettering Cancer Ctr, New York)
Pain 81:85-93, 1999   10–28

Objective.—The antinociceptive effects of parenteral and intrathecal ketamine are well known; however, little information is available on the antinociceptive effects of oral ketamine. The oral efficacy and bioavailability of ketamine; its antinociceptive effects; and the plasma and brain levels of ketamine and its major metabolite, norketamine, were studied in the rat.

Methods.—Ketamine (30, 60, 100 or 180 mg/kg) or saline was administered orally to fasted male Sprague-Dawley rats. CNS depression and formalin-induced behaviors were recorded, and ketamine and norketamine brain and plasma levels were measured by high-performance liquid chromatography. The effects of intrathecal ketamine and norketamine on the formalin test were analyzed. Binding affinities of ketamine and norketamine for the noncompetitive site of the N-methyl-D-aspartate receptor in brain and spinal cord were determined.

Results.—No CNS depression was observed at doses of 30 to 100 mg/kg of ketamine at 30 to 60 minutes after administration. At a ketamine dose of 180 mg/kg, 89% of rats lost their righting reflex and were unable to negotiate the 60° mesh until 90 minutes after administration. Within 90 minutes of pretreatment with ketamine, doses of 100 and 180 mg/kg significantly reduced formalin-induced flinching behavior. Plasma ketamine and norketamine concentrations (area under the curve for norketamine/ketamine = 6.4) were highest at 10 and 45 minutes, respectively, after administration and had declined by more than 80% at 90 minutes. The average brain levels of ketamine and norketamine (area under the curve for norketamine/ketamine = 2.9) peaked at 10 minutes and had declined by 85% and 32%, respectively, at 90 minutes. Spinal administration of ketamine resulted in no CNS depression or delayed flinching. Ketamine had a twofold to fourfold higher affinity for the noncompetitive N-methyl-D-aspartate site than did norketamine. Both ketamine and norketamine had a threefold to fourfold higher affinity for forebrain than for spinal cord receptors.

Conclusion.—The antinociceptive effects of oral ketamine are dose dependent. Both oral ketamine and its major metabolite, norketamine, contribute to the antinociceptive effects observed.

▶ It is always encouraging to see experimental results in animal models reproduced in clinical trials. Both of these studies demonstrate analgesic or antinociceptive activity of ketamine, and both studies attest to the efficacy of oral administration. The results of the rat formalin test suggest that, at lower doses, oral ketamine blocks spinal sensitization but is not antinociceptive. Shimoyama et al (Abstract 10–28) suggest that the oral administration of ketamine results in the biotransformation of much of the administered drug to norketamine, which appears to have an antihyperalgesic effect similar to that of ketamine. An important message from Rabben et al (Abstract 10–27) is the fact that ketamine is effective for opioid-unresponsive pain.

S. E. Abram, MD

Subcutaneous Infusion of Lidocaine Provides Effective Pain Relief for CRPS Patients
Linchitz RM, Raheb JC (Pain Alleviation Ctr, Jericho, NY)
Clin J Pain 15:67-72, 1999   10–29

Objective.—Successful pain relief is difficult to achieve for patients with complex regional pain syndrome (CRPS). Subcutaneous infusion of lidocaine has been demonstrated to relieve neuropathic pain. The preliminary successful use of subcutaneous lidocaine infusion for CRPS in an outpatient setting is reported.

Methods.—Nine patients (6 women), aged 37 to 63 years, with refractory CRPS pain received a subcutaneous infusion of lidocaine (100 mg/mL) via an ambulatory infusion pump for 4 to 8 weeks. The outcome measures were serum lidocaine level (SLL) and pain as scored on a 10-cm visual analogue scale.

Results.—Four patients did not complete the study. All the other patients reported a significant decrease in mean pain scores after lidocaine treatment compared with baseline pain scores (3.8 vs 8.4). Other signs and symptoms eliminated or alleviated included burning, allodynia, hyperpathia, muscle spasm, atrophy, temperature changes, hair/nail growth changes, skin color changes, impaired range of motion or ambulation, sleep disorders, depression, and impaired quality of life. The average SLL was 3.69 γ/mL. All patients experienced minor side effects during infusion but achieved sufficient pain relief to reduce or discontinue medication.

Conclusion.—Continuous subcutaneous infusion of 10% lidocaine solution is an effective treatment for pain control in selected patients with CRPS.

▶ It is not unusual for symptoms of CRPS to improve during active therapy, eg, during a series of sympathetic blocks. The most important aspect of this study, ie, the ability to maintain the symptomatic improvement, has not previously been reported. One might consider the use of oral lidocaine for the treatment of neuropathic pain states. The oral bioavailability is fairly high

(0.35), but the drug's oral use is limited by its high first-pass liver metabolism, with transformation to monoethyl glycine xylidide, a metabolite that may produce CNS irritability.

S. E. Abram, MD

Analgesic Effects of Nonsteroidal Anti-inflammatory Drugs in Cancer Pain Due to Somatic or Visceral Mechanisms

Mercadante S, Casuccio A, Agnello A, et al (SAMOT, Palermo, Italy; La Maddalena Clinic, Palermo; Univ of Palermo)
J Pain Symptom Manage 17:351-356, 1999   10–30

Objective.—Nonsteroidal anti-inflammatory drugs (NSAIDs) produce their analgesic effect by inhibiting peripheral prostaglandin synthesis and appear to be more effective in combatting somatic than visceral pain. To test this observation, NSAID efficacy was prospectively evaluated in cancer pain resulting from somatic or visceral mechanisms.

Methods.—NSAIDs, with or without opioids, were administered to 32 advanced cancer patients with somatic (S) (n = 17) or visceral (V) (n = 15) pain. Diclofenac was used in 10 S patients and 8 V patients, naproxen in 3 S patients and 2 V patients, and ketorolac in 4 S patients and 5 V patients. All patients received either misoprostol or ranitidine. Pain intensity was measured on a 10-cm visual analogue scale at baseline, 3, 7, and 14 days and by patient self-report 2 or 3 times a week. The average opioid dose, reported as oral morphine equivalents, was reported at baseline and on days 3, 7, and 14. The average dose of opioid, patient self-reported symptoms, and side effect intensity were recorded.

Results.—There was no significant difference in pain intensity between the somatic and visceral groups. Patients with visceral pain required significantly higher opioid doses on days 7 and 14 than on day 3. Opioid consumption and symptom rating were similar for both groups regardless of NSAID used. Adverse event reporting was similar for both groups.

Conclusion.—NSAIDs can provide effective relief for both somatic and visceral pain. Additional studies are needed regarding long-term NSAID use, risk factors for NSAID use, coadministration with steroids, and individual variability.

▶ A recent study has suggested that treatment with combinations of NSAIDs and opioids produces more adverse effects and no better analgesia than treatment with opioids alone. This study used either misoprostol or ranitidine, which may have improved tolerance to gastrointestinal side effects. COX-2 inhibitors should be considered in selected patients, both as sole therapy for mild to moderate pain and in combination with opioids for moderate to severe pain. They may not be more effective than conventional NSAIDs, but they will probably be better tolerated by cancer patients, who often have low platelets and other reasons for gastrointestinal and renal dysfunction.

S. E. Abram, MD

The State of Implantable Pain Therapies in the United States: A Nationwide Survey of Academic Teaching Programs
Fanciullo GJ, Rose RJ, Lunt PG, et al (Dartmouth-Hitchcock Med Ctr, Lebanon, NH; Brigham and Women's Hosp, Boston)
Anesth Analg 88:1311-1316, 1999   10–31

Objective.—Although the use of implantable pain management devices is increasing, little is known about the number of academic teaching programs that are implanting them and instructing in these techniques. A questionnaire addressing the questions of whether anesthesiologists alone or anesthesiologists and surgeons are implanting pain control devices, what implantation devices are being used, and what drugs are being prescribed by pain specialists was sent to pain fellowship programs accredited by the Accreditation Council for Graduate Medical Education.

Methods.—A 34-item questionnaire was mailed to 95 anesthesiology pain fellowship programs and directors identified from the 1998-1999 Graduate Medical Education Directory.

Results.—Responses were received from 76 program directors (80%). Of the 422 anesthesiologists practicing in the 76 programs, 177 (42%) implant spinal cord stimulators (SCSs) and 171 (41%) implant opioid infusion devices (OIDs). In 13% of centers, no anesthesiologist implanted SCSs, and in 16% of centers, no pain specialists implanted OIDs. The average number of SCSs and OIDs implanted per program in the previous year was 12.4 and 9.2, respectively. All programs performed trials on all their implanted patients. The average duration of SCS trials was 6.6 days, and 49% of programs admitted patients overnight. Although most non-revision SCS patients (83%) received cylindrical leads, 17% received resume leads. In OID trials, 52% of programs used continuous infusion, 31% employed bolus administration, and 16% used both. The method of administration was intrathecal in 59%, epidural in 17%, and both in 22% of programs. The specific drugs used in the programs included morphine (95%), bupivacaine (64%), hydromorphone (60%), baclofen (57%), clonidine (41%), sufentanil (35%), ketamine (7%), ropivacaine (5%), and other (16%). Implantations were performed by physicians alone in 54% of programs and by physicians and surgeons in 46% of programs. When surgeons performed the implantation, anesthesiologists placed the electrode or catheter 89% of the time, performed the tunneling 49% of the time, and created the pocket 27% of the time.

Conclusion.—There is little agreement with regard to the technical aspects of implantation of pain control devices, although most programs report admitting patients undergoing opioid trials overnight, and most conduct the trials intrathecally. Morphine is the drug of choice for most programs. Because few implantation guidelines are available, there are abundant opportunities for investigation into the technical aspects of the procedure.

▶ This study provides useful information to pain management program directors and prospective fellows about the prevalence of training in the use of implantable devices. It is clear that most program directors feel that fellows should have at least some training in the use of these devices. Some trainees may feel that they do not wish to incorporate these treatments into their practices, and will be content to train in a program that does not offer such experience.

Ethical questions emerge in every practice that incorporates implantable treatment. Once a stimulator or intrathecal drug delivery device is implanted, someone must be available to provide ongoing care of the patient, particularly those with pumps. What if the physician providing these services retires or leaves the community? What if a patient needs to move to a community where support services are unavailable? What happens when maintenance of patients with implanted devices uses so much of the practitioner's time that few new patients can enter the practice?

S. E. Abram, MD

A Randomized Comparative Trial of Acupuncture Versus Transcutaneous Electrical Nerve Stimulation for Chronic Back Pain in the Elderly
Grant DJ, Bishop-Miller J, Winchester DM, et al (Liberton Hosp, Edinburgh, Scotland)
Pain 82:9-13, 1999   10–32

Objective.—An increasing number of elderly patients are requesting physical therapies such as acupuncture for back pain relief. Because double-blind, placebo-controlled acupuncture trials are difficult to perform, the effects of acupuncture on chronic back pain relief in the elderly was compared with that of transcutaneous electrical nerve stimulation (TENS).

Methods.—Sixty patients, aged 60 to 90 years, with back pain of more than 6 months' duration, were randomly allocated to 4 weeks of acupuncture for 2 sessions/wk (n = 32, 30 women) or 4 weeks of TENS as required daily for up to 30 minutes per session for a maximum of 6 h/d (n = 28, 24 women). Patients were allowed to continue existing medication but were not permitted to start new analgesic drugs during the trial. Outcomes measures were pain as measured on a Visual Analogue Scale (VAS), pain as measured on the 38-item Nottingham Health Profile Part I (NHP), and number of analgesic tablets consumed in the previous week. Spinal flexion between C7 and S1 was measured by a blinded observer at baseline, 4 days after treatment, and at the 3-month follow-up visit.

Results.—There were 2 withdrawals in the acupuncture group and 1 in the TENS group. Three acupuncture patients reported dizziness, and 3 TENS patients reported skin reactions. At baseline, compared with TENS

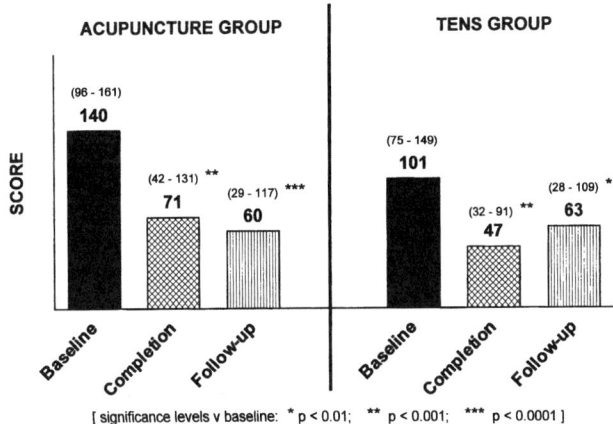

FIGURE 1.—Median (interquartile range) VAS scores. Significance levels vs baseline: *P < .001, †P < .001, ‡P < .0001. (Courtesy of Grant DJ, Bishop-Miller J, Winchester DM, et al: A randomized comparative trial of acupuncture versus transcutaneous electrical nerve stimulation for chronic back pain in the elderly. *Pain* 82:9-13, 1999.)

patients, acupuncture patients had higher VAS and NHP scores, reduced spinal flexion, and lower analgesia consumption (Figs 1 and 3). Both groups had a significant reduction in average VAS score by the end of the trial which was maintained at the 3-month follow-up visit. The acupuncture group demonstrated a nonsignificant improvement trend after the trial. Compared with baseline values, analgesic tablet consumption was significantly reduced by 50% in the acupuncture group and by 33% in the TENS group. The reduction was maintained during follow-up. Spinal flexion improved significantly by 10% at completion in the acupuncture

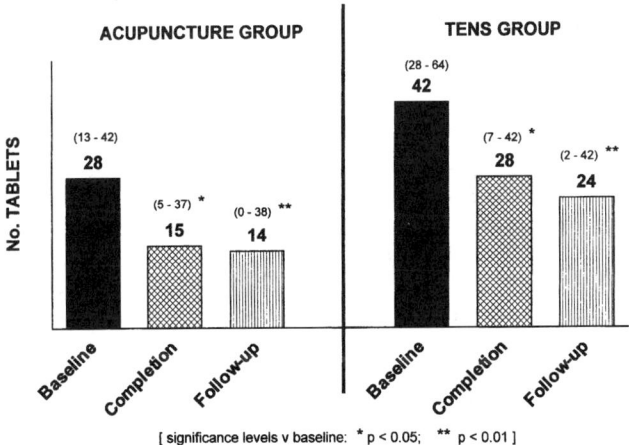

FIGURE 3.—Median (interquartile range) tablets consumed in previous week. Significance levels vs baseline: *P < .05, †P < .01. (Courtesy of Grant DJ, Bishop-Miller J, Winchester DM, et al: A randomized comparative trial of acupuncture versus transcutaneous electrical nerve stimulation for chronic back pain in the elderly. *Pain* 82:9-13, 1999.)

group. The improvement was not maintained at follow-up. Spinal flexion did not improve significantly in the TENS group.

Conclusion.—Although results are highly variable, both acupuncture and TENS are effective for treatment of chronic back pain in the elderly and should be used more widely.

▶ There have been relatively few recent studies of the use of either TENS or acupuncture for chronic pain management. This study provides some reaffirmation that these low-risk modalities provide measurable benefits and some potential for cost savings in patients with low back pain. TENS has the advantage over acupuncture of allowing more patient control and less need to travel to the health care provider. This is a major benefit in elderly patients, who are often homebound. This study may provide some leverage in our efforts to convince our regional Medicaid HMO that its refusal to provide reimbursement for TENS is shortsighted and mean-spirited.

S. E. Abram, MD

The Safety and Efficacy of Intrathecal Adenosine in Patients With Chronic Neuropathic Pain
Belfrage M, Segerdahl M, Arnér S, et al (St Görans Hosp, Sweden; Karolinska Hosp, Stockholm; Huddinge Univ Hosp, Sweden)
Anesth Analg 89:136-142, 1999   10–33

Objective.—Adenosine and adenosine receptor analogues have been shown to moderate pain in animal studies. Intrathecal (IT) adenosine was administered to 14 patients with chronic intractable neuropathic pain involving tactile hyperalgesia and/or allodynia.

Methods.—The safety and efficacy of 500 µg (n = 9) and 1000 µg (n = 5) IT adenosine was evaluated in an open study in 14 patients (10 women), aged 26 to 62 years, with peripheral neurogenic, central neurogenic, and/or nociceptive pain of 8 months' to 27 years' duration. Spontaneous and stimulus-evoked pain intensity were measured on a 100-mm visual analogue scale before and 60 minutes after adenosine administration.

Results.—Four patients receiving 500 µg and 1 patient receiving 1000 µg experienced pain after injection. There were no other adverse reactions. Spontaneous pain scores were reduced from 65 to 24 in 9 of 14 patients, and evoked pain scores were reduced from 71 to 12 in 9 of 12 patients (Fig 1). Areas of allodynia and hyperalgesia were reduced by at least 50% in 13 patients and by 30% in 1 patient. Only 2 patients reported no benefits of treatment.

Conclusion.—IT administration of adenosine provides effective, long-lasting pain relief in patients with chronic neuropathic pain.

▶ The preliminary finding that IT adenosine produces analgesia in patients with neuropathic pain is encouraging. Results of several animal mononeuropathy studies suggest that such a response is likely. I am somewhat

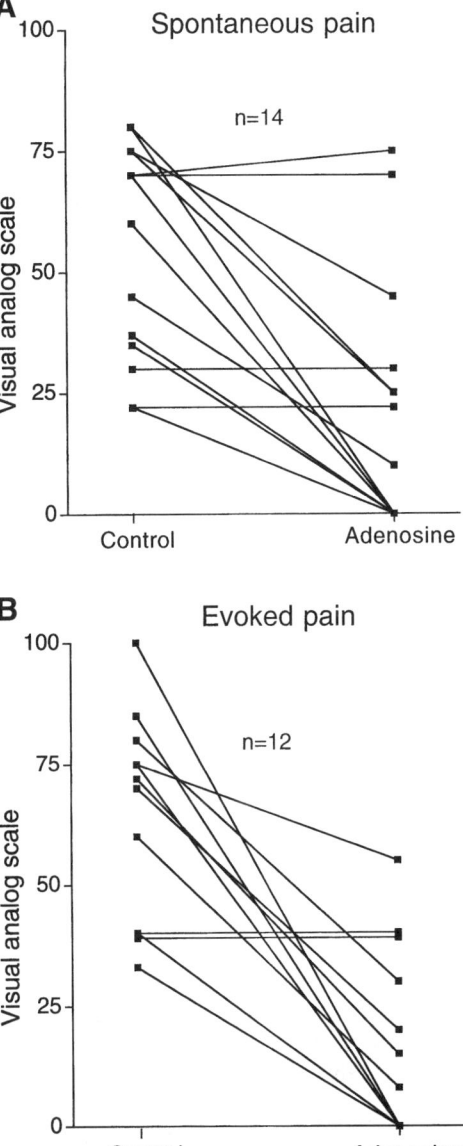

FIGURE 1.—Individual pain ratings of spontaneous (**A**) and evoked (**B**) pain before and 60 min after IT adenosine injection. (Courtesy of Belfrage M, Segerdahl M, Arnér, S, et al: The safety and efficacy of intrathecal adenosine in patients with chronic neuropathic pain. *Anesth Analg* 89[1]:136-142, 1999.)

disturbed, however, that the study was begun without more-rigorous animal testing of the safety of IT adenosine. The only investigation cited was an unpublished rodent study. The pain on injection experienced by some patients was a bit disturbing as well.

S. E. Abram, MD

A Trial of Intravenous Lidocaine on the Pain and Allodynia of Postherpetic Neuralgia
Baranowski AP, De Courcey J, Bonello E (Univ College London; Cheltenham Gen Hosp, England; St Thomas's Hosp, London)
J Pain Symptom Manage 17:429-433, 1999   10–34

Background.—Postherpetic neuralgia, a chronic pain syndrome, can develop after an acute herpes zoster infection. The effects of IV lidocaine in doses of 1 and 5 mg/kg, administered over 2 hours, on pain and allodynia in patients with postherpetic neuralgia were compared.

Methods.—Twenty-four patients were enrolled in a randomized, double-blind, within-patient crossover study. Each patient received saline, 0.5 mg/kg per hour, lidocaine and 2.5 mg/kg lidocaine per hour for 2 hours.

Findings.—The Visual Analogue Scores for ongoing pain were significantly reduced after all the infusions. Saline did not affect the Visual Analogues Score for dynamic pressure-provoked pain, whereas the 2 lidocaine doses reduced these scores at an equal significance level. In addition, both lidocaine doses decreased the area of allodynia, as mapped by brush stroke (Fig 3). Saline did not affect the area of allodynia.

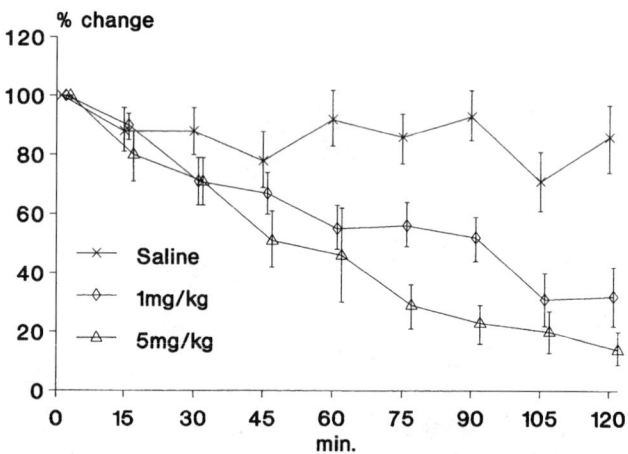

FIGURE 3.—Area of allodynia expressed as percentage change, plotted against time. (Reprinted by permission of Elsevier Science, from Baranowski AP, De Courcey J, Bonello E: A trial of intravenous lidocaine on the pain and allodynia of postherpetic neuralgia. *J Pain Symptom Manage* 17:429-433. Copyright 1999 by the US Cancer Pain Relief Committee.)

Conclusions.—Brief IV infusions of lidocaine positively affect pain and allodynia in patients with postherpetic neuralgia. The higher dose may result in plasma levels in the toxic range without significantly increasing the response.

▶ There is clearly a beneficial effect, at least on allodynia, from short-term administration of lidocaine. The question remains, what is the potential long-term benefit? Long-term infusion of low doses may be an option for some patients, especially those with extremely severe pain for whom other options have not helped. Some patients may benefit from repeated inter-mittent infusion therapy, whereas others may benefit from oral sodium channel blockers such as mexiletine.

S. E. Abram, MD

A Mixed Model for Factors Predictive of Pain in AIDS Patients With Herpes Zoster
Harrison RA, Soong S-j; Weiss HL, et al (Univ of Alabama, Birmingham)
J Pain Symptom Manage 17:410-417, 1999   10–35

Background.—Demographic and clinical variables reportedly affect quality-of-life variables in patients with herpes zoster. Intraindividual and interindividual quality-of-life measures among patients with HIV infection in the first month after herpes zoster disease onset and during the subsequent 12 months were investigated.

Methods.—One hundred sixty-six HIV-infected patients were enrolled in a randomized, controlled study of antiviral therapy of herpes zoster comparing acyclovir with sorivudine. In a "mixed model," predictors of pain severity, activity impairment, and sleep interruption were assessed.

Findings.—In the first month, the mean rate of change in acute pain was –0.04 unit pain per day. Chronic pain declined by 0.12 per month between 1 and 12 months. Acute pain severity was positively associated with the number of new skin vesicles, analgesic use, and baseline pain. It was negatively correlated with the percentage of lesion healing and crusting. Postherpetic neuralgia was associated with baseline pain, pain at 1 month, and the duration of lesions. Changes in pain severity were unrelated to treatment group, sex, race, and CD4 count.

Conclusions.—Baseline pain significantly predicted pain resolution, and mean pain severity predicted return to normal daily activities and sleep. The severity of acute pain at initial evaluation and 1 month later significantly predicted chronic pain.

▶ This study confirms the findings of previous studies indicating that the severity of acute herpes zoster pain predicts the likelihood of developing postherpetic neuralgia. In this cohort, there was no correlation between age and severity of pain at onset. There is continuing controversy over the issue of efficacy of nerve blocks performed early in the severe phase. It seems logical that early deafferentation of the neuropathic pain generator would block the development of central sensitization and reduce the likelihood of having long-term pain. On the other hand, there also appears to be some correlation between viral injury to spinal cord structures and long-term pain. Perhaps patients with the most severe pain at onset of the disease are those who have spinal gray matter involvement.

This study paves the way for useful outcome studies. If patients with severe early pain and an extensive rash are randomly assigned to receive or not receive aggressive regional blockade, the utility of such treatment could be assessed in a population with a high likelihood of having postherpetic neuralgia.

S. E. Abram, MD

Basic Science

The Analgesic Potency of Dexmedetomidine Is Enhanced After Nerve Injury: A Possible Role for Peripheral α_2-Adrenoceptors

Poree LR, Guo TZ, Kingery WS, et al (Stanford Univ, Calif; VAPAHCS, Palo Alto, Calif)
Anesth Analg 87:941-948, 1998   10–36

Introduction.—Animal studies have shown that morphine is less effective in models of neuropathic hyperalgesia and allodynia. This suggests that spinal nerve ligation might cause a rightward shift in the analgesic dose response to systemically administered $\alpha_2$adrenoreceptor (α_2AR) agonists. The effects of systemic dexmedetomidine, a selective α_2AR agonist, on mechanical and heat nociceptive withdrawal thresholds were studied in normal and neuropathic rats.

Methods.—The L5-6 spinal nerves of Sprague-Dawley rats were ligated to induce chronic mechanical and thermal neuropathic hyperalgesia. Hindpaw mechanical and heat withdrawal thresholds were then measured with the use of von Frey fibers and a thermoelectric Peltier device, respectively. The dose-response effect of systemic dexmedetomidine on these thresholds was investigated. Atipamezole, a selective α_2AR antagonist, was given to confirm that the analgesic effects of dexmedetomidine were mediated by the α_2AR. The inhibitory effects of a peripherally restricted α_2AR antagonist, L-659,066, were assessed as well.

Results.—Dexmedetomidine, administered intraperitoneally, increased both mechanical and thermal thresholds in dose-dependent fashion. Fifty-percent effective doses (ED_{50}) were 144 µg/kg for the mechanical threshold and 180 µg/kg for the thermal threshold. These ED_{50} values were significantly lower for nerve-injured rats: 52 and 29 µg/kg, respectively. According to assessments of activity, the sedative effects of dexmedetomidine were similar in control and neuropathic animals. In both groups of rats, atipamezole blocked both the analgesic and sedative effects of dexmedetomidine. In contrast, L-659,066 blocked the analgesic but not the sedative effects only in nerve-injured rats and blocked neither effect in control rats.

Conclusions.—The α_2AR agonist dexmedetomidine shows heightened analgesic potency in neuropathic rats, with an extra-CNS site of action.

The nerve injury induced in this model results in sensitization to α_2 analgesia while shifting the site of α_2 analgesic action outside the blood-brain barrier. The results suggest a promising role for peripherally restricted α_2 agonists in treatment of neuropathic pain.

▶ It is encouraging to learn that α_2 adrenergic agonists may have beneficial effects in certain types of neuropathic pain, which typically respond poorly to opioids. There has been considerable recent interest in the proliferation of $\alpha_{2A}AR$ in the dorsal root ganglia of nerve-injured animals. These receptors are coupled to calcium channels and may play an important role in the development of allodynia and hyperalgesia. This study provides evidence that α_2 adrenergic agonists may reduce allodynia at a peripheral rather than a central site. The observation that transdermal clonidine is more efficacious when placed directly over areas of hypersensitivity in patients with reflex sympathetic dystrophy supports this hypothesis.

S. E. Abram, MD

Interaction of Intrathecally Infused Morphine and Lidocaine in Rats (Part I): Synergistic Antinociceptive Effects
Saito Y, Kaneko M, Kirihara Y, et al (Shimade Med Univ, Japan)
Anesthesiology 89:1455-1463, 1998   10–37

Introduction.—Opioids and local anesthetics are commonly given together by infusion to treat various types of pain. Previous animal studies have demonstrated that opioids and local anesthetics have synergistic antinociceptive effects when given in bolus injections. However, the synergistic effects that occur when these drugs are given by continuous infusion are not known. A study was performed in rats to evaluate the synergistic somatic and visceral effects of morphine and lidocaine given by intrathecal infusion.

Methods.—Rats received intrathecal infusions of morphine 0.3 to 10.0 µg/kg per hour, lidocaine 30 to 1000 µg/kg per hour, morphine plus lidocaine, or placebo. The infusions continued at a constant rate of 1 µL/h for 6 days. Somatic antinociceptive effects were measured by the tail flick test and visceral effects by the colorectal distention test; motor function tests were performed as well. The magnitude of the synergistic interaction between drugs was evaluated by isobolographic analysis of the results of the tail flick test.

Results.—Somatic and visceral antinociceptive effects occurred in dose-dependent fashion in response to intrathecal infusion of both agents alone. The peak percentage maximum possible effect of morphine was lower in the colorectal distention (visceral) test than in the somatic (tail flick) test. At the 1000 µg/kg per hour dose, lidocaine caused motor impairment. On their own, morphine 0.3 µg/kg per hour and lidocaine 200 µg/kg per hour had no effects. When infused together, however, these two doses had a significantly higher percentage of maximum possible effects. The antinoci-

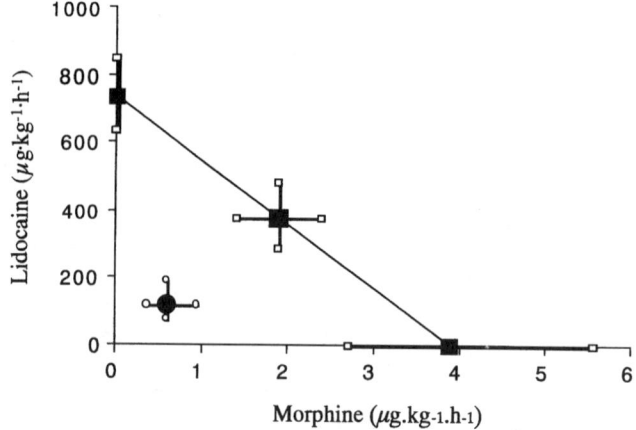

FIGURE 5.—An isobologram of antinociceptive median effective dose (ED_{50}) values and 95% CIs for morphine (*horizontal*), lidocaine (*vertical*), or a combination of morphine and lidocaine (point in the dose field). The *heavy lines* represent the CIs. The *dashed diagonal* line connecting the morphine and lidocaine ED_{50} values (*closed square* on the axes) is the theoretical additive line, and the point on this line (*large closed square*) is the theoretical additive point. The fact that the experimental points (*closed circle*) evaluated fell below the theoretical additive points indicates that the antinociceptive effects produced by the combination were synergistic. (Courtesy of Saito Y, Kaneko M, Kirihara Y, et al: Interaction of intrathecally infused morphine and lidocaine in rats [part I]: Synergistic antinociceptive effects. *Anesthesiology* 89:1455-1463, 1998. Copyright American Society of Anesthesiologists, Inc. Used with permission of Lippincott-Raven Publishers.)

ceptive effects of morphine were significantly potentiated in terms of duration and magnitude by lidocaine coinfusion. The synergistic effects of morphine and lidocaine were confirmed by isobolographic analysis (Fig 5).

Conclusions.—This animal study confirms that morphine and lidocaine have synergistic antinociceptive effects when given by continuous intrathecal infusion. Whereas morphine on its own has little visceral antinociceptive effect, coinfusion with lidocaine results in a sharp increase in visceral antinociception. Various combinations of opioids and local anesthetics may prove useful in long-term treatment of visceral and somatic pain.

▶ This study confirms previous data that suggest a synergistic analgesic effect between neuraxially administered local anesthetic opioids. The effect is demonstrated for both visceral and somatic pain. Isobolographic analysis shows a robust and statistically significant synergistic effect as measured by the tail flick test. As the authors point out, supra-additive effects are more difficult to demonstrate in clinical models of postoperative pain. However, it is clear that local anesthetic/opiate combinations are associated with fewer adverse effects and less functional impairment than either local anesthetics or opioids alone.

S. E. Abram, MD

Loperamide (ADL 2-1294), an Opioid Antihyperalgesic Agent With Peripheral Selectivity

DeHaven-Hudkins DL, Burgos LC, Cassel JA, et al (Adolor Corp, Malvern, Pa; Univ of California, La Jolla)

J Pharmacol Exp Ther 289:494-502, 1999

10–38

Background.—The potential value of an opiate agonist that antagonizes the hyperalgesia resulting from inflammation is clear. The in vitro profile of loperamide at cloned human opioid receptors and the potent antihyperalgesia produced by loperamide administered in various in vivo models of inflammatory pain were reported.

Methods and Findings.—Various inflammatory pain models in rodents were investigated. Loperamide showed potent affinity and selectivity for the cloned μ compared with the δ and κ human opioid receptors. Loperamide was a potent stimulator of [^{35}S]guanosin-5'-O-(3-thio)-triphosphate binding and inhibitor of forskolin-stimulated cAMP accumulation in Chinese hamster ovary cells transfected with the human μ opioid receptor. Injection of 0.3 mg of loperamide into the intra-articular space of the inflamed rat knee joint was associated with potent antinociception to knee compression antagonized by naloxone. Injection of loperamide into the contralateral knee joint or intramuscularly did not inhibit compression-induced changes in blood pressure. Although loperamide potently inhib-

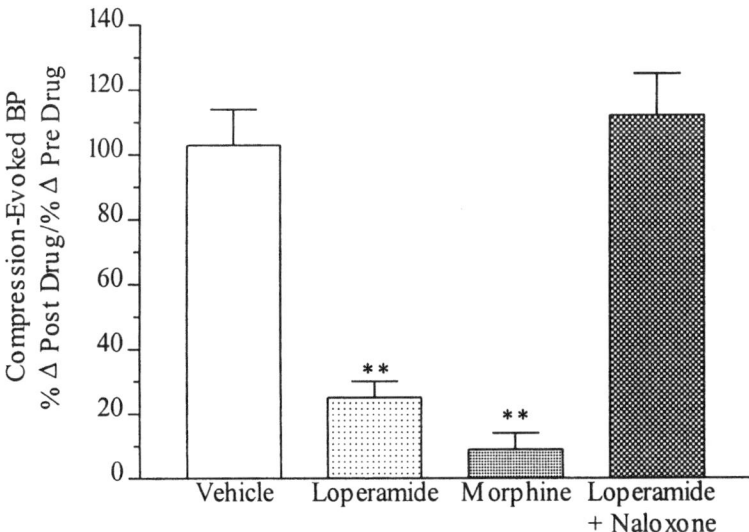

FIGURE 3.—Effect of intra-articular loperamide or morphine on blood pressure changes evoked by compression of the inflamed knee joint. Loperamide (0.3 mg) or morphine (3 mg) was injected by the intra-articular route at 3 hours after the induction of inflammation (n = 4 per group). Naloxone was injected intraperitoneally at a dose of 1 mg/kg (n = 4). **Significantly different from vehicle, Dunnett's test, P < .01. *Abbreviation: BP,* Blood pressure. (Courtesy of Dehaven-Hudkins DL, Burgos LC, Cassel JA, et al: Loperamide [ADL 2-1294], an opioid antihyperalgesic agent with peripheral selectivity. *J Pharmacol Exp Ther* 289:494-502, 1999.)

ited late-phase formalin-induced flinching after intrapaw injection, it was not effective against early-phase flinching or after injection into the paw contralateral to the formalin-treated paw. Local loperamide injection also resulted in antinociception against hyperalgesia induced by Freund's adjuvant or by tape stripping, shown by increased paw pressure thresholds in the inflamed paw. In all rodent models, local administration of loperamide was as potent as morphine or more so (Fig 3).

Conclusions.—Loperamide has potential as a peripherally selective opiate antihyperalgesic agent. This agent does not have many of the adverse effects usually associated with centrally acting opiates.

▶ This drug, widely used orally as an antidiarrheal, appears to have substantial antihyperalgesic effects when injected into inflamed tissues. This study illustrates that the peripheral analgesic effects of opiates are seen in inflamed but not intact tissues.

S. E. Abram, MD

Intrathecal Administration of mGluR Compound, (S)-4CPG, Attenuates Hyperalgesia and Allodynia Associated With Sciatic Nerve Constriction Injury in Rats

Fisher K, Fundytus ME, Cahill CM, et al (Clinical Research Inst of Montreal; McGill Univ, Montreal; Astra Research Centre Montreal; et al)
Pain 77:59-66, 1998
10–39

Objective.—The effect of intrathecal treatment with the group I metabotropic glutamate receptor antagonist, (S)-4-carboxyphenylglycine [(S)-4CPG], and the noncompetitive N-methyl-D-aspartate (NMDA) antagonist, dizocilipine maleate (MK-801), on mechanical allodynia and cold hyperalgesia associated with chronic constriction injury of the sciatic nerve in rats was examined. The effect of early or late treatment with (S)-4CPG on injury-related mechanical allodynia and cold hyperalgesia was also evaluated.

Methods.—A chronic constriction injury was produced in 76 male rats. (S)-4CPG and MK-801 were administered intrathecally by lumbar puncture. Early treatment with (S)-4CPG consisted of injections twice a day on days 0 to 3; late treatment consisted of injections twice a day on days 8 to 11. Mechanical allodynia and cold hyperalgesia testing were performed at baseline and on days 4, 8, 12, and 16 after surgery.

Results.—Eight-day treatment with (S)-4CPG decreased mechanical allodynia up to day 12 and cold hyperalgesia up to day 8. Eight-day treatment with MK-801 decreased mechanical allodynia up to day 16 and cold hyperalgesia up to day 16. Early treatment with (S)-4CPG significantly decreased the development of mechanical allodynia and cold hyperalgesia. Late treatment with (S)-4CPG did not decrease nociceptive behaviors in either task.

Discussion.—These findings indicate that the NMDA receptor is involved in chronic nociception and that group I metabotropic glutamate receptor antagonists have a more critical role in the development, not the maintenance, of mechanical allodynia and cold hyperalgesia associated with chronic constriction injury in rats. The effect of treatment with (S)-4CPG may result from antagonism of group I metabotropic glutamate receptors, because activation of these compounds causes production of second messenger systems important in persistent and chronic nociception.

▶ The excitatory amino acids glutamate and aspartate are capable of producing activation or sensitization of dorsal horn cells following release from primary afferent nociceptors. Their effects are mediated through multiple receptors, including the ionotropic α-amino-3-hydroxy-5-methyl-4-isoxazoleproprionic acid (AMPA) and NMDA receptors and the G-protein-linked metabotropic receptors. Investigation of the phenomena surrounding post-injury hyperalgesia has previously focused mainly on the NMDA receptor. However, the AMPA receptor, which gates a sodium ion channel, appears to be involved in the development of noxious stimulus-induced hyperalgesia. Similarly, Fisher et al have shown that 1 subtype of the metabotropic glutamate receptors is also important in the initiation, though not the maintenance, of spinal sensitization. Perhaps agents, such as (S)-4CPG, will be useful in reducing the development of post-operative hyperalgesic states, such as intercostal neuralgia or post-amputation pain.

S. E. Abram, MD

Surgical Pain Attenuates Acute Morphine Tolerance in Rats
Ho ST, Wang JJ, Liaw WJ, et al (Natl Defence Med Centre, Taipei, Taiwan)
Br J Anaesth 82:112-116, 1999   10–40

Objective.—Animals show tolerance to morphine after long-term administration, but patients do not. It has been hypothesized that noxious stimuli during administration of morphine may interfere with the development of tolerance. Upper and lower abdominal surgery procedures in Sprague-Dawley rats were used to test the effect of postoperative pain on prevention of acute tolerance to morphine administration.

Methods.—Rats were divided into 6 groups of 12 rats each. Group 1 had lower abdominal surgery, group 2 had lower abdominal surgery and IV infusion of saline solution, group 3 had upper abdominal surgery and IV infusion of morphine, group 4 had upper abdominal surgery and IV infusion of saline solution, group 5 had IV infusion of morphine and group 6 had IV infusion of saline solution. The antinociceptive effect was tested by means of the infrared thermal tail flick. Tail flick latencies were measured 10 minutes before and 30 minutes after administration of medication and hourly thereafter for 8 hours. Plasma concentrations of morphine were measured 1 minute before infusion and at 1, 2, 4, and 8 hours after the start of infusion.

Results.—Only the groups that received morphine showed analgesic effects, which reached a maximum at an average of 2 hours after infusion. Whereas analgesic effects diminished gradually after infusion in group 5, effects in groups 1 and 3 decreased more slowly, and those groups had significantly larger area under the curve values (34,556 and 32,548, respectively) than did group 5 (18,759). There were no significant differences in groups 1 and 3. Plasma morphine concentrations at 8 hours were similar for groups 1, 3, and 5 (179.9, 182.7, and 170.9 ng/mL, respectively).

Conclusion.—In the rat model, morphine tolerance that developed rapidly after IV infusion of morphine was attenuated significantly by surgical pain.

▶ Information derived from animal models of tolerance that involve opioid administration in the absence of ongoing pain is often extrapolated to clinical situations. As this study indicates, this may be inappropriate. In such animal models, nearly complete loss of analgesic effect occurs in about 1 week. Such rapid development of tolerance is rarely seen in patients with acute or chronic pain. Increased levels of protein kinase C are found in dorsal horn cells of opioid-tolerant animals and animals rendered hyperalgesic by experimental neuropathy. The interactions between the nociceptive, as opposed to neuropathic, pain state and the opioid receptor have not been elucidated.

S. E. Abram, MD

Acute Amitriptyline in a Rat Model of Neuropathic Pain: Differential Symptom and Route Effects

Esser MJ, Sawynok J (Dalhousie Univ, Halifax, Nova Scotia)
Pain 80:643-653, 1999   10–41

Objective.—Medical interventions have shown limited utility for treating neuropathic pain. Tricyclic antidepressants have demonstrated some efficacy against neuropathic pain. The mechanism and drug treatment of neuropathic pain using tricyclic antidepressants were investigated in the rat model.

Methods.—Spinal nerve ligation of the fifth and sixth spinal nerves was performed on male Sprague-Dawley rats. Tactile allodynia and thermal hyperalgesia were evoked in the rat paw. Amitriptyline was administered in a blinded fashion systemically by intraperitoneal injection, spinally through chronically implanted intrathecal cannulas, or locally in the dorsal surface of the paw.

Results.—Systemic administration of amitriptyline produced an antihyperanalgesic effect in the injured paw; intrathecal administration produced a partial reversal of thermal hyperalgesia; and local injection resulted in a marked local antinociceptive effect. Amitriptyline had no effect on allodynia in the injured paw regardless of route of administration.

Conclusion.—Although spinally, locally, and intraperitoneally administered amitriptyline relieves thermal hyperalgesia in the rat model, it is ineffective against allodynia.

▶ Previous explanations of the pain-relieving effects of amitriptyline (inhibition of serotonin and norepinephrine uptake) are clearly incomplete. There appear to be multiple, complex actions at both central and peripheral sites. These include *N*-methyl-D-aspartate receptor antagonism and potentiation of endogenous opioid-induced analgesia. Peripheral effects may be related to interference with adrenergic, histaminergic, or neurokinin 1 (substance P) receptors. With all of these potentially beneficial pharmacologic properties, it is disappointing that only a third of patients with neuropathic pain are likely to respond.

S. E. Abram, MD

---

d-Methadone Blocks Morphine Tolerance and *N*-Methyl-D-Aspartate–induced Hyperalgesia

Davis AM, Inturrisi CE (Cornell Univ, New York)
J Pharmacol Exp Ther 289:1048-1053, 1999   10–42

Objective.—*d*-Methadone has been shown to be an N-methyl-D-aspartate (NMDA) receptor antagonist. Whether systemic and/or intrathecal methadone can block morphine tolerance was investigated in the rat and mouse models.

Methods.—The percentage of analgesia was tested in mice and rats on days 1 and 5 after morphine (7 mg/kg) and either saline or systemic *d*-methadone (160 μg) was administered. Tail-flick tests established that morphine tolerance had developed by day 5.

Results.—Administration of *d*-methadone and morphine prevented development of tolerance to morphine, whereas saline plus morphine did not (Fig 1). Escalating doses of morphine given subcutaneously 3 times daily produced a threefold increase in the mouse tail-flick test, and intrathecal morphine created a 38-fold increase in the rat tail-flick test. Coadministration of *d*-methadone completely prevented both increases. Pretreatment with *d*-methadone blocked the NMDA-induced decrease in the thermal paw withdrawal test.

Conclusion.—The NMDA receptor antagonist *d*-methadone prevents the development of morphine tolerance in rats and mice and, possibly, can be used to treat neuropathic pain and improve the analgesic effectiveness of chronically administered morphine.

▶ Several opioids, including oxycodone and propoxyphene, have NMDA receptor–blocking actions, which may augment their efficacy in hyperalgesic conditions such as peripheral nerve injury and complex regional pain syn-

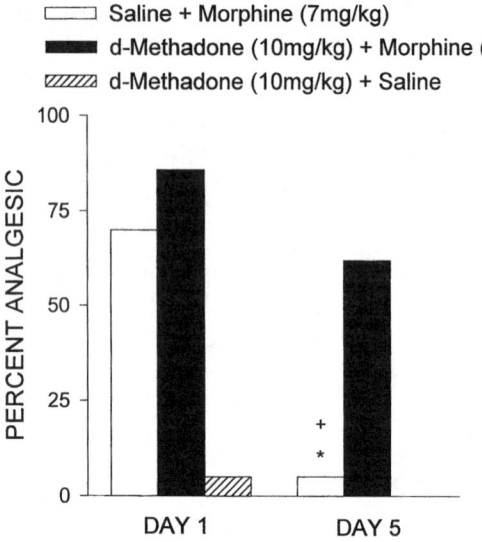

☐ Saline + Morphine (7mg/kg)
■ d-Methadone (10mg/kg) + Morphine (7mg/kg)
▨ d-Methadone (10mg/kg) + Saline

FIGURE 1.—Attenuation of morphine tolerance by pretreatment with d-methadone. d-Methadone at a dose of 10 mg/kg or saline was administered subcutaneously 30 minutes before each morphine injection (7 mg/kg) on days 1 to 5. The percentage of analgesic responders in the d-methadone plus morphine group was significantly different (*asterisk* indicates $P < .01$) from the saline plus morphine group on day 5. The saline plus morphine group response on day 5 was significantly different (*asterisk* indicates $P < .005$) from the saline plus morphine group response on day 1. The saline plus saline treatment group had no analgesic response or change in tail-flick values on day 1 or 5 (data not shown). (Courtesy of Davis AM, Inturrisi CE: d-Methadone blocks morphine tolerance and N-methyl-D-aspartate-induced hyperalgesia. *J Pharmacol Exp Ther* 289:1048-1053, 1999.)

drome and delay or reduce the incidence of opioid tolerance. NMDA antagonists have antihyperalgesic and antitolerance properties, both spinally and systemically. It is logical, therefore, to select these agents when other opioids are relatively ineffective. On the other hand, systemic administration of known NMDA antagonists such as dextromethorphan and amantadine are of limited clinical efficacy in patients with neuropathic pain or opioid tolerance.

S. E. Abram, MD

Poor Antibacterial Effect of Ropivacaine: Comparison With Bupivacaine
Pere P, Lindgren L, Vaara M (Helsinki Univ)
Anesthesiology 91:884-886, 1999   10–43

Background.—Ropivacaine, a long-acting aminoamide local anesthetic, was recently introduced as a replacement for bupivacaine. The antibacterial effects of these 2 agents were compared.

Methods and Findings.—Eight bacterial strains were used. Bupivacaine more strongly inhibited the growth of all bacteria studied except *Klebsiella pneumoniae.* The highest concentration of bupivacaine (3.75 mg/mL) fully inhibited the growth of *Escherichia coli*, *Psuedomonas aeruginosa*, and *Staphylococcus epidermidis.* Even the lowest concentration of this agent (0.938 mg/mL) significantly inhibited the growth of *P aeruginosa*, *S epidermidis*, and *Streptococcus pyogenes.*

Conclusions.—At clinical concentrations, bupivacaine was stronger than ropivacaine in inhibiting the growth of all bacteria studied, except for *K pneumoniae.* Bupivacaine's antibacterial effect increased with increasing concentrations.

▶ The antibiotic effects of local anesthetics may explain the low rate of serious intraspinal infections associated with long-term epidural analgesia. The greater antibacterial effect of bupivacaine may represent a potential advantage over ropivacaine for long-term infusion. On the other hand, at concentrations commonly used for prolonged analgesia, minimal effects were noted for either drug.

S. E. Abram, MD

Effects of Lamotrigine on Pain-Induced Chemo-somatosensory Evoked Potentials

Klamt JG, Posner J (Univ of São Paulo, Brazil; BIOS Ltd, London)
Anaesthesia 54:774-777, 1999   10–44

Background.—Lamotrigine is a sodium channel blocker that selectively inhibits the neuronal release of glutamate and produces analgesia in acute and chronic rat pain models without causing noticeable sedation. Administered orally, it also decreases pain scores in volunteers, as assessed by the cold-pain test. In the current study, the analgesic effect of lamotrigine given by mouth to healthy volunteers was analyzed by changes in chemosomatosensory evoked potentials.

Methods.—Twelve volunteers were given placebo or lamotrigine, 300 mg, on separate occasions in a double-blind, randomized, crossover design. The factors measured were latency to N_1 and P_{100} peak (ms), amplitude between the N_1 and P_{100} peak (μV), and visual analog pain intensity scores.

Findings.—At 2 hours after treatment, lamotrigine produced a significantly greater latency to P_{100} values than placebo. However, lamotrigine did not significantly affect the other factors.

Conclusions.—Lamotrigine, 300 mg, given orally did not have an analgesic effect in this acute pain model. This finding is not consistent with that of previous studies using the cold-pain test.

▶ Lamotrigine is currently being used to treat neuropathic pain. Its theoretical advantage is its capability to block the release of noxious stimulus-induced excitatory amino acids, particularly glutamate. Although this study failed to demonstrate analgesia from a brief noxious stimulus, it does not rule out its usefulness in patients with tonic, neuropathic pain. Studies of lamotrigine should focus on its capability to provide analgesia for patients whose treatments with other anticonvulsants have failed.

S. E. Abram, MD

11 Preoperative Evaluation

Preoperative Assessment of Cardiac Risk in Noncardiac Major Vascular Surgery
Roghi A, Palmieri B, Crivellaro W, et al (Niguarda Hosp, Milan, Italy)
Am J Cardiol 83:169-174, 1999   11-1

Introduction.—There is debate over the optimal evaluation of cardiac risk in patients requiring vascular surgery. A prospective study sought to determine whether a preoperative algorithm combining clinical and rest echocardiographic data would allow an adequate stratification of cardiac risk in patients unable to exercise. The predictive value of dipyridamole thallium-201(^{201}Tl) scintigraphy for postoperative adverse cardiac outcomes was assessed in patients at intermediate risk.

Methods.—Included in the study were 320 patients referred for elective major vascular surgery between January 1995 and December 1996. The patients were prospectively stratified into low-, intermediate-, and high-risk groups. Those considered to be at low or intermediate risk for adverse outcome underwent vascular surgery without further treatment. Of the 65 patients in the high-risk group, 49 underwent vascular surgery with perioperative intensive care treatment, 9 underwent presurgical revascularization, and 7 had the vascular procedure canceled. Rest echocardiography was performed before surgery in all intermediate- and high-risk patients and in 28 low-risk patients with mild hypertension. Ninety-nine patients were examined with dipyridamole ^{201}Tl scintigraphy.

Results.—Thirteen patients (3.8%) died within 30 days of surgery; 8 of these deaths were attributed to noncardiac causes. Cardiac mortality and morbidity were 1.5% and 10.4%, respectively. The 3 risk groups differed significantly in the distribution of "hard" adverse events (death, myocardial infarction, pulmonary edema, major arrhythmias) and "soft" ones (myocardial ischemia, minor arrhythmias). Multiple logistic regression analysis showed previous pulmonary edema to be a predictive variable of cardiac outcomes. In the group of 99 intermediate-risk patients who randomly underwent dipyridamole ^{201}Tl scintigraphy, 37 had redistribution, 10 had persistent, and 52 had no defects. Seven of 13 soft and hard cardiac events occurred in those with no defects. The sensitivity, specificity, and positive and negative predictive values of redistribution defects for postoperative adverse outcomes were 38%, 63%, 14%, and 87%, respectively.

Conclusion.—The vascular surgical protocol described in this study, in which known risk factors were used for stratification of patients, may provide a safe and cost-effective approach to the question of cardiac risk. Results do not support the routine use of dipyridamole ^{201}Tl scintigraphy for screening of patients considered at intermediate risk.

▶ I must have missed it: this study tried to define intermediate versus low and high risk patients, and whether intermediate patients would benefit from dipyridamole thallium by retrospective design, but with prospective allocation by a preoperative clinical algorithm. I must have missed it, because I can't find the algorithm anywhere in the study. How could editors let that slip by? Well, I've read the article three times and can't find it. Several places in the study they referred to the algorithm, and a simple algorithm. Nevertheless, we are led to believe by the data that routine use of dipyridamole thallium scintigraphy for screening of intermediate-risk patients may not be the best strategy. What is an intermediate-risk patient? Good luck reading this article and finding out, because I couldn't.

M. F. Roizen, MD

Impact of New Guidelines on Physicians' Ordering of Preoperative Tests
Mancuso CA (Cornell Univ, New York)
J Gen Intern Med 14:166-172, 1999   11–2

Objective.—The number and types of preoperative tests ordered for patients undergoing elective ambulatory surgery were compared for the 2 years before and 2 years after the establishment of new hospital testing guidelines.

Methods.—The preoperative testing and outcome of all orthopedic patients undergoing ambulatory surgery referred to 1 medical consultant 2 years before (n = 361) and 2 years after (n = 279) the establishment of new guidelines (August 1, 1991 through December 31, 1995) were reviewed for perioperative complications.

Results.—The number of tests ordered declined significantly by 30%, from an average of 8.0 before the guidelines to 5.6 after the guidelines. Decreases occurred for all patient groups and for patients with lower comorbidity scores but not for patients with higher comorbidity scores. Test ordering decreased for patients receiving all types of anesthesia with the exception of those receiving general anesthesia. According to multivariate analysis, only time and type of surgery were significant for all comparisons. Comorbidity and age were significantly correlated. When surgeons ordered fewer tests, medical consultants did not increase the number of tests they ordered. Most patients had no adverse intraoperative or postoperative events, and the percentage of patients admitted before and after the guidelines was not significantly different. The ordering of preoperative tests decreased by 23% to 44%, saving about $34,000 during the study, or $650,000 during the first 2 years.

Conclusion.—Changing guidelines for preoperative testing resulted in a decrease of 30% in ambulatory surgery patients and a 2-year savings of $650,000.

▶ This study shows a remarkable decrease in preoperative tests by just issuing a memo saying that the required tests have been changed. It was clear from the article that no educational program, no set of detailed guidelines, no research study, and no other major system change was made to cause the change in test order. Nevertheless, it is also clear that the patients in this orthopedic hospital have a different system than most patients. Not only is there surgeon involvement in preoperative preparation, and the involvement of an anesthesiologist, but there also appears to be an invariable medical consult. This invariable medical consult insures that patients with systemic disease have appropriate management of their chronic disease before being accepted for surgery. And another important point to remember in examining the data from this study is that these were outpatient operations. Thus, many of the patients were presumably being operated on to remedy sport injury–type events. Nonetheless, this should not diminish our enthusiasm for reducing tests to those appropriately needed, and this study demonstrates another process toward effecting that goal.

M. F. Roizen, MD

Expiratory and Inspiratory Chest Computed Tomography and Pulmonary Function Tests in Cigarette Smokers
Kubo K, Eda S, Yamamoto H, et al (Shinshu Univ, Matsumoto, Japan; Tokyo Women's Med College)
Eur Respir J 13:252-256, 1999   11–3

Objective.—A high resolution CT (HRCT) scan obtained at full expiration (E) compared with a scan obtained at full inspiration (I) allows the calculation of E/I, the amount of air trapped in small airways. The possibility that this measure might detect early signs of small airway dysfunction and emphysematous destruction in cigarette smokers was investigated.

Methods.—Pulmonary function tests and chest HRCT scans were performed on 10 normal nonsmoking volunteers (group A) and on 63 consecutive male smokers or ex-smokers between April 1994 and September 1997. The amount of emphysematous destruction was evaluated by visual scoring (VS), the Brinkman smoking index (BI) was used to calculate cigarette-years/d, and the E/I value was calculated. On the basis of pulmonary function tests, smokers were divided in 3 groups: group B1 (n = 7) had normal pulmonary function test results; group B2 (n = 21) had a lung diffusing capacity for carbon monoxide of at least 80% of that predicted, a forced expiratory volume in 1 second (FEV_1) of less than 80% of levels predicted, and/or a residual volume greater than 120% of predicted; and group B3 (n = 35) had a lung diffusing capacity for carbon monoxide of less than 80% of predicted levels, a FEV_1 of less than 80% of predicted levels, and/or a residual volume more than 120% of predicted volume. Fifteen smokers were classified as mild (BI < 600) and 48 as heavy smokers (BI ≥ 600).

Results.—E/I and VS were significantly higher in heavy smokers than in mild smokers or nonsmokers. There were no significant differences between the E/I and VS of mild smokers and nonsmokers. E/I was significantly higher for groups B2 and B3 than for groups A and B1. VS was significantly higher in group B3 than in group B2.

Conclusion.—The results of the E/I and VS measures of emphysema were significantly higher in heavy smokers. Although E/I was significantly higher in groups B2 and B3 compared with group B1, VS was not significantly different between groups B2 and B1. E/I may be a measure of hyperinflation and airway obstruction regardless of the degree of emphysematous destruction.

▶ The finding that HRCT is not as useful in determining functional classification when analyzed by VS, as opposed to an E/I ratio when pulmonary functions are used as the gold standard, is an important finding—one that will gain increasing importance as more HRCT maneuvers are done in smokers to detect the early presence of cancer. How common will these tests be? I don't know, but it looks like if we're going to avoid pulmonary function tests, and still gauge functional capacity as if we did pulmonary function tests in patients who have had HRCTs, we will need to have a HRCT number, a full expiration and full inspiration, or the E/I ratio provided.

M. F. Roizen, MD

Effect of Obesity and Erect/Supine Posture on Lateral Cephalometry: Relationship to Sleep-Disordered Breathing

Brander PE, Mortimore IL, Douglas NJ (Univ of Edinburgh, Scotland)
Eur Respir J 13:398-402, 1999   11–4

Objective.—Bony craniofacial abnormalities may be more of a risk factor for sleep apnea/hypopnea syndrome (SAHS) in nonobese patients than in obese patients. The relationship between apnea/hypopnea index (AHI) severity and lateral cephalometric measurements and the effect of body position on cephalometric measurements were assessed in obese and nonobese individuals.

Methods.—Lateral cephalometric radiographs of patients with SAHS were obtained with 31 obese and 42 nonobese males in both the erect and supine positions. The cephalograms were analyzed by a blinded investigator. Relationships between AHI, body mass index, lowest arterial oxygen saturation during sleep, and cephalometric measurements in both supine and erect positions were analyzed using the Pearson correlation and multiple regression for obese and nonobese patients.

Results.—AHI and hyoid to pharyngeal wall (H-PW) distances were significantly higher in obese patients than in nonobese patients. For obese patients, the H-PW distance was significantly larger than for nonobese patients in both the supine and erect postures. For nonobese patients, the H-PW distance was larger in the supine position. According to multivariate regression analysis, upper airway dimensions were significantly correlated with AHI. Body mass index was significantly correlated with H-PW in both erect and supine postures.

Conclusion.—Upper airway size is significantly correlated with AHI. Upper airway size differences between obese and nonobese patients are the result of soft tissue rather than bony abnormalities.

▶ While this was a needed study, its results confirm what most of us believe: bone structure is not the same as soft tissue structure, and it appears to be soft tissue and muscle tissue changes that causes obstruction in airways, not just the position of bones. And while these are loosely related, there is no hard and fast test. This study confirms that what is needed when one cares for a patient is a good anesthesiologist, not a good radiologic review in advance to see if a good anesthesiologist is needed.

M. F. Roizen, MD

Cephalometric Abnormalities in Non-Obese and Obese Patients With Obstructive Sleep Apnoea
Sakakibara H, Tong M, Matsushita K, et al (Fujita Health Univ, Toyoake, Japan)
Eur Respir J 13:403-410, 1999   11–5

Objective.—Although some studies have found cephalometric abnormalities in patients with sleep disordered breathing, the effect of body mass index and age on these measurements have not been established. The cephalometric features of patients with normal and obstructive sleep apnea (OSA) were evaluated, and the relationship between cephalometric variables and apnea severity in nonobese and obese patients with OSA was clarified.

Methods.—Polysomnography was performed in 114 male Japanese patients with OSA (average age, 49 years) and in 19 of 37 normal male control subjects (average age, 36 years). Among the OSA patients, 60 were obese. Lateral cephalograms were obtained for all participants, and 48 cephalic variables were measured. Intra- and interobserver reliability were determined.

Results.—Compared with non-obese control subjects, obese OSA patients had thicker soft tissue in the nasopharynx area, increased tongue length and thickness, an anteriorly displaced hyoid bone, larger soft palate, increased craniocervical angulation, and decreased cervical-horizontal angulation. Intra- and interobserver reliability were high. There were no correlations between cephalometric variables and age. Compared with obese patients, nonobese patients had a shorter G-VL, a shorter cranial base, and a narrower bony nasopharynx and oropharynx. The obese group had more extensive and severe soft tissue abnormalities than bony abnormalities. Cephalometric measurements were correlated with apnea severity in obese and nonobese patients. Anterior cranial base length and mandibular length were significantly related to apnea severity in nonobese OSA patients. Distance between the anterior vertebra and the hyoid bone was significantly correlated with soft tissue measurements in obese OSA patients.

Conclusion.—Although obese patients with OSA tend to have soft tissue abnormalities, which may contribute to the sleeping disorder, nonobese OSA patients appear to have the apnea because of bony structure abnormalities.

▶ This study shows that, while there are differences from normal in cephalometric measurements in patients with OSA, none of these were of a great enough difference to create a definitive preoperative test.

M. F. Roizen, MD

"One-Stop" Surgery: Implications for Anesthesiologists of an Expedited Pediatric Surgical Process
Overdyk FJ, Burt N, Tagge EP, et al (Med Univ of South Carolina, Charleston)
South Med J 92:308-312, 1999   11–6

Introduction.—The traditional time line for pediatric patients undergoing simple outpatient procedures is 3 days: 1 day for preoperative testing, 1 for surgery, and 1 for postoperative follow-up. "One-stop surgery," (OSS) an innovative program that consolidates this process into 1 day, is described.

Methods.—Physicians referring pediatric patients for umbilical hernia repair, circumcision, or central venous catheter removal were sent a questionnaire by facsimile asking for details regarding the patients' present condition and medical history. The questionnaire was returned by facsimile to the anesthesia department for review by an anesthesiologist on the OSS team. If there were no medical contraindications, patients were placed on the operative schedule during a time period dedicated to OSS. The first 2 patients were scheduled to arrive at the same time, and the remaining patients were scheduled at the usual operative intervals. On the eve of their surgery, an OSS perioperative nurse gave directions and preoperative instructions by telephone. The surgeon and the anesthesiologist gave medical clearance on the morning of surgery if surgery was considered appropriate. After surgery, the physician and the nurse made separate follow-up telephone calls on postoperative days 7 to 14 to inquire about the child's recovery and the family's satisfaction with this approach. Average times for OSS and non-OSS procedures were calculated and compared.

Results.—Of 99 pediatric patients (class I or II by American Society of Anesthesiologists criteria) referred for OSS procedures, 3 had co-morbidity that precluded OSS. Two patients refused suggested surgery, 2 did not require surgery, and 12 did not keep their appointments. Eighty patients underwent surgery with no complications. The average total time for OSS compared to non-OSS was significantly less for circumcision (120 vs 142 minutes) and for umbilical hernia repair (139 vs 165 minutes). Times were nonsignificantly different for catheter removal. All patients' families reported complete satisfaction with the OSS process and the anesthetic care.

Conclusion.—OSS may be considered a safe, efficient, and conventional alternative to the traditional pediatric surgical process.

▶ The authors are to be commended, both for their honesty in revealing a 20% no-show rate, and the efficiency that they have induced. But one of the important things that can get overlooked here is that patients have a physical examination by a pediatrician before being referred for an OSS procedure. That is clearly an important step and allows the evaluation of relatively healthy patients on the morning of surgery. The inefficiency of the program before OSS, and the increased efficiency since OSS has started is impressive and dictates that those of us who happen to be in inefficient practices (and don't just read "academic" here) should read this article.

M. F. Roizen, MD

Gene Expression Profile of Aging and Its Retardation by Caloric Restriction
Lee C-K, Klopp RG, Weindruch R, et al (Univ of Wisconsin, Madison; VA Hosp, Madison, Wis)
Science 285:1390-1393, 1999   11–7

Introduction.—Most multicellular organisms experience a progressive and irreversible physiologic decline (aging), the molecular basis of which remains unknown. The gene expression profile of the aging process was examined in the skeletal muscles of mice.

Findings.—Oligonucleotide-based arrays were used to assess the molecular events in skeletal muscle related to aging in mammals. A comparison of the gastrocnemius muscle from adult (5 months) and old (30 months) mice showed that aging is associated with changes in messenger RNA (mRNA) levels, which may reflect alterations in gene expression. Of 6347 genes surveyed in the oligonucleotide microarray, 58 (0.9%) showed a greater than 2-fold rise in expression levels as a function of age. Fifty-five (0.9%) had a greater than 2-fold reduction in expression. These findings are in agreement with an earlier display analysis of gene expression of aging mice. This suggests that the aging process is not likely to be caused by large, widespread alterations in gene expression. Functional classes were assigned to genes revealing the largest alterations in expression. Of 58 genes that intensified in expression with age, 16% were mediators of stress responses. The greatest differential expression between the adult and aged mice (a 3.8-fold induction) was seen for the gene encoding the mitrochondrial sarcomeric creatine kinase, an important target for inactivation induced by reactive oxygen species. Fifty-five genes (0.9%) displayed a higher than 2-fold age-related reduction in expression. Genes involved in energy metabolism were responsible for 13% of these alterations. Aging was also characterized by big decreases (2-fold or more) in the expression of biosynthetic enzymes. Most alterations could be completely or partially prevented by caloric restriction, which is the only intervention known to slow aging in mammals.

Conclusion.—Transcriptional patterns of calorie restriction in mammals indicates that caloric restriction slows the aging process by causing a metabolic shift toward increased protein turnover and diminished macromolecular damage.

▶ Although there are many hypotheses of how and why we age, and at least 8 theories of what the molecular basis of aging is, this study used magnificent combinations of chip technology in gene analysis and interventions to show how we can control how well and how long we live. The authors used 5-month-old mice (about age 13 in human years) and 30-month-old mice (age 80 in human years). Analysis of the gastrocnemius muscle RNA and DNA revealed that aging is associated with alterations in mRNA levels, which may reflect changes in gene expression, mRNA stability, or both. Of the roughly 6400 genes surveyed, 58 displayed a greater than 2-fold increase in expression as a function of age and 55 displayed a greater than 2-fold decrease in expression. What the authors found was that, with calorie restriction, these differences caused by aging were minimized. Of all the studies that I have read this year, this one may be the most important for our future. Does that mean I'll go home and diet? Well, not because of this article, and it's tough to chronically have 15% to 30% fewer calories than you need. I don't think man was made that way. But maybe, just maybe, we'll find out a lot about the molecular basis of aging from studies like this and be able to improve the quality and length of our life without having to go through the pain of near starvation.

M. F. Roizen, MD

12 Clinical Trials

The Utility of Routine Postoperative Chest Radiography in the Post-anesthesia Care Unit
Barak M, Markovits R, Guralnik L, et al (Rambam Med Ctr, Haifa, Israel)
J Clin Anesth 9:351-354, 1997   12-1

Background.—It is common procedure to obtain chest radiographs after anesthesia and surgery to assess the positioning of chest tubes or an endotracheal tube and central venous catheter, or to determine whether there are any immediate surgical or postanesthetic complications. However, these radiographs rarely change the management of the patient, so their clinical significance is uncertain. In addition, the performance of each radiograph requires several persons, including one or more postanesthesia care unit nurses and a radiology technician. The performance of these radiographs has not been demonstrated to be cost-effective and may be painful and inconvenient to the patient. The clinical significance and cost-effectiveness of routine chest radiographs performed in the postanesthesia care unit, and whether additional information and therapeutic actions would result from review of the radiographs by a chest radiologist after the radiograph had been earlier evaluated in the postanesthesia care unit by a staff anesthesiologist were investigated.

Methods.—Researchers evaluated 100 routine postoperative chest radiographs performed in the postanesthesia care unit after thoracotomy (30 patients), thoracoscopy (7 patients), central vein catheterization (75), pulmonary artery catheterization (3), and mechanical ventilation (36). Radiographs were taken from an anteroposterior position, with the patient in either a supine or semirecumbent position. A staff anesthesiologist in the postanesthesia care unit evaluated each radiograph after examining the patient. Preoperative chest radiographs were also available to the anesthesiologist for comparison as warranted. After the physical examination and review of the postoperative radiograph, the anesthesiologist decided on any additional treatment based on the radiographic findings. Each radiograph was then reviewed several days later by a chest radiologist, and the radiologist's interpretation was compared with that of the anesthesiologist. The cost of each radiograph at the study facility was about $34 (US), including the costs for materials, radiology technician, radiologist, maintenance, and insurance.

Results.—Abnormal findings were discovered by the staff anesthesiologist in 8% of the radiographs. These findings directly affected management in 4% of cases. The anesthesiologist's findings were confirmed by the radiologist, who found 4 additional abnormalities. The total cost of the radiographs performed in this study was $3400.

Conclusions.—Routine chest radiographs performed in the postoperative care unit yield little data that affect patient management; in this study, abnormal findings resulted in medical management changes for only 4% of the patients. Decreases in work load and cost may be achieved by performing chest radiographs for specific indications instead of routinely. Staff anesthesiologists can safely and accurately evaluate postoperative chest radiographs.

▶ Like many articles from the *Journal of Clinical Anesthesia*, this article is a superb one for what it tells us about clinical practice. While the data are solid, however, one might have to differ with the conclusion. Is misplacement of a central venous catheter into the right atrium or ventricle, or knowing about a small pneumothorax in another 3% to 4% of patients, worthwhile and worth the expense of getting the routine test? Especially when one can't predict which patients have the problem? I think the risk of complications of central venous catheterization are great enough that, although one has to applaud this study, one has to question the conclusion that specific indications for getting a chest radiograph (such as central venous catheter placement) are inappropriate.

M. F. Roizen, MD

Waste Anaesthetic Gases Induce Sister Chromatid Exchanges in Lymphocytes of Operating Room Personnel

Hoerauf KH, Wiesner G, Schroegendorfer KF, et al (Univ of Vienna; Univ of Regensburg, Germany)
Br J Anaesth 82:764-766, 1999   12–2

Objective.—Chronic exposure to waste anesthetic gases is suspected of causing DNA mutations. The frequency of sister chromatid exchange (SCE) in peripheral lymphocytes was measured in operating room personnel exposed to trace amounts of isoflurane and nitrous oxide.

Methods.—Venous blood samples were obtained from 27 nonsmoking anesthetists (exposed for at least 3 months to 11.8 ppm nitrous oxide and 0.5 ppm isoflurane expressed as an 8-hour time-weighted average) and 27 non–anesthesia-exposed, nonsmoking physicians at the University Hospital of Regensburg, Germany. The frequency of sister chromatid exchange in peripheral lymphocytes was measured after 30 complete second metaphases.

Results.—Sister chromatid exchange rates were significantly higher in exposed personnel than in control subjects (9.0 vs 8.0). The significant remained for exposed (n = 13) and nonexposed (n = 18) men but not for exposed (n = 14) and nonexposed (n = 9) women. Age and sister chromatid exchange rate were not correlated.

Conclusion.—Exposure to low concentrations of waste anesthetic gases can result in increased risk of sister chromatid exchange.

▶ Boy, how they got an 11% change in sister chromatid exchanges, with the variation they found of 15%, to be statistically significant, and how they compared the stress and other components of those physicians' lives and came to the conclusion that it was the exposure rate to waste anesthetic gases that was significantly different that caused the problem—these conclusions elude me, even after I reread this study.

M. F. Roizen, MD

Hemorrhagic Transformation in Acute Ischemic Stroke: The MAST-E Study
Jaillard A, for the Multicenter Acute Stroke Trial–Europe Group (Univ Hosp, Grenoble, France; et al)
Stroke 30:1326-1332, 1999   12–3

Objective.—The risk factors for hemorrhagic transformation (HT) following the administration of streptokinase after stroke has not been well studied. The occurrence and the late predictors of cerebral HT in both streptokinase and placebo group was investigated in a post hoc analysis of data from the double-blind, controlled Multicenter Acute Stroke Trial-Europe (MAST-E) Study.

Methods.—Three hundred ten patients received either 1,500,000 units of streptokinase (n = 156) or placebo (n = 154), administered intravenously, within 6 hours of the onset of stroke symptoms. Mortality and severe disability were assessed at 6 months' follow-up, safety was evaluated at 10 days, and asymptomatic HT and symptomatic HT (SHT) were evaluated by CT within 5 days.

Results.—HT was diagnosed in 96 (61%) patients in the streptokinase group (37 with SHT) and in 61 (31%) patients in the placebo group (4 with SHT). Patients with SHT were significantly more likely to have diabetes mellitus, atrial fibrillation, no heparin use, streptokinase treatment, and early CT signs. According to multivariate analysis, early CT signs, streptokinase treatment, diabetes mellitus, hemispheric sulcus attenuation, and interaction between a decreased level of consciousness and streptokinase treatment predicted HT. In the streptokinase group, diabetes mellitus, hemispheric sulcus attenuation, and decreased level of consciousness predicted HT. The sensitivity, specificity, positive and negative predictive values, and efficiency for SHT were 19%, 99%, 78%, 89%, and 89%, respectively. Rates of HT and SHT in this study were higher than in previously published studies.

Conclusion.—Early CT signs were strong predictors of HT and SHT in stroke patients, particularly in streptokinase-treated patients. Patients with a decreased level of consciousness were at higher risk for SHT.

▶ Many anesthesiologists will be involved in the treatment of acute ischemic stroke now that thrombolytics are becoming more popular and now that the use of the tissue plasminogen activator has almost become routine. This study shows a large transformation from ischemic stroke to hemorrhagic stroke with use of streptokinase in the same range and perhaps even greater than those used with the tissue plasminogen activator. This article is excellent at helping to quantify those risks for us and to understand the situation and the baseline characteristics of the patients with whom we will be dealing.

M. F. Roizen, MD

The Effect of Graded Postischemic Spinal Cord Hypothermia on Neurological Outcome and Histopathology After Transient Spinal Ischemia in Rat
Kakinohana M, Taira Y, Marsala M (Univ of California, San Diego; Univ of the Ryukyus, Okinawa, Japan)
Anesthesiology 90:789-798, 1999   12–4

Objective.—Localized spinal cord cooling may protect against transient spinal cord ischemia. Localized cooling was tested in a rat model to study whether a protective effect is exerted after ischemia begins.

Methods.—Spinal cord ischemia lasting 10 minutes was induced in anesthetized male Sprague-Dawley rats by aortic occlusion. Spinal cord hypothermia was induced using a heat exchanger and cold water. Animals were divided into 3 groups: in group 1, cooling to 34°C, 30°C, or 27°C was initiated immediately and maintained for 2 hours; in group 2, cooling was initiated immediately and maintained for 15 or 120 minutes; and in group 3, cooling was initiated at 5, 60, or 120 minutes after ischemia and maintained for 2 hours. Neurologic function was assessed for 2 to 3 days. Then the animals were killed, and a histopathologic analysis was performed on the spinal cords.

Results.—In group 1, motor scores improved as spinal cord temperature decreased. In group 2, spinal cord cooling for 120 minutes provided better protection than cooling for 15 minutes. In group 3, delayed cooling afforded no protection. Loss of motor and sensory function was correlated with the extent of histopathologic changes in spinal cord. Neuronal damage was correlated with spastic paraplegia. Most neurons had a normal appearance in animals that made a nearly compete recovery.

Conclusion.—Spinal neuron degeneration is dependent on temperature, with the greatest protection afforded at the lowest temperature (27°C) and the longest period of hypothermia (120 minutes).

▶ This may be a classic study. We've known for a long time that cold or hypothermia prior to ischemic events decreases the magnitude of ischemic damage. But now we know that cold induced immediately after the injurious interval of normothermic ischemia also provides significant protection. This investigation was especially well done because the authors studied and found that if you waited to induce cold into the reperfusion interval, cold was less beneficial—in fact, it was not beneficial at all—as opposed to cold induced immediately after the ischemia and maintained for 2 hours of reperfusion. Perhaps the most interesting implication of the study is that if we can find the mechanism of hypothermia-induced protection, maybe we can pharmacologically manipulate it to cause the same effect without having to induce hypothermia.

M. F. Roizen, MD

The Effect of Anesthetic Patient Education on Preoperative Patient Anxiety
Bondy LR, Sims N, Schroeder DR, et al (Mayo Clinic Rochester, Minn)
Reg Anesth Pain Med 24:158-164, 1999   12–5

Introduction.—The increase in outpatient surgery and same-day admission for surgical patients has reduced the preoperative time spent with patients. Previous studies have shown that anesthetic patient education before surgery can decrease anxiety and reduce the need for sedation to relieve anxiety and pain. In an attempt to reduce anxiety, patients in this study received 2 pamphlets and a VHS video describing general and regional anesthesia before admission.

Methods.—Patients included in the study were scheduled for an elective total hip arthroplasty or total knee arthroplasty. The patients were randomly assigned to the usual care, which consisted of a visit with the anesthesiologist/anesthetist in the preoperative waiting area, or to an intervention group in which patients were additionally sent the pamphlets and video. All patients were mailed a preoperative demographic questionnaire and a State Trait Anxiety Inventory. The questionnaires were completed at least 96 hours before admission and again preoperatively on the day of surgery.

Results.—Of the 200 patients assigned to the usual-care group or to the intervention group, 134 completed both sets of questionnaires. The 2 study groups were similar in surgery type distribution, age, sex, and time from baseline assessment to surgery (median, 16 days). All patients had at least 1 prior surgery. In the usual-care group, there was a significant increase in state anxiety score from baseline to immediately prior to surgery. The change in their score was significantly greater than that for the group who received the educational information. Nearly half (47%) of the patients who were sent pamphlets and a video reported that the information influenced their choice of anesthesia technique. Most patients (71% of the usual-care group and 70% of the interventional group), however, reported that anesthesia options had not been discussed with them before meeting with anesthesia personnel just before surgery. Forty-nine percent of those in the usual-care group would have liked to have received additional information.

Conclusion.—Preoperative anxiety can be reduced in patients when they are provided with additional anesthesia information before surgery. Patients in the intervention group recommended both the educational video and pamphlets to other patients undergoing outpatient and same-day admission procedures.

▶ Have Bondy and coworkers played with statistics? Both groups had the same level of state anxiety and trait anxiety before surgery, and no significant difference. It's only when one looks at the change that there's a difference. Yes, it sounds like I'm saying gibberish, and maybe that's what the authors are feeding us. The authors went to look at whether patient education decreased preoperative anxiety, and of course, were able to find it with statistical techniques and statistical processes that my statisticians, at least, say are open to questions.

Despite those statistical ploys, this is an important article to read and understand, because it tells us a lot about what patients think they want preoperatively.

M. F. Roizen, MD

Hygienic Practices of Consultant Anaesthetists: A Survey in the North-West Region of the UK
El Mikatti N, Dillon P, Healy TEJ (South Manchester Univ, England)
Anaesthesia 54:13-18, 1999   12–6

Introduction.—Despite modern hygienic protocols, operations still continue to be complicated by postoperative wound sepsis. The morbidity and surgical failure attributable to sepsis indicate a need to identify factors responsible for sepsis and to reduce the rate of wound infection. There is evidence that precautions recommended by the Association of Anaesthetists of Great Britain and Ireland in 1988 have not been universally implemented by anesthetists in the United Kingdom. Questionnaires were distributed to all consultant anesthetists in the northwest region of the United Kingdom to assess the hygienic precautions taken to reduce the potential for transmission of infectious agents.

Methods.—The questionnaire, distributed to 213 consultant anesthetists, was designed to be completed anonymously. Respondents were asked to characterize the frequency of their use of face mask, gloves, and hand-washing between cases. Other items in the survey addressed aseptic technique for IV cannulation, scrub for spinal/epidural block, and the reuse of syringes.

Results.—Questionnaires were returned by 145 (68%) consultant anesthetists, 35% of whom had the job for more than 15 years and 41% for between 5 and 15 years. Face masks were used frequently by 33.1% of respondents and always by 35.2%. A large proportion of anesthetists (42.1%), however, rarely used gloves. Hand-washing was a frequent practice for 47.5% and always performed by 36.4%. Eighty percent of respondents never reused syringes, 71.8% always scrubbed for spinal/epidural block, and 54.2% always used aseptic technique for IV cannulation. Most have changed their practice since the recognition of the transmission of HIV (74.8%) and hepatitis B and C (69.8%). A high proportion of anesthetists reported administering anesthesia despite suffering from respiratory (94%), gastrointestinal (42.9%), or herpes simplex (32.6%) infections. A third of respondents changed the disposable anesthetic breathing system at the end of each day or after a high-risk case.

Discussion.—Although anesthetists are well informed about occupational hazards and proper hygienic practices, many do not follow recommendations designed to protect patients, other surgical personnel, and themselves. The anesthetists rated their potential for transmitting or contributing to patient infection as a median of 3 on a scale of 0 to 10 (10 = significant).

▶ The performance of consultant anaesthetists in this region of the United Kingdom can only be called poor, as aseptic technique for IV cannulation was rarely used by 39%, reuse of syringes was present in 20% of cases, face masks were reused without cleaning by 65%, gloves were not used by 80%, and even hand-washing was incredibly scarce between cases. Is the poor hygienic processes because the British just don't believe Listeur's theories (he was French, was he not after all?) Or do they believe that infectious disease transmission to physicians doesn't exist? Are they just sloppy due to the time pressures? Or maybe they didn't understand the questions. No, I think that we are creatures of habit, habits developed when we grew up, and the new generation will hopefully do better than these current and older generations of anaesthetists still practicing.

M. F. Roizen, MD

Extent and Practicalities of Filter Use in Anaesthetic Breathing Circuits and Attitudes Towards Their Use: A Postal Survey of UK Hospitals

Atkinson MC, Girgis Y, Broome IJ (Royal Infirmary of Edinburgh, Scotland; Kettering Gen Hosp, England; Falkirk and District Royal Infirmary, Scotland)
Anaesthesia 54:37-41, 1999   12–7

Introduction.—The Blood Borne Viruses Advisory Panel (BBVAP) of the Association of Anesthetists of Great Britain and Ireland recommends placement of an appropriate filter or use of a new breathing system for each patient. The current use of electrostatic and pleated hydrophobic membrane filters in anesthetic breathing systems in the United Kingdom was examined, and anesthetists' opinions of the value of filters were requested.

Methods.—Questionnaires were mailed to 120 randomly chosen hospitals throughout the United Kingdom. Diagrams and manufacturers' product names of the different types of filter were mailed with the questionnaires. Anesthetists were asked to score their reasons for using filters in the order of importance and to indicate whether filter use is worthwhile or cost-effective.

Results.—The response rate was 76%. The survey revealed that 77.2% of anesthetic departments in the United Kingdom use a new filter for every patient. Filters were used by 6.5% of the respondents for selected patients only, 8.7% changed filters only at the end of each day, and 6.5% did not use filters in the anesthetic breathing system. The filter gas sampling port was used for both adult and pediatric patients. Seventy-eight percent of the respondents used either an angle connector or a catheter mount distal to (on the patient's side of) the filter. These devices were either reusable (33.9% of catheter mounts and 55.7% of angle pieces) or disposable (66.3% and 44.3%, respectively) after single use. Nearly 35% reported that perceived extra efficiency of pleated hydrophobic membrane filters outweighed their extra cost and should be used for all patients; 55.4% disagreed and thought that the money could be used elsewhere; 9.8% were not sure. Use of various filters was similar. Electrostatic filters were the most commonly used.

Conclusion.—Most respondents (77.2%) questioned the use of a new filter. Departments with policies of changing filters at the completion of each day or for selected patients only may protect the anesthetic breathing system, the anesthetic machine, or the ventilator from contamination and yet do little to protect the individual patient. One of the primary responsibilities of anesthetists is to protect patients from hazards. It is suggested that anesthetists follow BBVAP recommendations for single-use filters.

▶ The United Kingdom in general has been wonderful at having these surveys that let you know how others practice anesthesia. For those of us locked in a room all day, who don't get to see what other hospitals and other people are doing, this is a wonderful way of looking at it. However, it is clear, from cognitive interviewing, that the questions you ask may not be the questions that are answered. One deficit of many articles, whether in *Anaesthesia* (a British journal), in *Anesthesiology*, or even in *Anesthesia and Analgesia*, is the lack of validation of the surveys at eliciting responses to the questions that you think you are asking. That deficiency is present here as well. As for the subject matter, the transmission of contamination from one patient to another is indeed a worthwhile topic, especially as we go to the anesthesia machine and circuit being used to deliver only oxygen and not the virus-killing volatile agents.

M. F. Roizen, MD

The Effects of Prostaglandin E$_1$ on Intraoperative Temperature Changes and the Incidence of Postoperative Shivering During Deliberate Mild Hypothermia for Neurosurgical Procedures

Kawaguchi M, Inoue S, Sakamoto T, et al (Nara Med Univ, Japan)

Anesth Analg 88:446-451, 1999   12–8

Introduction.—Prostaglandin E$_1$ (PGE$_1$) is a potent vasodilator that affects vascular smooth muscle. Because of its minimal effects on cerebral dynamics, it has been used in patients undergoing neurosurgery. The effects of PGE$_1$ on intraoperative changes in core temperature and the rate of postoperative shivering were examined in 83 patients undergoing neurosurgery and deliberate mild hypothermia.

Methods.—Patients were randomly allocated to 1 of 3 groups: 0.02 µg/kg per minute PGE$_1$ (PG20), 0.05 µg/kg per minute PGE$_1$ (PG50), and no PGE$_1$ (control subjects). Administration of PGE$_1$ was initiated immediately after induction of anesthesia and was continued until completion of anesthesia. Anesthesia was sustained with nitrous oxide in oxygen, sevoflurane, and fentanyl. A water blanket and a convection device were used to cool patients. Tympanic membrane temperature was kept at 34.5°C. Patients were rewarmed during wound closure. Groups were compared for intraoperative changes in tympanic membrane and skin temperatures and for the rate of postoperative shivering.

Results.—Groups were similar in demographic and intraoperative variables and in tympanic temperatures. Skin temperatures at 30 minutes after rewarming were significantly higher in the PG50 group than in the PG20 group. The rate of postoperative shivering was 43%, 13%, and 17%, respectively, for the PG20, PG50, and control groups.

Conclusion.—No benefit was realized from intravenous PGE$_1$ administration during deliberate mild hypothermia in patients undergoing neurosurgery. Since skin temperatures tended to be lower and the incidence of postoperative shivering was notably higher in patients receiving 0.02 µg/kg per minute PGE$_1$, it is recommended that this dose not be used in patients undergoing neurosurgery with deliberate mild hypothermia.

▶ PGE$_1$ may be the best drug for pulmonary hypertension when one is coming off of bypass—as good as nitric oxide, according to recent studies. This study looks at another potential use of PGE$_1$ and the side effects of it. I believe that we need to familiarize ourselves with the use of this potent vasodilator, as it is likely to have much more use in perioperative care.

M. F. Roizen, MD

Neurologic Complications After Placement of Cerebrospinal Fluid Drainage Catheters and Needles in Anesthetized Patients: Implications for Regional Anesthesia

Grady RE, and the Mayo Perioperative Outcomes Group (Mayo Clinic, Rochester, Minn)

Anesth Analg 88:388-392, 1999   12–9

Introduction.—Neurosurgical injury produced by needle insertion into the central neuroaxis is frequently forecast by pain, paresthesias, or movement. These warning signs can be masked by general anesthesia, making needle insertion in anesthetized patients controversial. The neurologic consequences of insertion of lumbar subarachnoid drains were retrospectively examined in anesthetized patients who underwent neurosurgery to determine the types and incidence of neurologic complications attributable to spinal drainage.

Methods.—The medical records of 530 consecutive patients who had undergone transsphenoidal surgical procedures performed with lumbar CSF drainage were reviewed. The postoperative records were examined for information regarding evidence of new neurologic changes characterized by sensory or motor disturbances in the buttocks, perineum, groin, pelvic region, or lower extremities. The presence of postdural puncture headaches and need for an epidural blood patch were also noted. One-year follow-up visits were reviewed for possible neurologic dysfunction.

Results.—Every patient was anesthetized during CSF drain placement. A 19-gauge malleable needle was used in 473 patients (89%). Twenty- or 16-gauge subarachnoid catheters, respectively, were placed with 18- or 14-gauge epidural needles in 17 (3%) of the patients. The type of drain could not be determined in 40 patients (8%). No new neurologic deficits attributable to spinal drain insertion were observed in the immediate postoperative period or in the first year after surgery. Thirteen patients (2.5%) experienced postdural puncture headaches, and 7 (1.3%) needed an epidural blood patch.

Conclusion.—The low incidence (0%) of neurologic injury from spinal drain insertion in anesthetized patients in this cohort is in agreement with the medical literature with respect to both CSF drain insertion and spinal anesthesia.

▶ There are several things to emphasize in this study by the Mayo Perioperative Outcomes Group. First, the lower incidence of complications is remarkable and is to be applauded, but even at the Mayo Clinic the notes aren't perfectly kept, and in 8% of the patients the type of drain wasn't noted in a chart or noted in a way that someone could read it. The second thing to comment on is the outstanding follow-up of the patients. We in anesthesia are very lucky that the Mayo Clinic has such an outstanding department and research process from which the rest of us can benefit substantially.

M. F. Roizen, MD

No Risk of Metal Toxicity in Combined Spinal-Epidural Anesthesia
Holst D, Möllmann M, Schymroszcyk B, et al (Ernst Moritz-Arndt-Univ, Greifswald, Germany; St Franziskus, Münster, Germany; Westfalian Wilhelm's Univ, Münster, Germany)
Anesth Analg 88:393-397, 1999   12–10

Introduction.—Combined spinal-epidural (CSE) anesthesia may be accomplished reliably and quickly by the needle-through-needle technique. It has been suggested that tiny metal particles that may pass into the epidural or spinal compartments are abraded from the inner edge of the epidural needle by the spinal needle during this procedure. The needle-through-needle technique was simulated with the use of an in vitro model to determine whether (1) metal particles can be abraded from both types of needle and (2) the catheter can be inadvertently passed intrathecally through the hole in the dura created by the spinal needle.

Methods.—The needle-through-needle technique was simulated with the use of a test tube flushed free of metal, closed with an inert plastic foil, and then perforated with an 18-gauge Tuohy needle. The CSE procedure was simulated through the lumen of the Tuohy needle with a 27- or 29-gauge Quincke spinal needle. The presence of abraded metal particles was assessed by means of atomic absorption spectrography (AAS). Needles were also examined under an electron microscope.

Results.—Metal particles were not observed by means of AAS after performance of the needle-through-needle technique or with the electron microscope. With intentional rough handling and caudal orientation of the spinal needle tip, minimal scratches were viewed with the electron microscope; no metal particles were detected by AAS.

The possible passage of the epidural catheter anesthetic through the dural puncture hole into the cerebrospinal fluid compartment was examined endoscopically in a cadaver model. Endoscopy did not reveal passage of dyed epidural local anesthesia or penetration of the epidural catheter into the cerebrospinal fluid compartment.

Conclusion.—The needle-through-needle procedure is acceptable for CSE anesthesia. When an in vitro model was used, it did not seem likely that patients could be endangered by an unintentional intrathecal misplacement of the epidural catheter with small 27- or 29-gauge needles.

▶ This is a very innovative article that makes one feel somewhat safe. The safety of the combined needle-through-needle technique for spinal epidural anesthesia was investigated for potential fraying of the needles rubbing one against the other. No such metal particle break-down was seen by the most sensitive technique known to man. This publication is another example of how innovative research can be, and the novice, as well as the experienced investigator, will do well to read this article to examine how innovative and important some seemingly simple investigations can be.

M. F. Roizen, MD

Risk Factors for Post-carotid Endarterectomy Hematoma Formation

Self DD, Bryson GL, Sullivan PJ (Ottawa Hosp, Ont)
Can J Anesth 46:635-640, 1999   12–11

Introduction.—Carotid endarterectomy (CEA) is considered the gold-standard treatment for patients with severe symptomatic or asymptomatic carotid stenosis. One of the surgical risks of CEA is airway compromise secondary to post-CEA hematoma formation. Reports of incidence rates range from 1% to 3% to as high as 26%. Reduction in airway cross-sectional area and volume may be observed radiographically after CEA. Identification of risk factors may help prevent and manage these events. A retrospective review of all patients who underwent CEA was performed to identify risk factors for post-CEA hematoma formation and to determine the incidence of this complication at the participating institution.

Methods.—Medical records of all patients who underwent CEA at one hospital between Jan 1, 1996, and Dec 31, 1997, were reviewed for information regarding demographics, surgeon, anesthesiologist, anesthetic technique, and general outcome data. All patients with post-CEA wound hematoma were matched for age and sex from within the cohort. These matched pairs were examined for 31 potential risk factors, including demographic details, coexisting medical conditions, preoperative medications, intraoperative management, and postoperative parameters.

Results.—From the 249 charts reviewed, 29 patients (12%) with post-CEA hematoma were identified. Six of 31 potential risk factors for hematoma formation were identified on univariate analysis: general anesthesia, carotid shunt placement, intraoperative hypotension, nonreversal of heparin, neurosurgery service, and preoperative use of aspirin. After logistic regression, only nonreversal of heparin, intraoperative hypotension, and carotid shunt placement remained as multivariate predictors of post-CEA hematoma formation. Patients in the hematoma group spent more time in critical care settings ($P < .01$) and had a higher perioperative mortality rate ($P = .04$).

Conclusion.—Post-CEA hematoma formation was correlated with increased morbidity and mortality. The identified risk factors for post-CEA hematoma formation may prompt re-examination of current anesthetic and surgical practice patterns, especially the relationships between heparin reversal versus nonreversal and post-CEA hematoma formation and regional versus general anesthesia for CEA.

▶ The surprising thing in this study is that preoperative use of aspirin and postoperative hypertension were not determinants of hematoma formation. But perhaps the most surprising thing is that, in this study of 278 patients, post-CEA hematoma severe enough to call for anesthesia observation or intervention occurred in 12% of the cases. There were cases in which airway compromise was detected by nurses in the recovery room. That figure seems incredibly large, but maybe I just have had the privilege of working with too many outstanding surgeons. I'll always believe that the main risk factor for post-CEA hematoma formation is lack of silk.

M. F. Roizen, MD

Perioperative Strokes After 1001 Consecutive Carotid Endarterectomy Procedures Without an Electroencephalogram: Incidence, Mechanism, and Recovery
Hamdan AD, Pomposelli FB Jr, Gibbons GW, et al (Harvard Med School, Boston)
Arch Surg 134:412-415, 1999   12–12

Introduction.—The use of shunting during carotid endarterectomy (CEA) may prevent postoperative stroke. Cerebral monitoring is usually performed with an electroencephalogram (EEG) or with regional anesthesia in an awake patient. Some patients may experience significant cerebral hypoperfusion, measured by EEG changes, on carotid clamping. The EEG monitoring necessitates additional equipment and expertise and generates a cost. Another method that eliminates the need for cerebral monitoring is general anesthesia with routine shunting. A computerized vascular registry established in 1990 was used to identify patients who underwent CEA without the use of EEG.

Methods.—The 7-year retrospective review used data from 1001 patients who underwent CEA (without EEG monitoring) under general anesthesia with routine shunting. Information was gathered regarding overall stroke and mortality rates and causes and consequences of postoperative strokes.

Results.—Fourteen patients had nonfatal strokes (1.4%) and 2 died within 30 postoperative days, for a combined stroke and death rate of 1.6%. Eleven patients (1.9%) and 3 patients (0.7%), respectively, who experienced postoperative stroke had symptomatic and asymptomatic stenosis. Eleven of the 14 patients (79%) underwent general endotracheal anesthesia with shunting, and the remainder underwent regional anesthesia. Causes of stroke varied in 9 patients who underwent re-exploration for ipsilateral postoperative neurologic deficits: 5 internal carotid artery thromboses or the presence of fresh clot without an intimal flap, 2 distal intimal flaps with clot flow, 1 distal kink with obstruction of flow, and 1 embolus or hypoperfusion. The remaining 5 patients did not undergo re-exploration. Available information indicated that 1 patient had heparin-induced thrombocytopenia and complete thrombosis of the internal carotid artery after a subsequent peripheral bypass graft 14 days after CEA, 1 patient had intracerebral bleeding on postoperative day 8, and the 3 remaining patients with radiographically patent internal carotid arteries had emboli or hypoperfusion. Thus, of 14 postoperative strokes, 9 (64.3%) may have been caused by technical error. Seven patients (50%) experienced mild deficits and 7 required inpatient rehabilitation. Twelve patients (86%) returned home without needing additional assistance.

Conclusion.—Most postoperative strokes in this cohort were caused by technical errors. This result suggests that more effort should be directed toward performing precise endarterectomy and less toward the method of cerebral monitoring. When strokes occur, most patients can make a reasonable recovery and return to a level of functioning sufficient for living at home.

▶ It's always interesting to me that if people try to get 1000 patients, they never make it exactly and always have 1 extra. For instance, Hurtzer, Beven, Young et al,[1] in their study, "Coronary Artery Disease in Vascular Patients: A Classification of 1000 Coronary Angiograms and Results of Surgical Management," had 1001, not 1000—patients. This article reports another study that goes just a little too far, in that they got 1001 consecutive patients. This group of surgeons might be outstanding, as they have a very low complication rate, or it may be that they didn't routinely seek complications and the complications weren't included in the record. Nevertheless, the death rate, which should be reliably detected, was very low—2 deaths in 1001 patients. But were these just the deaths attributed to stroke? What about other complications and the deaths associated with myocardial infarction? How were complications sought? How were they recorded? How routinely were signs of physchomotor dysfunction sought? None of these questions are answered by the review. Unfortunately, like quite a few good articles, this one leaves us with more questions than answers.

M. F. Roizen, MD

Reference

1. Hurtzer NR, Beven EG, Young JR, et al: Coronary artery disease in vascular patients: A classification of 1,000 coronary angiograms and results of surgical management. *Ann Surg* 199:223-233, 1984.

Perioperative ST-Segment Depression and Troponin T Release: Identification of Patients With Highest Risk for Myocardial Damage
Rapp H-J, Rabethge S, Luiz T, et al (Univ of Heidelberg, Germany)
Acta Anaesthesiol Scand 43:124-129, 1999   12–13

Introduction.—Patients undergoing major vascular surgery are at high risk of perioperative complications, particularly myocardial infarction. Compared with the various techniques used in ST segment analysis, cardiospecific troponins have better sensitivity and specificity in identifying both reversible myocardial damage and irreversible infarction. Troponin T may be useful in determining ischemic myocardial damage in the perioperative period. The role of cardiac troponin T was examined in patients undergoing major vascular surgery in whom ST segment analysis was performed in the perioperative setting.

Methods.—Twenty patients scheduled for elective aortic resection were assessed by Holter ECG (including ST segment analysis) from the evening before surgery until the third postoperative day. During this time, serum levels of cardiac troponin T were obtained at 8 time points.

Results.—Of 20 patients evaluated, 8 (40%) had significant ST depression without any clinical symptoms. The median number of episodes was 9 (range, 2-24). Three patients with repetitive episodes of ST depression had elevated troponin T levels. The remaining patients had no troponin T release or cardiac events. No relationship was observed between troponin T release and the magnitude of ST depression or the number of episodes of ST depression.

Conclusion.—Repeated and long-lasting episodes of ST segment depression may cause myocardial damage, as demonstrated by the release of troponin T. There was a stronger relationship between duration of ischemia and myocardial cell damage than with the number of episodes or maximal ST depression. The ability to identify myocardial damage by repetitive troponin T determination should lead to an earlier and more aggressive therapeutic approach.

▶ The strength of this study is that troponin T release was measured in all patients. Thus, in fact, we find that ST segment depression has 100% negative predictive value; ie, its specificity is 100%, whereas its sensitivity is only around 40%. Nevertheless, the change in ST segments might be used as a screen to designate which patients to select for troponin T studies. Which is more expensive? Which is easier to get? Which is easier to read? And did these patients have other clinical signs of myocardial dysfunction perioperatively? That is, did they have problems clinically, and could clinical signs be as good as ECG signs at identifying these patients? This might prove true. Perhaps Mary Charlson's old formula of the way to follow such patients, that is, with an ECG on day 1 and follow-up, may still be the best approach.

M. F. Roizen, MD

▶ This was a very small study, and it would be interesting to perform a larger epidemiologic/population study in vascular surgical patients. This study suggests that the postoperative period is important, and that prolonged periods of ST depression may not be well tolerated and require measurement of cardiac troponin T levels.

M. Wood, MD

Craniotomy Procedures Are Associated With Less Analgesic Requirements Than Other Surgical Procedures
Dunbar PJ, Visco E, Lam AM (Univ of Washington, Seattle)
Anesth Analg 88:335-340, 1999   12–14

Introduction.—The common belief that patients who undergo neurosurgical procedures require less analgesia has recently been challenged. The anesthesia and postanesthesia care unit (PACU) records for all patients who underwent major intracranial and selected extracranial procedures during 1995 were reviewed and compared.

Methods.—Patients were grouped according to the procedure performed: group E, open fixation of mandible or maxilla; group I, clipping of aneurysms or excision of tumors; or group L, lumbar laminectomy. Medical records were reviewed for data regarding weight, operative time, time in the PACU, intraoperative and postoperative opioid use, PACU pain scores, and level of consciousness.

Results.—The 78 patients in group I received less fentanyl in the operating room than the 134 patients in group E and the 21 patients in group L. They also received less morphine in the PACU, reported lower pain scores, and spent less time in the PACU than patients in group E and group L. These findings remained similar when only patients with Glasgow Coma Scale scores of 14 or higher were used in a subset analysis.

Conclusion.—Patients who underwent intracranial procedures had less pain and used fewer opioids in the PACU than patients who underwent facial reconstruction or lumbar laminectomy. There was a small subset of patients, several of whom underwent frontal craniotomies, who needed aggressive treatment of postoperative pain.

▶ This article seemed to be a well-done epidemiologic study. It confirmed one of the biases that I have been taught and have adopted, namely, that craniotomy procedures require less pain relief than do noncraniotomy procedures. The implication is clear that, with this knowledge, we should be able to have less postoperative nausea, vomiting, and sluggishness, but the implication is also important from another one of the points the authors make that patients with frontal craniotomies may need more aggressive pain management than those with other types of craniotomy. The authors are to be applauded for doing this study so well.

M. F. Roizen, MD

Simultaneous Aortic Aneurysm Repair and Colonic Surgery
Oshodi TO, Abraham JS, Kelly JF (Royal Lancaster Infirmary, England)
Br J Surg 86:217-218, 1999   12–15

Introduction.—Although the surgical treatment of abdominal aortic aneurysms larger than 5 cm in diameter is accepted, there is a lack of consensus on the management of serious concomitant colonic lesions. In most reported cases, surgeons have chosen to treat the majority of patients sequentially. Yet perioperative morbidity and mortality is increased when patients are managed in 2 stages. The 9 patients reported in this study underwent a combined procedure.

Methods.—Since 1979, patients at the study institution who had a significant aortic aneurysm and an intra-abdominal lesion requiring surgery had the 2 procedures performed simultaneously. Fifty-three patients underwent combined aortic and gastrointestinal procedures between 1979 and 1998, and 9 of these patients had colonic pathology. In 8 of these 9 cases, the aortic aneurysm was performed first. All patients received broad-spectrum antibiotic prophylaxis for 5 days.

Results.—The mean duration of the combined procedure was 150 minutes, and the median postoperative stay was 10 days. Two patients, both with infarcted colon, died in the hospital. Superficial wound infection developed in 2 patients and an incisional hernia developed in 2. No patient had evidence of graft infection. Two of the patients were alive at 3 and 5 years, respectively, after surgery, and the remaining 5 patients died at periods ranging from 3 to 10 years after surgery. Myocardial infarction was the most common cause of late death.

Discussion.—Many surgeons faced with a coexisting aortic aneurysm 5 cm or more in diameter and serious colonic pathology advise a staged treatment to minimize the potential risk of graft infection. In the authors' experience, however, simultaneous gastrointestinal and aortic surgery can be performed without an obvious increase in the risk of graft infection. The risk of delayed treatment of either lesion, such as aneurysm rupture immediately after colonic resection alone, may outweigh the potential risks of the combined procedure.

▶ This report of combined aortic and colonic procedures is noteworthy in that the surgeons report an almost 25% perioperative mortality among patients who had their abdomens prepared. One wonders what might have happened if they had not had bowel preps and cleansing procedures beforehand. The compelling combination of this procedure is still not clear to me. What should happen with the patient who presents for abdominally aortic aneurysm repair and has a serious colonic lesion? Well, we'll leave that for board exams, as we don't think that there is a definitive answer at this time.

M. F. Roizen, MD

13 Technology Assessment

The Cuffed Oropharyngeal Airway vs the Laryngeal Mask Airway: A Randomised Cross-Over Study of Oropharyngeal Leak Pressure and Fibreoptic View in Paralysed Patients
Brimacombe J, Keller C (Univ of Queensland, Cairns, Australia; Leopold-Franzens Univ, Innsbruck, Austria)
Anaesthesia 54:683-702, 1999   13–1

Background.—The cuffed oropharyngeal airway (COPA) was designed to form a seal in the proximal laryngopharynx, providing a clear airway by elevating the epiglottis away from the posterior pharyngeal wall by means of a pointed anterior cuff. By contrast, the current "gold standard," the laryngeal mask airway (LMA), is designed to form a seal around the periglottic tissues. Previous studies comparing the COPA and LMA have shown that the LMA is more effective for apneic patients as well as those nonparalyzed patients who can breathe spontaneously. However, to date there have been no studies with paralyzed patients and no data has been gathered regarding the fiberoptic view. The aims of this study were to test the hypothesis that there is a difference in both the fiberoptic view and the oropharyngeal leak pressure between the COPA and LMA in paralyzed patients, and to determine whether inflation of the cuff on the COPA produces elevation of the epiglottis.

Methods.—The study group comprised 10 men and 10 women, all consecutive patients who were undergoing minor peripheral surgery. The mean age of the group was 37 and 38 years for the men and women, respectively. The mean height and weight for the men were 177 cm and 76 kg, 162 cm and 70 kg for the women. Patients who were at risk for aspiration or were for some other reason unsuitable for the LMA or COPA were not included in the study. Standard anesthesia protocol and routine monitoring were used. Insertion of the COPA and LMA was performed in random order, with a size 10 COPA or size 4 LMA used for the women and a size 11 COPA or size 5 LMA used for the men. For the LMA, measurements were made with the head and neck in the neutral position, using a pillow; COPA measurements were made with the head flexed and the neck extended, using a pillow and a chin lift. The oropharyngeal leak volume was then assessed at zero volume and again for every 10 mL up to maximums for the COPA and LMA. Assessment of the fiberoptic view of the epiglottis and vocal cords were done at 0.5 cm within the distal end of the device. Any position change of the epiglottis in relation to the posterior pharyngeal wall as the cuff was inflated was noted as unchanged, elevated, or depressed. Statistical comparison of the data was done at overall, minimum, and maximum oropharyngeal leak pressure.

Results.—Oropharyngeal leak pressure and fiberoptic scores were significantly higher for the LMA than for the COPA in both men and women. The vocal cords were visible in 96% of the LMA observations, versus 39% of the COPA observations. With the COPA, the epiglottis was not elevated away from the posterior pharyngeal wall.

Conclusions.—The LMA is more effective in sealing and provides a better fiberoptic view of the glottic inlet than the COPA in paralyzed patients.

▶ This is a wonderful study that gives credence to the reason that many use the LMA as a bridge to fiberoptic intubation. I always like studies that support what we do, so I'm clearly biased. But this is an excellent study of a random allocation of a group of 20 patients.

M. F. Roizen, MD

Does the Murphy Eye Reduce the Reliability of Chest Auscultation in Detecting Endobronchial Intubation?

Sugiyama K, Yokoyama K, Satoh K, et al (Kagoshima Univ, Japan)
Anesth Analg 88:1380-1383, 1999   13–2

Background.—Serious complications can result from inadvertent endobronchial placement of an endotracheal tube (ETT). Chest auscultation in particular has been routinely used in both the operating room and emergency department to determine the proper positioning of an ETT. However, studies have demonstrated the poor diagnostic value of auscultation for endobronchial intubation, possibly relating to the structure of the tip of the ETT. The Murphy tube is an ETT with a beveled tip and a hole (commonly called the eye) opposite the bevel. The Murphy tube and its possible relation to the diagnostic unreliability of auscultation in detecting endobronchial intubation were investigated.

Methods.—The study group included 20 Japanese women scheduled for elective oral and maxillofacial surgery under general anesthesia. Patients with pulmonary diseases evidenced by chest radiographs were excluded from participation in the study. Half of the study group was intubated with a Magill tube (with a simple beveled tip) and the other half with a Murphy tube, both assigned in a random manner. A fiberoptic bronchoscope was inserted through the ETT after inflation of the cuff. A mark was made on the ETT after confirmation with the fiberoptic bronchoscope that the tip of the tube had reached the carina of the trachea. The fiberoptic bronchoscope was then removed. The ETT was withdrawn several centimeters and then advanced while bilateral breath sounds were auscultated with a stethoscope and manual compression of the reservoir bag. Second and third marks were made on the ETT when the quality of the breath sounds changed and then disappeared completely. The distances from the carina to the tube tip were then calculated at the change and disappearance of breath sounds. Data were analyzed using paired and unpaired Student's *t*-tests.

Results.—There was not a difference between the two groups in the distance the tube tip was inserted before auscultatory changes in breath sounds. With the Magill tube, unilateral change in auscultated breath sounds was not observed until the tip of the ETT was advanced beyond the carina and 1.5 ± 0.4 cm into the right mainstem bronchus. With the Murphy tube, unilateral change in auscultation was not observed until the tube tip was advanced beyond the carina and 2.0 ± 0.4 cm into the right mainstem bronchus. When the tip was advanced to 3.2 ± 0.3 cm from the carina, the breath sounds disappeared completely. The distal end of the cuff at that time was 2.5 cm from the tip of the ETT and 0.7 cm below the carina, suggesting that the inflated cuff interrupted the gas supply to the opposite bronchus and precluded ventilation of the left lung.

Conclusions.—The results suggest that the Murphy eye plays a significant part in disappearance of breath sounds on auscultation. Breath sounds could be heard until the Murphy tube was inserted more deeply than the Magill tube into the right mainstem bronchus. Thus, the eye of the Murphy tube reduces the reliability of auscultation as a means of detecting endobronchial intubation.

▶ This is an important article, as it says that the Murphy eye can help mislead you in auscultation—but is the Murphy eye really misleading you, or are you getting stuck going the other way and, thus, the misleading concept isn't misleading you about ventilation, but is telling you about ventilation that is actually occurring? While that's probably a confusing enough sentence, I guess the basic message is this: how accurate is auscultation of the lungs anyway? And since it isn't really very accurate, does a Murphy eye make it less accurate?

M. F. Roizen, MD

An Assessment of the Luminance and Light Field Characteristics of Direct Laryngoscopes

Crosby E, Cleland M (Univ of Ottawa, Ontario)
Can J Anesth 46:792-796, 1999   13–3

Background.—Light field characteristics and luminance, as well as the effect of residual battery potential and luminance on light color temperature in fiber-light and bulb-light laryngoscopes at one institution were studied. Direct laryngoscopy requires adequate illumination of the airway tissues by the laryngoscope. The illumination is determined in part by the intensity and color of the light that is cast and the area (light field) over which the light is cast. The color of the light and its intensity, as well as the nature and dimensions of the light field, are influenced by the type of bulb, the potential of the power source, and, in fiberoptic systems, the characteristics of the fiber bundle. In the study of light measurement, the term *luminance* is used to describe the amount of light emitted or re-emitted per unit area of a surface in a given direction. In laryngoscopy, luminance determines the examiner's perception of the brightness of the field. The color of the light can influence both the illumination and perceived sharpness of an image. A hotter light that has a higher temperature and is less red is likely more desirable because less of the light will be absorbed by the tissues under view, affording a better appreciation of the laryngeal anatomy. However, to date there has been no determination of the optimal color for laryngoscopy.

Methods.—Used Macintosh #3 and #4 fiber-light and bulb-light laryngoscopes were studied and compared with respect to luminance and bright-field characteristics. After the residual battery potentials in the laryngoscope handles were determined, a power supply was used to eliminate the effect of variable battery potentials. New bulbs were installed in the handles of the fiber-light laryngoscopes before testing, but the bulbs in the bulb-light laryngoscopes were not replaced. Measurements were made using a Pentax brand digital spotmeter for luminance and a Minolta brand Color III color temperature meter for light color under controlled, constant conditions. For light color, measurements were made at 0.1 V increments, and the power source potential was increased from 2 to 3 V. A millimeter-increment ruler mounted on the base of the test fixture was used for the light field measurements.

Results.—The #4 fiber-light laryngoscope produced significantly higher luminance values than the #3 fiber-light scope at both 2.5 and 2.8 V. Luminance values increased with increases in potential. The bulb-light laryngoscope produced higher luminance values than those produced by fiber-light laryngoscopes in all comparisons. Light temperature decreased with decreasing potential and luminance values. No differences in light field dimensions were observed in any comparisons.

Conclusions.—The minimum luminance for laryngoscopy of 100 cd/m^2 was met with much greater frequency by the bulb-light laryngoscopes in this study than by the fiber-light laryngoscopes. The minimum luminance standard was not met by 15% of the bulb-light laryngoscopes, compared with 92% of the fiber-light laryngoscopes that did not meet the criterion for minimum luminance.

▶ This is a fascinating article, especially useful because it reviews how the minimum required luminance for laryngoscopy was determined by Skilton and colleagues in 1996.[1] These authors then used that gold standard and found that 15% of the bulb-light laryngoscopes did not meet the standard for minimum required luminance for laryngoscopy. Perhaps the technique that is proposed here can be used to assess our bulb strength, or perhaps just opening the laryngoscope to see whether it works and is bright is good enough; no clinician-judged test was evaluated—that would be a useful addition to this study.

M. F. Roizen, MD

Reference

1. Skilton RWH, Parry D, Arthurs GJ, et al: A study of the brightness of laryngoscope light. *Anaesthesia* 51:667-672, 1996.

Prediction of Movement at Laryngeal Mask Airway Insertion: Comparison of Auditory Evoked Potential Index, Bispectral Index, Spectral Edge Frequency and Median Frequency

Doi M, Gajraj RJ, Mantzaridis H, et al (HCI International Med Centre, Clydebank, Scotland; Law Hosp, Carluke, Scotland; Royal Infirmary, Glasgow, Scotland)

Br J Anaesth 82:203-207, 1999

13–4

Introduction.—A monitor of depth of anesthesia must predict movement caused by stimuli. No published study has assessed how well the auditory evoked potential (AEP) index can predict movement to any noxious stimuli or the ability of the bispectral index (BIS), median frequency (MF), or 95% spectral edge frequency (SEF) to predict movement on insertion of the laryngeal mask airway (LMA). A simultaneous recording of the 4 variables (AEP index, BIS, SEF, and MF) in patients undergoing general anesthesia was designed to assess the ability of these variables to predict movement in response to insertion of the LMA.

Methods.—Forty-six patients with a mean age of 51 years (range, 16-86 years) took part in the study. Anesthesia was induced in all cases with target-controlled infusions of propofol and alfentanil. The LMA was inserted without the assistance of a laryngoscope or neuromuscular blocker after loss of eyelash reflex and the establishment of adequate jaw relaxation. "Movers" were patients who showed any visible spontaneous muscle movement within 1 minute of LMA insertion. Each of the 4 variables was recorded simultaneously and averaged values for 15 seconds were obtained 5 times, from before the induction of anesthesia to 30 seconds before surgical incision. Prediction probability was used to evaluate the efficacy of each variable to predict movement in response to insertion of the LMA. A prediction probability value of 1 means that the values of the indicator always correctly predict movement in response to LMA insertion.

Results.—Only the AEP index, with a prediction probability of 0.872, discriminated between the 14 movers and the 32 nonmovers. The prediction probabilities of BIS, SEF, and MF were 0.547, 0.549, and 0.587, respectively. Thus prediction probability values for BIS, 95% SEF, and MF were not significantly different from 0.5 (no better than a 50% chance of a correct prediction).

Conclusion.—Only the AEP index discriminated between movers and nonmovers in response to insertion of the LMA. The reason may be that the AEP reflects subcortical as well as cortical brain activities. Variables that did not discriminate were BIS, 95% SEF, MF, heart rate, systolic arterial pressure, and predicted blood propofol concentration.

▶ No one said that sleep and arousal to pain were the same things, although with this anesthetic combination, one would think they would be. Thus, it is surprising to me that with this technique, neither the BIS, nor any of the other transformations of the EEG, were able to predict depths of anesthesia with the propofol-alfentanil infusion technique. On the other hand, it's impressive that the AEP did predict it. And it looks like the auditory AEP is as easy to obtain by this technique as is the BIS reading. Those of us interested in depth of anesthesia—and what anesthesiologist isn't—are encouraged to read this carefully done and important study.

M. F. Roizen, MD

The Effect of Steam Sterilisation at 134°C on Light Intensity Provided by Fibrelight Macintosh Laryngoscopes
Bucx MJL, Veldman DJ, Beenhakker MM, et al (Univ of Amsterdam)
Anaesthesia 54:875-878, 1999   13–5

Introduction.—Decontamination of laryngoscopes begins with rigorous mechanical cleaning. There is controversy regarding whether this cleanup should be followed by high-level disinfection or sterilization. One of the possible disadvantages of steam sterilization at 134°C is that it may be detrimental to fiberlight blades. There are no known data regarding the effects of steam sterilization on fiberlight laryngoscope blades. The effect of automated machine washing and subsequent steam sterilization at 134°C was examined in various fiberoptic laryngoscope blades and handles, with a focus on the effect on light intensity provided by the blades.

Methods.—New reusable fiberoptic Macintosh size 3 laryngoscopes from Heine, Medicon, Penlon, Riester, and Upsher were evaluated. All blades were examined with 2.5 V bulbs provided by the manufacturer. Light intensity was measured with a light meter, and measurements were expressed in lux. Two methods were used to determine light intensity. For the first method, the blade was introduced into a tubular laryngoscope holder and the light was shined on the sensor positioned at the end of the tube. For the second method, the tip of each laryngoscope blade was positioned against the edge of the sensor. Measurements were not taken in a photographer's darkroom, so ambient light had an effect on the measurements. Measurements were taken before cleaning and sterilization procedures and after each series of 25 until a total of 200 cycles had been completed. A new 1.5 V battery was installed for each series of measurements.

Results.—For the laryngoscope holder, the values before cleaning and sterilization cycles began ranged from 400 to 1400 lux. After 200 cycles, these values were 0 light emission to 950 lux. With the manual method, these values before cleaning and sterilization were 1200 to 6000 lux. After 200 cycles, the range was 0 light emission to 5200 lux. The decrease in light intensity after 200 cycles, compared with the intensity before cleaning and sterilization, ranged from 37% to 100% (method 1) and from 13% to 100% (method 2).

Conclusion.—There were significant differences between fiberlight blades in terms of the detrimental effects of steam sterilization at 134°C on light intensity. The Riester and Medicon blades had the most favorable results and offered excellent light intensity after 200 cycles of cleaning and sterilization. The Penlon blade did not transmit any light after 100 cycles. The lifetime of a fiberblade depends on the number of cleaning and sterilization cycles and on the way it is used by the handler.

▶ It appears that the old method of soaking the laryngoscope in a sterilizing solution may be the best, at least for light intensity. One wonders whether, if infection rates are so great, one should have steam sterilization, or whether we are causing more problems with the steam sterilization. One also wonders whether the allergic reactions to the uncleaned sterilization materials in the cold sterilization process cause more problems than the infection rate. I wish we had better data, and the study paradigm used by the authors is a good start.

M. F. Roizen, MD

Swift Conversion From Laryngoscopic to Fiberoptic Intubation With a New, Handy Fiberoptic Stylet
Saruki N, Saito S, Sato J, et al (Gunma Cancer Ctr, Ota, Japan; Gunma Univ, Maebashi, Japan)
Anesth Analg 89:526-528, 1999   13–6

Introduction.—It is difficult to predict a difficult airway during preoperative assessment. Fiberoptic endotracheal intubation is a reliable approach for management of a difficult airway; yet it is not always available for immediate use. Handy fiberoptic stylets have a flexible shaft that can accommodate a bundle of fiberoptics. A physician acting alone can easily operate this device. A tracheal tube may be advanced through the vocal cords in airways that are easy to intubate. Using a direct laryngoscopic approach, the physician can identify a difficult airway by looking through the eyepiece on top of the stylet. It takes only a few seconds to change the approach and use the fiberoptic approach. The fiberoptic stylet was examined for its usefulness in the clinical setting.

Methods.—A custom model fiberoptic stylet was tailor made. The stylet was 482 mm long, and the flexible shaft was 395 mm long and 5.4 mm in diameter. This device was used in 18 patients with airways graded Cormack's I or II and 16 patients with airways graded III or IV. After induction of anesthesia, a Macintosh direct laryngoscope was inserted in the mouth and visualization of the vocal cords was attempted by a standard procedure. The final view taken by the direct laryngoscope was classified according to Cormack's criteria, and tracheal intubation was attempted and completed according to standard procedure when there was direct visualization. When direct visualization was not possible, the tracheal tube set on the fiberoptic stylet was inserted beyond the tongue along the blade of the tracheal tube. Viewing of the vocal cords was attempted again through the eyepiece. Location of the vocal cords was ascertained by moving the top of the tracheal tube. When the vocal cords were aligned with the center of the field of view, the tube was passed through the vocal cords until the tracheal cartilage rings were seen through the eyepiece. Patients with grade III or IV airways were subdivided further into grades IIIa, IIIb, and IVa, based on the first view through the fiberoptic stylet. Patients with grade IIIb airways and no distance between the epiglottis and the posterior wall of the pharynx required movement and rotation of the upper stylet and further lifting of the jaw with the laryngoscope to visualize the vocal cords.

Results.—Mean intubation time with a fiberoptic stylet was 28 seconds for patients with grade I and II airways and 30 seconds for patients with grade IIIa airways. Airway insertion time ranged from 44 to 64 seconds for the 3 patients with grade IIIb airways and was 19 seconds for the 1 patient with a grade IVa airway.

Conclusion.—The mean intubation time ranged between 20 and 30 seconds (in patients with grade I, II, and III disease) with a fiberoptic stylet, nearly the same time needed for routine direct laryngoscopic intubation.

▶ This looks like a great technique. I can't wait to try it myself. I wonder how it compares with the success rate of the standard fiberoptic processes? I wish there were more data comparing the two techniques, and I hope that this article, like all good ones, will lead to more study and further refinement.

M. F. Roizen, MD

Passive Sampling and Head Space Analysis for Quantitative Determination of Nitrous Oxide Exposure
Kumagai S, Koda S (Osaka Prefectural Inst of Public Health, Japan; Kochi Med School, Kohasu Oko-Cho, Nankoku, Japan)
Am Ind Hyg Assoc J 60:458-462, 1999   13–7

Introduction.—Nitrous oxide (N_2O) may be a chronic health hazard in hospital operating theaters. It is necessary to monitor and control the N_2O exposure of those who staff the operating theater. A new technique for determining the time-weighted average personal exposure to N_2O gas is described.

Methods.—N$_2$O gas was passively collected on a molecular sieve enclosed in a glass tube and partially desorbed in a vial to attain solid-gas equilibrium at 100°C. The N$_2$O concentration in the head space air in the vial was measured with a gas chromatograph equipped with an electron capture detector. Three sets of 5 tubes each were placed in an atmosphere of 50 ppm of N$_2$O in a Tedlar bag for 4 hours and then instantly placed in vials after sampling. One set was evaluated within 24 hours, and the remaining 2 sets were stored at around 4°C and 25°C for 2 weeks before undergoing analysis.

Results.—N$_2$O concentration in the head space was proportional to both the N$_2$O concentration in the test atmosphere and the sampling time up to 1600 ppm/h, producing a coefficient of variance of less than 10%. The performance of the sampler was not influenced by water vapor or carbon dioxide in the atmosphere or by air currents.

Conclusion.—The passive sampler described may be used in the quantitative determination of N$_2$O exposure. The performance of the sampler was not affected by water vapor, carbon dioxide, or air currents. This device may be stored for 2 weeks at either 4°C or 25°C. Because the device is small and light, it may be used to determine exposure to N$_2$O during surgical procedures.

▶ This article shows that the passive sampler developed by the authors can be used for quantitative determination of N$_2$O exposure, even in small places like the operating room. The passive nature of this and the high degree of quantitation mean that it can be used inexpensively. Does this matter in the United States, where we have a high number of operating room air changes per hour, scavenging systems, and small use of N$_2$O? The answer is that we don't know. We don't know what dangers lurk with N$_2$O in truth, and we don't know whether, with modern technology it matters whether N$_2$O exposure is sampled. My own bet is that it doesn't matter in the concentrations we have now, but I still also bet that we should do things carefully and keep the operating room as free of pollution as possible. Then we won't need to develop such devices as the British and perhaps the Japanese need to develop if they have operating rooms that are less than perfectly scavenged. Perhaps this device is important for office operatories, which are now increasing, rather than the type of operatory that most of us use in a hospital or ambulatory facility.

M. F. Roizen, MD

Low-Dose Succinylcholine Facilitates Laryngeal Mask Airway Insertion During Thiopental Anaesthesia
Yoshino A, Hashimoto Y, Hirashima J, et al (Nihon Univ, Tokyo)
Br J Anaesth 83:279-283, 1999   13–8

Background.—This study was designed to determine whether use of succinylcholine in low doses can aid in the insertion of the laryngeal mask airway (LMA) without causing significant myalgia during anesthesia using thiopental. Important obstacles to correct insertion and positioning of a LMA are adverse responses such as gagging, coughing, and laryngospasm. A variety of drugs have been tried and recommended to minimize these adverse reactions and to ease insertion of the LMA, including thiopental and propofol. Thiopental produces less satisfactory conditions for insertion than propofol; however, in one study, the rate of easy insertion of the LMA was only 62%. In addition, propofol is a relatively expensive drug. Some researchers have speculated that succinylcholine, given in low doses to avoid significant myalgia, may prove efficacious.

Methods.—Sixty patients undergoing elective surgery were randomly assigned to one of three groups of 20 patients each: group 1 received normal saline, group 2 received succinylcholine 0.25 mg/kg, and group 3 received succinylcholine 0.5 mg/kg. There were no significant differences among the groups in terms of patient characteristics. Patients were premedicated with hydroxidine 1 hour before surgery. Thiopental was used to induce anesthesia, and then the succinylcholine or placebo was administered by a single researcher when the patients lost consciousness. Assessments were made of jaw relaxation, gagging or coughing on insertion, and presence of fasciculations. Patient interviews both later on the day of surgery and 3 days later assessed muscle pain. An analysis of variance was the statistical analysis performed.

Results.—Jaw opening scores did not differ significantly between the groups. However, groups 1 and 2, with saline and 0.25 mg/kg succinylcholine, respectively, did experience significantly more gagging and coughing than group 3. Insertion conditions overall were better for group 3 than for the other two groups. Postoperative myalgia on the day of surgery was not significantly different among the three groups, but the incidence of myalgia 3 days after surgery was significantly higher in group 3 compared with group 1, although similar to group 2. There were no differences in the degree of fasciculations between groups 2 and 3, but the degree of fasciculations was much higher in both of these groups than in group 1. Group 3 also had a much longer duration of apnea than group 2.

Conclusions.—Succinylcholine provides adequate depression of laryngeal reflexes but has a number of adverse effects, including prolonged apnea and anaphylaxis. Myalgia is also a minor adverse effect. The reduction of the succinylcholine dose to 0.5 mg/kg provided satisfactory conditions for LMA insertion in this study, whereas a dose of 0.25 mg/kg succinylcholine did not. Further studies should be done regarding the use of the propofol-alfentanil combination and thiopental. The use of propofol combined with opioids for induction of anesthesia may be more efficacious than use of low-dose succinylcholine and thiopental.

▶ One wonders if the side-effect of this low-dose succinylcholine treatment would have been diminished if one had pretreated the patients with either a defasculating dose of non-depolarizing muscle relaxant, or something like lidocaine or atropine. Nonetheless, one has to question whether the extra time of apnea is worth the improvement in insertion conditions for the LMA.

I would conclude that this study indicates the need for more study, rather than that low-dose succinylcholine should or should not be used, depending on one's belief of the relative risks versus benefits.

M. F. Roizen, MD

Capnography Monitoring During Neurosurgery: Reliability in Relation to Various Intraoperative Positions
Grenier B, Verchère E, Mesli A, et al (Univ Hosp, Bordeaux, France)
Anesth Analg 88:43-48, 1999   13–9

Introduction.—Capnography may be helpful in providing an estimate of $PaCO_2$ in patients undergoing general anesthesia. It can be a reliable estimate of $PaCO_2$ only if the arterial to end-tidal CO_2 partial pressure difference (P[a-ET]CO_2) remains constant over time. This assumption has been questioned, particularly during long procedures, including neurosurgery. The only known report regarding the effects of intraoperative position on P(aET)CO_2 evaluated patients undergoing renal surgery in the lateral decubitus position. The accuracy of $PETCO_2$ in estimating $PaCO_2$ during neurosurgical procedures longer than 3 hours was prospectively examined, along with the effect of surgical positioning on P(a-ET)CO_2 over time.

Methods.—One hundred four patients, with a mean age of 49 years and a mean weight of 64 kg, undergoing intracranial or spinal procedures were grouped according to surgical positioning: supine (SP), lateral (LT), prone (PR), or sitting (ST). Measurements of $PaCO_2$, $PETCO_2$, and P(a-ET)CO_2 were taken after induction of anesthesia (T0), after positioning (T1), at each following hour (T2, T3, T4), and at completion of the procedure after return to the SP position (T5).

Results.—The mean duration of surgery was 3.7 hours, and the mean duration of positioning was 4.1 hours. There was a mean P(a-ET)CO_2 of 6 mm Hg for 624 simultaneous measurements of $PaCO_2$ and $PETCO_2$. The P(a+ET)CO_2 was highest in the LT group because of a lower $PETCO_2$. Negative P(aET)CO_2 ($PETCO_2 > PaCO_2$) was observed 22 times only in the SP and ST groups (9 and 13 times, respectively). Changes in opposite direction of $PETCO_2$ and $PaCO_2$ between successive measurements were observed in 26% of the patients. Correlation coefficients for SP, LT, PR, and ST ($PaCO_2$ vs $PETCO_2$) were not in good agreement. The mean bias was between 5 and 7 mm Hg, and both the superior and inferior limits of agreement were too large to expect $PETCO_2$ to replace $PaCO_2$.

Conclusion.—It is recommended that capnography be performed with regular analysis of arterial blood gases for optimal ventilatory adjustment in patients undergoing neurosurgical procedures longer than 3 hours. Findings suggest that $PETCO_2$ cannot replace $PaCO_2$ because of scattering of individual values, the occurrence of negative arterial to end-tidal CO_2 gradient (P[a-ET]CO_2; $PaCO_2$ and $PETCO_2$ variations in opposite directions;

substantial changes in $P(a\text{-ET})CO_2$ between 2 samples; and instability of $P(a\text{-ET})CO_2$ over time.

▶ This is a fascinating article, and I only wish the authors had related the changes in arterial to end-tidal CO_2 on each patient over a prolonged period of time. The major question isn't whether the end-tidal CO_2 reflects arterial CO_2, although that is an important question, but whether there is a consistent relationship in any one patient between arterial CO_2 and end-tidal CO_2. Although the authors make the comment that arterial minus end-tidal CO_2 between two successive samples varies by more than 5 mm of mercury in 11% of the samples, it isn't clear whether these were errors that would have led to different therapies. Thus, I find it difficult to agree with the conclusion, as I haven't seen the full data set. Maybe the authors have better data to share with us than the editors of the journal allowed them to publish.

M. F. Roizen, MD

The Use of Side-Stream Spirometry to Assess Air Leak During and After Lung Volume Reduction Surgery
Robinson RJS (McGill Univ, Montreal)
Anesthesiology 91:571-573, 1999   13–10

Background.—In patients undergoing lung volume reduction surgery, a gas leak from surrounding bullous tissue occurs in 46% to 53% of patients. Another 13% of patients experience sudden rupture of the lung after surgery. Two cases demonstrate the use of intensive care ventilators and in-line side-stream spirometers in the operating room and postoperatively to measure the volume of gas leaking from the lungs.

> *Case Report 1.*—Man, 66, with severe emphysema underwent lung volume reduction surgery of the right lung apex by means of a left-sided, one-lung ventilation and left-sided, double-lumen endobronchial tube. A linear stapler loaded with bovine pericardial strips was used to staple 15% to 20% of the patient's right lung. After the collapsed lung was gradually reinflated, a large gas leak was observed in the flow volume loop of a side-stream spirometer. A tear in the bulla was observed close to the previous staple line, and additional bullous lung was then excised. On positive-pressure ventilation and gentle reinflation of the right lung, nearly complete closing of the flow volume loop was observed on the side-stream spirometer, with only a minimal gas leak. Bronchospasm and persistent gas leak from the right lung complicated the patient's postoperative care. He was discharged 21 days after surgery.
> *Case Report 2.*—Man, 72, underwent bilateral apical lung volume reduction surgery for severe bullous emphysema. He had bilateral air leaks and subcutaneous emphysema on the first postoperative day. Chest radiography revealed incomplete reexpansion

of his right lung, which was treated by increasing chest suction. A PaO_2 of 50 to 60 mm Hg was maintained for 2 days on controlled ventilation; he needed cardiac support with norepinephrine and dopamine to increase venous oxygen saturation. However, the bilateral gas leaks continued. Early closing of the expiratory loop was observed on the flow volume loop of a side-stream spirometer. Chest suction to the right pleura was removed, and the leak from the lungs diminished. The patient's lungs were ventilated on postoperative day 3 to 15-cm pressure support and 10-cm positive end-expiratory pressure to trigger the ventilator. Within the next 2 days, the gas leak from the right chest tube stopped, but an increasing leak from the left lung was observed on side-stream spirometry, despite reduction of pressure support. On postoperative day 6, the surgeon repaired a large tear in the bulla of the left lung. Low pressure pulmonary edema developed in the left lung, along with significant arterial desaturation, and the patient died 9 days after surgery.

Summary.—These two cases demonstrate use of continuous monitoring of flow volume loops to both detect and quantify air leaks during lung volume surgery and postoperatively. It is likely that a postoperative gas leak after lung volume reduction surgery prolongs hospital stay and increases hospital morbidity rates; the routine use of side-stream spirometry may be of value in determining the best means of managing postoperative gas leaks.

▶ For those involved in lung reduction surgery, this article seems a must.

M. F. Roizen, MD

Adenosine: A Sensitive Indicator of Cerebral Ischemia During Carotid Endarterectomy
Weigand MA, Michel A, Eckstein H-H, et al (Univ of Heidelberg, Germany)
Anesthesiology 91:414-421, 1999   13–11

Background.—Evidence suggests that adenosine may act to protect from certain pathogenetic mechanisms involved in cerebral ischemia. However, little is known about the role of adenosine and its metabolites in the process of human cerebral ischemia. Adenosine was compared with hypoxanthine and lactate as indicators of cerebral ischemia in patients undergoing carotid endarterectomy.

Methods.—Intraoperative monitoring of arterial and jugular venous blood was performed during carotid endarterectomy in 41 patients. Changes in adenosine, hypoxanthine, and lactate were assessed throughout the operation. In addition, somatosensory-evoked potentials were used to monitor cerebral oxygenation. Six patients received carotid artery shunts after somatosensory-evoked potentials were lost.

Results.—In patients who went on to have carotid artery shunting, mean jugular venous levels of the 3 biomarkers before carotid artery clamping were 229 nmol/L for adenosine, 1105 nmol/L for hypoxanthine, and 0.85 nmol/L for lactate. After clamping, adenosine increased significantly to 389 nmol/L and hypoxanthine to 1444 nmol/L, compared with no significant change in lactate. In identifying the presence of focal cerebral ischemia, the concentration of adenosine in jugular venous blood had a sensitivity of 83% and a specificity of 71%.

Conclusions.—For patients undergoing carotid endarterectomy, the levels of adenosine and hypoxanthine in jugular venous blood may help identify those with adequate collateral flow. In patients without adequate contralateral flow, adenosine and hypoxanthine levels increase significantly in response to carotid artery clamping. Thus, changes in adenosine, if they signal the presence of focal cerebral ischemia, may be a useful monitor for ischemia in clinical settings.

▶ This is an outstanding study, but it is too bad that somatosensory-evoked potential changes were used as the indicator of focal ischemia and the gold standard, rather than others. Nevertheless, I think this is a very, very important study, both for what it says about the mechanism of damage, and for what it says about the brain's protective events, as well as for what it says about monitoring techniques. Will we be able to develop an intraoperative adenosine monitor that will allow us to place an electrode on the skin and measure adenosine levels in venous affluent of the brain? Or even of other organs? While that is the major implication, there are other important implications of this article. I recommend that you read this because it is an extremely well-done study, especially for the young scientist who might consider doing technology assessments. This is an outstanding place to start.

M. F. Roizen, MD

Effect of Mild Hypothermia on the Vascular Actions of Phenylephrine in Rat Aortic Rings

Lagneau F, Kirstetter P, Bernard C, et al (Hôpital Beaujon, Clichy, France; Hôpital Bichat, Paris; Polyclinique de Savoie, Paris; et al)
Br J Anaesth 82:938-940, 1999   13–12

Background.—Mild hypothermia is a common occurrence during surgery and can alter the actions of phenylephrine. The changes induced by mild hypothermia in phenylephrine-induced contractions of aortic rings of rats were investigated.

Methods.—The thoracic aorta was removed from male Sprague-Dawley rats and placed in a modified HEPES buffer. The buffer was aerated with a mix of 95% oxygen and 5% carbon dioxide. The aorta was then divided into ring segments, suspended, and each segment placed in a 10-mL water-jacketed organ chamber. The organ chambers were maintained at a pH of 7.35 to 7.4 and aerated continuously with 95% oxygen and 5%

carbon dioxide. Isometric tension was measured at two temperatures, either 34°C or 38°C, using a data acquisition system. Increasing concentrations of phenylephrine, from 10^{-8} to 10^{-5} mol/L, were used to test vascular response to phenylephrine. Relaxation produced by addition of 10^{-6}-mol/L acetylcholine on 10^{-5}-mol/L phenylephrine precontracted aortic rings was used to assess the integrity of the endothelium. The endothelium was considered to be intact if the addition of acetylcholine effected vasodilation at a minimum of 30%. When the acetylcholine failed to produce vasodilation, the endothelium was considered to be removed. Assessment of the role of endothelium was done by comparing the phenylephrine-induced contractions in the presence or absence of the endothelium. The roles of nitric oxide and prostanoid endothelial pathways were assessed by comparing the phenylephrine-induced contractions in intact rings in the presence of indomethacin and *N*-nitro-L-arginine (L-NNA) and a combination of the two.

Results.—Emax, the maximum tension in response to phenylephrine, was significantly reduced at 34°C as compared with 38°C when the endothelium was present. EC_{50}, the concentration that produces 50% of Emax and resting tension, was also significantly increased. However, there were no significant differences between the two temperatures for both Emax and EC_{50} when the endothelium was removed. At 38°C there were no significant differences in Emax or EC_{50} with or without either L-NNA, indomethacin, or a combination of the two compounds. However, at 34°C the Emax increased significantly, and EC_{50} decreased significantly with indomethacin, L-NNA, or a combination of the two.

Conclusions.—Mild hypothermia was responsible for a significant reduction in phenylephrine-induced rat aortic contraction in vitro by means of endothelium-dependent mechanisms. It is likely that endothelium-dependent vasodilators—particularly, increased nitric oxide production or the response of nitric oxide to phenylephrine during moderate temperature decreases (common during surgery)—are probably involved.

▶ This is an important article because it tells us why we have to adjust the dose of drugs as the temperature of the patient changes over ranges that are commonly seen in perioperative care. Does it all relate to nitric oxide synthase inhibitor or nitric oxide production? Since we are seeing that more use of mild hypothermia can benefit organs, this study is important for us to understand, and perhaps this should start a whole new field looking at all of our vasoactive drugs under conditions of mild hypo- and hyperthermia.

M. F. Roizen, MD

The Bispectral Index: A Measure of Depth of Sleep?

Sleigh JW, Andrzejowski J, Steyn-Ross A, et al (Waikato Hosp, Hamilton, New Zealand; Dept of Physics and Electronic Engineering, Hamilton, New Zealand)
Anesth Analg 88:659-661, 1999   13–13

Introduction.—With the bispectral index (BIS), a measure of depth of anesthesia and sedation, increasing depth of anesthesia results in a decreasing cortical integration and a decreasing BIS score. During general anesthesia, BIS values typically range from 40 to 55. The effects by natural sleep on the BIS were investigated.

Methods.—Five volunteers ranging in age from 14 to 43 years took part in the study. Electroencephalographic (EEG) data was collected from participants during the early part of the night. The stages of sleep were recorded according to EEG patterns: light sleep (stages 1 and 2), characterized by a high-frequency/low-amplitude EEG signal, with the presence of sleep spindles or K complexes; slow-wave sleep (stages 3 and 4), with high-amplitude/low-frequency waves; and rapid eye movement (REM) sleep, with a low-amplitude/high-frequency EEG as in stage 1, but with co-existing hypotonia and eyeball movement artifacts. The changes in BIS were compared with the EEG stages of sleep.

Results.—All 5 study subjects exhibited dramatic and remarkably consistent changes in the BIS. Sleep spindles started to be seen in the EEG at BIS levels of 75 to 90. Slow-wave sleep was associated with BIS levels in the range of 20 to 70, and REM sleep occurred with the BIS in the range of 75 to 92. The minimal BIS in all cases was less than 47; with a brief awakening, the BIS abruptly increased to over 90. Both the BIS and 95% spectral edge frequency decreased significantly with increased depth of sleep.

Conclusion.—The effects of natural sleep on the BIS, as recorded in the study participants' home environments, were found to be similar to the effects of general anesthesia on the BIS. The BIS may have a role in monitoring depth of sleep.

▶ We, too, found similar results to those of Sleigh et al, with the induction of sleep occurring below 90. But rather than use the BIS, then, as a nonspecific measure of the level of consciousness or as a monitor for routine somnography, we found that it was an easy-to-use measure of induction of sleep. Maybe Chamoun and Aspect have created much more for us than just an easy-to-understand number as a transformation of an EEG and EMG signal.

M. F. Roizen, MD

Prevention of Needle-Stick Injury: Efficacy of a Safeguarded Intravenous Cannula

Asai T, Matsumoto S, Matsumoto H, et al (Kansai Med Univ, Osaka, Japan)
Anaesthesia 54:258-261, 1999   13–14

Objective.—The use of needleless devices or needles with safeguard mechanisms can reduce the incidence of needlestick injuries. The ease of use and the efficacy of the safeguard mechanism of the Insyte AutoGuard (Becton Dickson Infusion Therapy Systems, Sandy, Utah) IV cannula were evaluated in a randomized study.

Methods.—One hundred patients without bloodborne infections or bleeding disorders were randomly assigned to receive an 18-gauge conventional IV cannula (group 1) or the Insyte AutoGuard cannula (group 2) for IV infusion. In group 1 the needle was removed and a drip-infusion was started. In group 2, the button on the cannula was pressed to retract the needle into the safety barrel before the needle was removed from the cannula. The ease of insertion was evaluated, and any needle-stick injuries or blood contamination were recorded.

Results.—Cannulation was successful the first time in 35 (70%) group 1 patients and in 36 (72%) group 2 patients. There were no needle-stick injuries. Blood contamination of the patient's arm occurred in 7 group 1 patients and in 5 group 2 patients. The incidence of blood contamination, occurring most frequently where a withdrawn needle was placed, was significantly higher in group 1 than in group 2. There was no blood stain in group 2.

Conclusion.—The AutoGuard cannula mechanism for handling used needles makes it safer than the conventional IV cannula and does not affect ease of insertion.

▶ This article makes it seem like it is easy to switch from the old needles to the new ones, but is there a cost-benefit ratio, or even a benefit-risk ratio? Are there problems encountered with the new needle that wouldn't be encountered with the old needle? This article is a randomized comparison with many positives, but it seems to lack the discussion of any downside. I'd be interested in hearing from individuals who have found a downside with the new needles, because the safety needles appear to be beneficial, even if somewhat costly. Obviously, the benefits of their safety and their safe use depends on when most needle-stick injuries occur. According to the data I've seen, most needle-stick injuries occur when recapping a needle on a syringe, not at the time of IV cannula insertion. I would love to have good epidemiologic data showing, in a large number of patients, whether the use of such an IV cannula, which costs about $1 per patient more than the old devices, actually prevents any needle-stick injuries, or whether so many of the needle-stick injuries are really in recapping needles and syringes as has been implied. If one reads the other article in this 2-part set by Deniz

Akduman, MD, you'll see that protective equipment is not used very routinely by operating room personnel, even in a tertiary care university hospital, where it was stressed. Thus, it's unclear whether there are system changes that need to be made to allow us to use universal precautions and to make safety procedures easier so that we can use them to a greater degree.

M. F. Roizen, MD

Continuous Pulse Oximetry in the General Surgical Ward: Nellcor N-200 Versus Nellcor N-3000
Christensen M, Lie C, Rosenberg J (Hvidovre Univ Hosp, Denmark)
Anaesthesia 54:253-257, 1999   13–15

Objective.—Patient movement during pulse oximetry monitoring can cause artifacts resembling desaturations that can trigger alarms. New Nellcor pulse oximeters are designed to ignore motion-generated odd-shaped signals. The incidence of alarms and signal loss were recorded in the new Nellcor Symphony N-3000 and the Nellcor N-200 (Nellcor Puritan Bennet, Pleasanton, Calif) pulse oximeters during monitoring in the late postoperative period, when patients are often moving.

Methods.—Patients (N = 22, 10 men) were connected to both oximeters between 8 AM and noon and were monitored for 24 hours. The oximeters were connected to a computer that stored data.

Results.—One patient was excluded because only 1 oximeter recorded. Patients were monitored for a total of 275 hours with a median monitoring per patient of 16 hours for each oximeter. There was a median of 18 desaturations for the N-200 and 4 for the N-3000 and a median of 13 and 9 drop-out episodes, respectively. The N-200 and N-3000 recorded a median desaturation value of 96% and 97%, respectively. The N-200 registered significantly more episodes of desaturation than the N-3000. The N-200 and N-3000 registered a saturation alarm level of at least 85% 23% and 6% of the time, respectively.

Conclusion.—Compared with the N-200, the N-3000 had less alarm time and fewer alarms when used to monitor patients postoperatively.

▶ The authors of this article tried to establish whether a new generation of pulse oximeters has been developed, and they found that the Nelcor N-3000 is, in fact, better that the prior generation, the N-200. The main difference between the N-3000 and the N-200 appears to be a new algorithm that eliminates—or, at least, is purported to eliminate—many of the false alarms and time-in-alarm mode that is so common with the N-200 generation of pulse oximeters. The number of false alarms per hour was approximately 1.1 for the N-200, versus 0.25 for the N-3000. Is this too much? Well, if you're the patient who is woken up from a sound sleep by either false alarm or by having the sting of a blood gas drawn because of the false alarm, or any of the other myriad of options that could occur, you'd say that it was too many, even if it is 0.25 per hour. Does the Masimo SET pulse oximeter reduce this even further? Only head-to-head comparisons will tell with the Nellcor N-3000, as the Masimo SET uses another algorithm to screen out motion, artifact, and other sources of false alarms.

M. F. Roizen, MD

14 Cost Containment

Decrease in Case Duration Required to Complete an Additional Case During Regularly Scheduled Hours in an Operating Room Suite: A Computer Simulation Study
Dexter F, Macario A (Univ of Iowa, Iowa City; Stanford Univ, Palo Alto, Calif)
Anesth Analg 88:72-76, 1999   14–1

Objective.—Reducing the time a patient spends in surgery to increase the productivity of an operating room (OR) does not allow a surgeon to perform another operation unless the average duration for surgery was less than 1 hour. When more than 1 OR is available, decreases in surgical time may permit an additional operation to be scheduled. The possibility that decreasing the case duration of all cases performed in an OR suite with more than one OR could permit an additional surgery to be scheduled and completed during regularly scheduled 8 hours of surgery was investigated.

Methods.—A Monte-Carlo simulation was used to evaluate the effect of small decreases in surgical times on new open OR time that would permit the scheduling of another surgical procedure during regular working hours. Average surgical times used were 1, 2, and 3 hours, and the range of OR suite sizes used were 1, 2, 5, 10, and 15 rooms. Each surgery and each turnover time were randomly assigned. Each surgery was scheduled in the OR with the most time available. Each patient's surgery was performed to minimize the duration of the operation. Additional surgeries were scheduled if there was a 95% chance that the operation could be performed during the day. An iterative process was used to maximize the use of the ORs.

Results.—The required decreases in surgical times for 1-, 2-, and 3-hour operations to allow scheduling of another operation were 30 to 39, 79 to 110, and 105 to 206 minutes, respectively. The regularly scheduled OR hours were extended from 8 to 10 hours.

Conclusion.—Decreasing the OR time for individual patients' surgeries is unlikely to generate enough extra time to schedule an additional operation. OR time can be optimized by judicious scheduling.

▶ This is an article I have read many times, and although it is easy to understand its conclusions, they differ from what we actually find in practice. Does this mean that computer simulations don't work for our OR? Does it mean that real life practice is different than the computer "pictures," or just that our anecdotes of success overrun the science that says we can't really do what we do consistently. Anyone who has ever worked in an OR should read this article multiple times. It contains important ideas that explain OR functioning and management; but, despite reading it many times, I am unfortunately left with my biases of the successful anecdotes.

M. F. Roizen, MD

Anaesthesia Clinical Directors in the United Kingdom: Organisation, Objectives and Support Needs

Thoms GMM, McHugh GA, Pollard BJ, et al (Manchester Royal Infirmary, England; Arrowe Park Hosp, Merseyside, England)
Anaesthesia 54:753-760, 1999   14–2

Background.—Health care reforms in the United Kingdom in the early 1990s brought changes in the work of anesthesia services and the work of anesthesia clinical directors, as well as a growing body of literature relating to medical management. However, the literature has scant information concerning what is actually happening in operating theaters and anesthesia services. There is a critical need for better information regarding the daily work of anesthesia clinical directors for a number of reasons. Better information is needed to more effectively support clinical directors and to improve their effectiveness. There is much pressure in all areas of the medical profession to improve patient care and to restore public confidence, which has resulted in additional responsibilities for anesthesia clinical directors. This study gathered basic, timely information regarding anesthesia clinical directors and their daily work in light of the increasing demands on them.

Methods.—After a pilot study to confirm the most important issues faced by anesthesia clinical directors, information forms and questionnaires were sent to 269 acute hospital trusts in the United Kingdom. A second questionnaire was sent to nonresponders.

Results.—Responses of some kind, either initial responses, main survey, or nonresponder follow-ups, were received from 80% (215 of 269 sites). The majority of the clinical directors were men (82%) and ranged in age from 29 to 60 years. The mean time spent as clinical director was 3 years (range, 1-10 years). A total of 44 separate functions were reported as being within the purview of anesthesia clinical directors. Staffing varied significantly, as did directorate annual budgets. Directorates without operating theaters had smaller median directorate budgets and lower staff strength. Most clinical directors (57%) had no job description. There were no formal written objectives for 53% of the clinical directors, and 36% had neither formal job descriptions nor written objectives. The general trend was toward underfunding of the managerial time, and 20% of clinical directors had no funded managerial time. Managerial activity in three categories ranged from 5% to 95% for operational work time, 0% to 70% for clinical leadership, and 5% to 70% for managerial time. Support from secretarial staff was rated poor or very poor in 12% of sites, and support from information staff was rated as poor or very poor in 33% of sites. Support from trust board members was rated as poor or very poor in 26% of sites, and from purchasers, poor or very poor in 64%. Results of the survey also indicated a desire for more external education, training, and support.

Conclusions.—This appears to be the first in-depth investigation of anesthesia clinical directorates. Survey results reveal a need for written job descriptions and objectives for a majority of clinical directors, better funding of the managerial component, and improved support from information staff and at the trust board and purchaser levels. Greater networking for anesthesia clinical directors was also called for, as was increased training in several areas, particularly human resource management and monitoring of performance.

▶ This is an important article for every department chair to read. Clearly, there are many objectives that need be followed and a lot of unfunded time for clinical directors, both in Britain and in the United States, and my guess is throughout the world. I think this is a great article and I'm going to place it in my "repeatedly read" file.

M. F. Roizen, MD

Using Queueing Theory to Determine Operating Room Staffing Needs
Tucker JB, Barone JE, Cecere J, et al (Stamford Hosp, Conn)
J Trauma 46:71-79, 1999   14–3

Background.—Criteria from the American College of Surgeons mandate in-house operating room (OR) staff 24 hours per day for levels I and II trauma centers. However, there is a question as to whether a trauma center should automatically call in the second OR team to stand by whenever the first team is busy. Different procedures at various institutions mean that some institutions may be incurring unwarranted costs based on the criteria they use to determine when to bring in their backup OR teams. Queueing theory, a tool in operations research that was first developed in the early 1900s to determine the number of switches needed to handle telephone calls at a switchboard, offers an objective method for determining staffing needs.

Methods.—The essential variables for queueing theory are mean arrival rate and mean service rate. To determine the mean arrival rate, the number of actual cases (62) was divided by 2920 hours in a year (8 hours per night × 365 nights per year). The mean service rate was determined by averaging the length of the actual cases during the study period, the result being 0.7427 patients per hour. Queueing theory formulae were then applied to these two variables to determine the probability of two or more patients needing the OR at the same time, which was used to determine the probability of needing to activate the backup OR team. The results from the queueing model were then validated with simulation.

Results.—Application of queueing theory to the specific institution in this study indicated an arrival rate of 0.0212 patients per hour (one patient every 5.9 days), and an average service rate of 0.7427 patients per hour. Queueing theory formulae resulted in a probability of less than 0.1% for two or more patients needing the OR simultaneously at this institution.

Conclusions.—Queueing theory can be a valuable tool for institution administrators trying to determine staffing needs, not only for the OR but for many other departments. At the institution in this study, the activation of a second OR when the first team is busy on the night shift was deemed unnecessary because the likelihood of two cases occurring simultaneously is less than one in a thousand. Trauma centers should use queueing theory to determine the most cost-effective use of their resources.

▶ I love this article. It is logical and well written. Does the computer simulation reflect actual practice? I don't know because I haven't tried this, but I hope someone other than the original authors who tries this will E-mail me and tell me if the system works. I want all those involved in operating room staffing to read this article. The study was performed well enough, and the queueing theory is interesting enough that I think it has some value.

M. F. Roizen, MD

Use of Personal Protective Equipment and Operating Room Behaviors in Four Surgical Subspecialties: Personal Protective Equipment and Behaviors in Surgery

Akduman D, Kim LE, Parks RL, et al (Gazi Univ, Ankara, Turkey; Washington Univ, St Louis)

Infect Control Hosp Epidemiol 20:110-114, 1999   14–4

Objective.—The epidemiologic characteristics of bloodborne pathogens among surgical personnel were observed to evaluate compliance with universal precautions recommending the wearing of personal protective equipment.

Methods.—Between June and October 1996, orthopedic, general, gynecologic, and cardiothoracic surgery procedures were observed at one 1000-bed, tertiary-care hospital. Three trained observers studied randomly selected procedures, recorded patient and procedure information, documented the personal protective equipment worn by operating room staff, and recorded any risky behaviors. Hand surgery and procedures requiring no incision or only a small incision were excluded.

Results.—Observers viewed 76 procedures and 597 health care workers. With respect to eye protection, 39% wore goggles, 5% wore face shields, 32% wore regular glasses, and 24% worn no eye protection. General surgery personnel were most likely to wear eye protection (55%), followed by gynecologic and orthopedic surgery personnel (>40%), and then cardiothoracic surgery personnel (31%). Medical students, house staff, and scrub nurses used eye protection at least 60% of the time, attending physicians 27% of the time, and anesthesia personnel only 22% of the time. Only 28% of 344 health care workers that should have worn double gloves actually did so. Orthopedic surgery personnel, gynecologic surgery personnel, and cardiothoracic and general surgery staff wore double gloves 64%, 20%, and 9% of the time, respectively. House staff used double gloves 43% of the time, attending physicians 26%, medical students 26%, and scrub nurses 15% of the time. Sharps passages were not announced in 91% of procedures. Among the surgical procedures in which sharps passages were announced, 64% were gynecologic. The total exposure rate was 22% and included 2 scalpel injuries, 1 needle-stick, 14 cutaneous blood and body fluid exposures occurring in 8 orthopedic and 6 gynecologic procedures.

Conclusion.—Compliance of operating room personnel with universal precautions is poor. The observed exposure rate of 22% underscores the need for educational programs to increase compliance.

▶ Is it individual laziness, or is it so difficult to comply to universal precautions that we don't do so as routinely as we should? It's our own health at risk. Do we consider ourselves immortal, or is it that the system and the equipment is just too tough to use routinely? This article, like many similar to it, shows that we need to be more careful of our own health. But perhaps it says more than that. Perhaps the difficulty, and what the authors call "risk-taking behavior of the operating room staff" are caused by inadequate systems and inadequate equipment that make it hard to move efficiently and effectively while facilitating universal precautions.

M. F. Roizen, MD

Surgical Subspecialty Block Utilization and Capacity Planning: A Minimal Cost Analysis Model
Strum DP, Vargas LG, May JH (Univ of Arkansas, Little Rock; Univ of Pittsburgh, Pa)
Anesthesiology 90:1176-1185, 1999   14–5

Introduction.—The traditional measures of operating room (OR) utilization do not reveal inefficiencies in the use of ORs. The authors of this study define 2 new terms, underutilization and overutilization, which can be used to better detect OR operational inefficiencies. These new measures are illustrated in an evaluation of surgical subspecialty ORs. Capacity planning (optimizing surgical subspecialty block time allotments) is also described, using a minimal cost analysis (MCA) model.

Methods.—All surgeries performed at a large teaching hospital over a 6-year period were evaluated. Variables included in the analysis were patient age and sex, 9th International Classification of Diseases code, anesthesia start and end time, location (surgical suite), anesthesiologist, surgeon, and admission status (inpatient or outpatient). All cases were evaluated according to the surgical subspecialty blocks to which they were assigned. Surgical records were categorized relative to budgeted OR block time for each subspecialty. Cases were thus described as following the budgeted time (budgeted utilization), taking less than the budgeted time (underutilization), or as using time before/after the budgeted block (over-utilization). The authors used an MCA that minimized the cost of under- and overutilization to allot block time to surgical specialties. Actual costs of operation were computed as the sum of the cost of the actual block allocation plus the measured cost of overutilization. As an illustration of potential savings realized by implementation of MCA budgets, actual operational costs were compared with the estimated MCA budget costs. Savings were expressed as a percentage of actual costs.

Results.—Data were analyzed from 58,251 surgical cases and 10 surgical subspecialty blocks. Results were summarized for all 10 subspecialties, but detailed results were reported from only 3 blocks of varying size: cystoscopy, gynecology, and cardiothoracic (blocks consisting, respectively, of 1, 2, and 3 ORs). For each block-day by surgical subspecialty, classic utilization ranged from 44% to 113%. Overutilization ranged from 4% to 49%, and average daily block-specific underutilization ranged from 16% to 60%.

Conclusion.—The model presented in this study evaluates the use of OR time as a function of underutilization and overutilization and reveals the potential savings if either or both could be eliminated. Although neither can be totally eliminated, they can be quantified, and the effect of man-agement decisions aimed at reducing them can be measured.

▶ Anyone involved in OR management will want to read this article. It is logical and compelling. Yet, I have problems with its analysis. It's fine to say that my surgeons can have blocks of different durations, but can they have 30.4 hours? I live in a union environment. It's either 32 hours (four 8-hour days), or 30 hours (three 10-hour days)—to get 30.4 hours would be impossible. Balancing the cost of overtime versus usual utilization and the variants of any one surgeon doing any one case makes it unlikely that I'll be able to implement this strategy. If only patients were like widgets and we could cut and repair in 4-hour increments predictably. But, alas, they aren't. Some are thin, some are fat, and some surgeons have more coffee or less coffee in the morning, or soda, or faster or slower music. Some actually teach while operating, and some teach more or less depending on the quality of their assistants. I wish we could have a multivariable equation that could account for it all, but alas, I don't think we can. Nevertheless, I think this is a very important article and one worthy of your attention.

M. F. Roizen, MD

A Survey of Undergraduate Teaching in Anaesthesia

Cheung V, Critchley LAH, Hazlett C, et al (The Chinese Univ of Hong Kong, PRC)
Anaesthesia 54:4-12, 1999   14–6

Introduction.—Worldwide, many medical schools have undergone significant revisions in their teaching methods. Anesthesia has only recently been added to the medical curriculum, reflecting changes in the role of anesthesia within the hospital. Anesthesiologists are experts in several areas of patient care and therefore have much to offer to undergraduate education. Yet the role of anesthesia is not clearly defined within the undergraduate curriculum. There is little guidance in the literature. A survey of undergraduate anesthesia and intensive care courses was conducted to help formulate an undergraduate anesthesia curriculum.

Methods.—Of 73 university departments of anesthesia contacted, 65 (89%) replied from South-east Asia, Australia, New Zealand, the United Kingdom and Ireland, and Canada. Questionnaires were mailed to heads of anesthesia departments from all medical schools within each region. The questionnaire comprised 37 items, with a focus on experience in running a 4-week undergraduate course in anesthesia and intensive care. Surveyed items included organization of anesthesia within the medical facility, medical school curriculum in general, topics covered by the anesthesia department, teaching of practical clinical skills, resuscitation, critical care medicine and pain management, evaluation of student performance, and postgraduate teaching.

Results.—Significant regional differences were observed. Most departments taught pharmacology of anesthetic drugs (83%), preoperative evaluation (92%), care of the unconscious patient (77%), airway management and intubation (97%), IV cannulation (80%), basic life support (92%), and advanced life support (71%). Fewer than half of the schools offered advanced trauma support principles (44%). Critical care teaching was not as well defined. Respiratory failure and ventilation, management of circulatory shock, and principles of sepsis and multiorgan system failure were taught by a consensus of programs. Most students were educated in practical clinical skills in classes that used patients and simulators; 46% of the schools had a skills laboratory, and 6 had a resuscitation officer.

Conclusion.—It is recommended that anesthesia be taught in the latter years of medical school, with the following anesthesia core curriculum: anesthesia and perioperative medicine, practical clinical skills, critical care medicine, and optional elective curriculum.

▶ Although this survey is important in telling what is taught, it clearly does not tell how well it is taught or whether these subjects are viewed as important and well taught by the receiving medical students. It's interesting that this defines the level of teaching in Southeast Asia, Australia, New

Zealand, United Kingdom, Ireland, and Canada but skips the United States. Are we USA'ers that unimportant, are surveys in our area of the world poorly returned, or is the United States just considered to have too shabby a teaching program overall to merit surveying? It would be useful if an outcome measure of teaching and of student satisfaction relating to such were included in such a study.

M. F. Roizen, MD

The Ethics of Cost Containment From the Anesthesiologist's Perspective
Vogel WA, Manecke GR Jr, Poppers PJ (State Univ of New York, Stony Brook)
J Clin Anesth 11:73-77, 1999   14–7

Introduction.—Pressure to contain costs can force physicians into ethical dilemmas. Economic credentialing, year-end bonuses, capitated reimbursements, and the threat of termination of managed care contracts create conflicts for all providers, including anesthesiologists. Choosing of less expensive medications, optimizing operating room use, with emphasis on cost-efficient management of anesthesia personnel, and decreasing operating room turnover time between patients are important cost control targets.

The Ethical Continuum.—The ethical continuum extends from the white zone of ethically sound decisions through the gray zone of ethically questionable decisions into the black zone of ethically indefensible decisions where patient care is clearly compromised. Most decisions fall into the gray zone, where the outcomes are unclear and ethical conflicts can arise creating daily stress for health care workers.

Physicians' Rights and Business Obligations.—Although the welfare of patients is of primary importance, the rights and needs of the providers must also be considered. Thus the provider-employer contract is a social as well as an economic contract. The physician as business person must now consider the best interests of the insurer, in addition to those of the patient and the employing institution. With the expansion by the courts of the narrow employment-at-will doctrine, employees are now deemed to have certain moral entitlements. Although the degree of social responsibility required of business varies depending on the school of thought, recognition of the basic rights of health care workers is important to the ethical underpinning of the business.

Conclusion.—Anesthesiologists need to continually review and investigate the effects of cost containment on patients and physicians in an ethical light.

▶ This is a provocative article that all of us should read. It's important for what it says, as well as what it doesn't say. Many of us have been convinced that there is waste in medicine, and that doing the right thing to improve quality also reduces costs. This article takes a different perspective, but a very important one, and says that we have to examine cost-containment from a basic while keeping in mind the working conditions and the perspectives of patients and physicians alike.

M. F. Roizen, MD

Subject Index

A

Abdominal
  aortic surgery outcomes related to
    organization characteristics of
    ICUs, 140
  surgery
    in high-risk patients, dopexamine
      reduces incidence of acute
      inflammation in gut mucosa after,
      178
    major, epidural ropivacaine alone or
      with fentanyl after, 218
Acetaminophen
  morphine-sparing effect of, in pediatric
    day-case surgery, 104
Acidosis
  hyperchloremic, produced by rapid
    saline infusion in patients
    undergoing gynecologic surgery,
    171
  metabolic, cause in prolonged surgery,
    175
Acupuncture
  vs. transcutaneous electrical nerve
    stimulation for chronic back pain,
    in elderly, 236
Adenosine
  as indicator of cerebral ischemia during
    carotid endarterectomy, 291
  intrathecal, for chronic neuropathic
    pain, safety and efficacy of, 238
Adenotonsillectomy
  pediatric
    effects of anticholinergics on
      postoperative vomiting, recovery,
      and hospital stay in, 111
    preoperative oral dextromethorphan
      does not reduce pain or analgesic
      consumption after, 219
ADL 2-1294
  study of, 245
Adrenal
  surgery, laparoscopic, in obese patients,
    20
Adrenaline
  improves thoracic epidural analgesia
    produced by low-dose infusion of
    bupivacaine, fentanyl and
    adrenaline after major surgery, 203
Adrenoceptors
  α2-, analgesic potency after nerve injury
    (in rat), 242
Adverse drug events
  in ICU, and pharmacist participation on
    physician rounds, 141

Adverse events
  in day-case surgery, preexisting medical
    conditions as predictors of, 23
Aging
  gene expression profile of, and its
    retardation by caloric restriction (in
    mice), 259
AIDS
  patients with herpes zoster, mixed
    model for factors predictive of, 241
Air
  embolism, systemic, during positive-
    pressure ventilation, 162
  leak during and after lung volume
    reduction surgery, assessment with
    side-stream spirometry, 290
Airway
  laryngeal mask
    flexible reinforced, *vs.* tracheal
      intubation in intranasal surgery,
      125
    insertion, during thiopental
      anesthesia, effect of low-dose
      succinylcholine on, 287
    insertion, prediction of movement at,
      283
    recurrent laryngeal nerve injury due
      to, 126
    vs. cuffed oropharyngeal airway, 279
  management in critical care medicine,
    146
  obstetricians' ability to assess, in labor
    and delivery, 57
  oropharyngeal, cuffed, *vs.* laryngeal
    mask airway, 279
Alcoholic
  pancreatitis, chronic, natural history of
    pain in, 230
Alfentanil
  after head trauma, 195
  /propofol/nitrous oxide general
    anesthesia, women emerge faster
    than men from, 107
  vs. remifentanil, potency determination
    using ventilatory depression, 101
Allodynia
  associated with sciatic nerve
    constriction injury, intrathecal (S)-
    4CPG attenuates (in rat), 246
  of postherpetic neuralgia, IV lidocaine
    for, 240
Alopecia
  postoperative, after elective cosmetic
    surgery, 93
Alveolar
  concentration, minimum, of sevoflurane

Author Index